How to be One with God

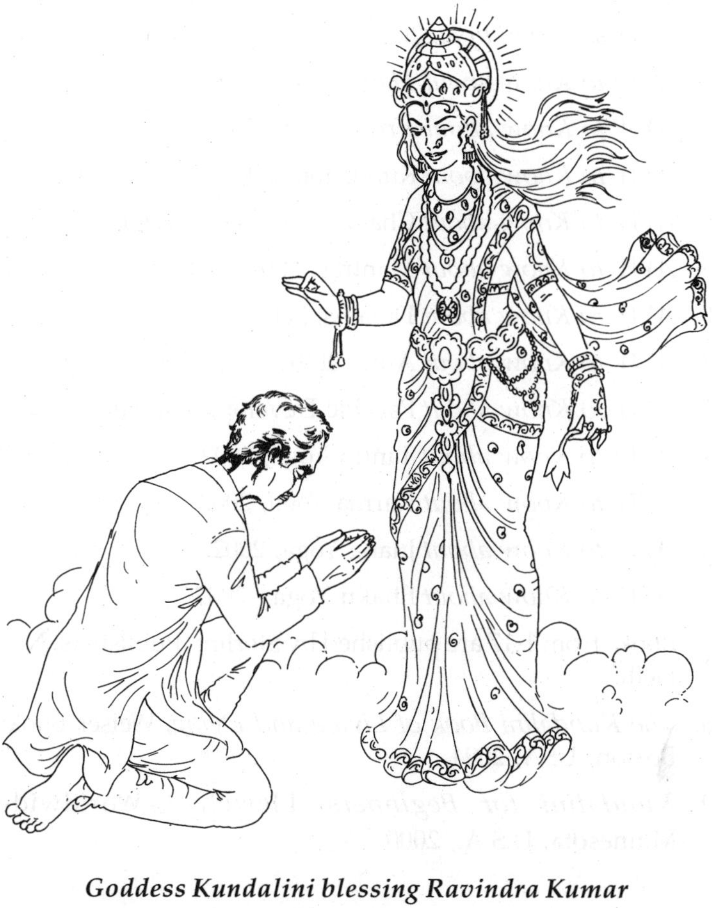

Goddess Kundalini blessing Ravindra Kumar

> Other books by the same author

1. *Secrets of Numerology*, 1992.
2. *Destiny, Science and Spiritual Awakening*, 1996.
3. *Kundalini—Journey Back to Our True Home*, 1999.
4. *Secrets of Kundalini Awakening*, 2003.
5. *Secrets of Shaktipat*, 2005.
6. *AYW to Know about Hatha Yoga*, 2000.
7. *AYW to Know about Kriya Yoga*, 2000.
8. *AYW to Know about* Kundalini, 2000.
9. *AYW to Know about* Chakras and Nadis, 2000.
10. *AYW to Know about* Mantras, 2001.
11. *AYW to Know about* Dreams, 2001.
12. *AYW to Know about* Aura, 2001.
13. *AYW to Know about* Psychic Development, 2001.
14. *AYW to Know about* Tantra Yoga, 2002.
15. *AYW to Know about* Karma Yoga, 2002.
16. *AYW to Know about* Jnana Yoga, 2002.
17. *AYW to Know about* Bhakti Yoga, 2002

    Books from 1-17 are published by Sterling Publishers, New Delhi.
18. *The Kundalini Book of Living and Dying*, Weiser Books, Boston, USA, 2004.
19. *Kundalini for Beginners*, Llewellyn Worldwide, Minnesota, U.S.A., 2000.

How to be One with God

(An Autobiography of a Scientist Yogi)

Ravindra Kumar
(Now Swami Ravindranand)

Sterling Paperbacks

STERLING PAPERBACKS
An imprint of
Sterling Publishers (P) Ltd.
A-59, Okhla Industrial Area, Phase-II,
New Delhi-110020.
Tel: 26387070, 26386209; Fax: 91-11-26383788
E-mail: sterlingpublishers@airtelbroadband.in
ghai@nde.vsnl.net.in
www.sterlingpublishers.com

How to be One with God
© 2008, Ravindra Kumar
ISBN 978-81-207-3733-4

All rights are reserved.
No part of this publication may be reproduced, stored in a retrieval system or transmitted, in any form or by any means, mechanical, photocopying, recording or otherwise, without prior written permission of the original publisher.

Printed and Published by Sterling Publishers Pvt. Ltd.,
New Delhi-110 020.

Dedicated to the loving memory of
my parents, grandparents
spiritual teachers and gurus
and my wife
Jytte Kumar Larsen
who has helped and supported me althrough

Contents

Preface	ix
The Aura of the First Author	xxiii
The Aura of the Second Author	xxv
The Divine Light, Sound and Touch	xxvi
Cosmic Consciousness	xxix
Introduction	xxxi

Chapter 1. The Autobiography—My Journey to Godhood ■ Introduction ■ Historical Background ■ Life in Africa ■ Observations ... 1

Chapter 2. We are all Gods in the Making ■ Introduction ■ The Spiritual Hierarchy ■ Initiation and Nature of Gods ... 100

Chapter 3. The Creation of Universe and Man: Cosmic Evolution ■ The Seven Races ■ Nature of Gods and Seven Rounds ■ God, Monad (Jiva) and Atom (The Creation of Man) ■ Venus ■ On Variety of Creators and the Process of Creation of Man ... 123

Chapter 4. The Liberation of Man ■ Blavatsky ■ Swami Sri Yukteswar ■ The Goal ■ The Procedure ■ The Revelation ■ Patanjali's Yoga Sutras ■ Srimad Bhagavata Mahapurana ■ The Process of Meditation ■ Sri Ishopanishad and Swami Prabhupada of ISKCON ■ Invocation ■ Mantras ... 175

Chapter 5. Quantum Jump into Divinity through Shaktipat ■ Introduction ■ Why There is Anxiety About Death? ■ How Shakti Replaces the Fear of Death with a Trust in Existence? ■ Shaktipat or Kundalini Mahayoga ■ Guru and the Initiate ■ Shaktipat Initiation ■ Liberation ■ Experiences on Awakening ■ Order of Experiences of Realization ■ My Own Experiences ■ What Help is Offered?   276

Afterword   301
Glossary   302
References   312
Bibliography   324
Index   327

Preface

Our universe came into being some 2000 million years ago. It took 300 million years to evolve mineral, vegetable and human existence. Therefore humans are walking on earth for the last 1700 million years. However, first human root race was ethereal, sexless, non-intelligent and highly spiritual; second was still ethereal but beginning to condense and was gigantic, less intelligent but still very spiritual; third became solid, intelligent, hermaphrodite and less spiritual. By the end of the third root race humans became very intelligent but little spiritual, the separation of sexes took place, and the 'Fall' into generations began. The fourth root race became very intelligent (rather cunning) and spiritually eclipsed; they were males and females, and their gigantic stature began to shorten. Lower gods produced our physical structure and higher gods gave us intelligence and spirituality, but both of them failed to give the desired results as expected by the Lord. Man was left to himself to grow out of phenomenal consciousness and achieve spiritual consciousness. We at present are at the middle of the fourth round out of seven rounds set from beginning to the end of creation. At this mid-point the reverse journey has begun as scheduled, and spirituality is increasing. Normal course will take another 2000 million years to bring the original order of spirituality, but the men of yoga are already on the path 'back to the Lord' through metaphysical practices, and they are teaching the same to others.

Only an initiate or 'twice-born' can comprehend the truth spoken in scriptures or anywhere. However great a scholar one may be, one cannot really appreciate the facts presented therein in the real sense. Why this is so and what is the way back to our original spirituality, is the subject matter of the present book. I have first presented my own autobiography giving details of the spiritual journey back to the Lord; then the details of the evolution of the universe, and then various methods of transcending normal consciousness and becoming a 'twice born'. Finally the method of Shaktipath in which the Guru can pass the 'spiritual energy' to the disciple directly and thus awaken his hitherto dormant 'serpent of wisdom' called Kundalini, and thus regain his lost 'original spirituality' in a short time is also dealt. In this manner, the chain of repeated births is broken and one finds a place to live on a spiritual planet forever.

My autobiography, the journey from dusk to dawn with experiences in full details, is the subject matter of Chapter 1. Authenticity of experiences is maintained through corroboration with scriptures and various faiths and traditions. I had been unknowingly following the 'eight-fold path of yoga.' Passage through three states is described: inner turmoil, experience of death (of ego), and resurrection. The turning point from material to spiritual comes through a 'crisis'—physical, emotional, moral, scientific or religious. The 'crisis' may come by accident, e.g., falling through a mountaintop and surviving, or more rationally and systematically, it can be created through yoga and meditation. After passing through the 'crisis' one becomes an Initiate or 'twice born,' and understands the meaning of scriptures. The 'twice born' enters the Kingdom of God, as was rightly said by Jesus Christ. At this level one experiences seeing divine lights, hearing sounds and at the end having visions of the 'divine child,' which signifies the completion of the process of individuation as described by Carl Jung. With the balance of masculinity and femininity in nature, inner marriage

Preface

takes place and the 'divine child' is born. The son of man becomes the son of God, and acquires the level of gods or angels or *devas*, or even surpasses the gods who are intransitive.

I have described seven major milestones I passed through in my spiritual journey and have elaborated on the three stages of realization: Brahman, paramatman and Lord Absolute. The factors that assisted me all my life were my loneliness, dreams, *bhakti* or devotion, *jnana* or knowledge through reading, and *karma* or action without any attachment to its fruits. Talking to my father, who died several years ago, and some Gurus living on higher realms, and my personal travels to higher realms provided me with the first hand knowledge of inner worlds, which is presented therein. Alchemists talking about the 'philosopher's stone' that converts iron (normal consciousness) into gold (spiritual consciousness) has also been discussed as well as details on the Academy of Kundalini and Quantum Soul and its centres worldwide all being founded by me.

We are all gods in the making, is the theme of Chapter 2. First an explanation is given about what we mean by God, and then the meaning of becoming God is explained. Every faith and tradition has a creator God (gods or *devas* in plural), which can be termed as the 'third order potency.' Above God is higher God or the planner, which is 'second order potency.' Still higher is the Unknowable Absolute Lord, who is the causeless cause of everything, and the 'first order potency.' Table 1 gives the names of these three potencies in different religions. Third order potency is Brahma or Jehovah having a team of creator gods or *devas*, collectively called God, who themselves are intransitive and can be surpassed by men of yoga. This is the meaning of becoming God. These are gods or *devas* of lower order, represented by spirit was nature, which are themselves desirous of incarnating on earth for their own evolution. The above creator gods are *rebellious gods* who refused to create men saying that they will never be happy. These *rebellious gods* provided the 'spark' of intelligence (*manas*) to humans who could evolve to Godhood, and hence are really our saviours. Through this 'spark' men could become 'twice born' and cross the ring 'Pass Not' created by angels or *devas* at the disappearance of the last Atlantean remnant (of Plato) some 12,000 years ago. Ring 'Pass Not' separated 'transcendental truth' from 'ordinary phenomenal intelligence' so that unworthy people could not know about it and make a mess of it. Jesus also said, 'Only the 'twice born' can enter the Kingdom of God.'

This chapter also explains some facts about the creation of the universe, initiation, nature of gods and Monad (*jiva*) or individual soul. The age of our universe is the same as the age of Brahma, which is 100 years, each year having 360 days and equal number of nights, and each day having 4,320 million years of earth.

The cosmic evolution or creation of the universe and man is described in Chapter 3. Seven groups of men emerge simultaneously from seven planets. Astral was born before the physical body. Four great races have lived and died before our Adamic race—five races on five continents: Imperishable sacred land, Hyperborean, Lemuria, Atlantis, and America. Gods and men arose from the same source. Like duality of Dhyani Chohans (spiritual and planet) every man has inner and outer principle. Creation from beginning to end is divided into seven rounds. Beings of the first round were ethereal, non-intelligent, super spiritual; second round were gigantic, and firmer and more condensed and less intelligent than spiritual; third round comprised compact bodies and gigantic apes, which were more intelligent (rather cunning) than spiritual; while the last half of the third round had the gigantic size decreasing and nationality increasing though more as apes. The fourth round projects an enormous development of intellect, and a decrease of spiritualism. We are now in the middle of the fourth round. Two thousand million years have passed till the present position. Human existence began some 1700 million years ago. From this middle point things are getting reversed, materialism is decreasing and spirituality is on the increase. Explanation is given about the spiritual principle of nature. Our *pitris* (ancestors and creators) were a group of seven—three in the higher group that was *arupa* or formless and spiritual, and four in the lower group that was *rupa* or with form, material and without intelligence. Correspondingly, human heart has seven cavities—three higher, and four lower. There are seven nervous plexuses, radiating seven rays. Human skin has seven distinct layers. It is observed that Poimandres, Vedas, Puranas, Mazdean scriptures and Kabala have talked about seven primitive men. Seven pillars of Scandinavian *Aesir*, seven Greek Kosmokratores, seven *rishis* and seven *pitris* in India, seven Chaldean gods and seven evil spirits, seven Kabalistic Sephirots, and seven planetary spirits and Christian mystics—all represent identical mythical facts. Details are given about shadows (men) created by seven groups of creators, which were inferior. Many creations came but failed. Lower group created man but failed. Higher group provided mind and spirituality to man but failed. The fruit of the tree of knowledge, dwelling as serpents of wisdom in men, and known as Kundalini, has remained forbidden. The poor material man was left to himself to grow.

Two falls are explained—the fall of angels and the fall of Adam and Eve. Fallen angels were the higher spiritual *devas*, who refused to create man to avoid the 'germ of sorrow.' They were cursed by Brahma to take repeated human births, were called demons by Christians, and the 'Spirits of Darkness' by the Zoroastrians. Christians forgot St. Michael who was the first to refuse to create, and was declared Satan. Truth is that the so called 'Fallen Angels' were our real saviours who gave us the spark of intelligence and discrimination, which alone had produced yogis going back to God. Gnostics recognized the lower group of creators including Jehovah, much before the laws of Moses came into being. These creators did not want man to become 'one of them' and so gave them ideas to commit mistakes even in worshipping the Lord, fighting among themselves, falling into sins and remain engaged in 'fruitless worship based on blind faith.' Chapter 3 also gives the details about the most mysterious symbol of Svastika revered by Indians, Chaldeans, Scandinavians and even Trojans, since it was found in the ruins of ancient Troy. The symbol represents the whole working of the universe and is the mid-point between heaven and man. It is unfortunate that the people did not value it, the understanding of which could have led to salvation. Details are also given about 'third Root Race' at the end of which separation of sexes took place and the 'Fall' into generation began.

Chapter 4 presents the procedure of liberation of man. Four outstanding methods are given there, which are advocated by Madam Blavatsky, Swami Sri Yukteswar, Srimad Bhagavatam, and Ishopanishad commented by Swami Prabhupad of ISKCON.

According to Blavatsky, the fathers (lower angels) are nature-spirits who created men, but the spark of intelligence (*manas*) was given by divine rebels, who are in reality our saviours. Because of this 'spark' men rebelled against the morbid activity of pure spirit and this gave men self-consciousness, and capabilities and attributes of God. This 'spark' is also known as 'spiritual fire' or 'higher self' without which liberation could never be possible and men would have always lived as animals. Two forces—*Monad (Jiva)*, acting unconsciously as inherent force, and lower astral body or the personal sell—are responsible for forcing evolution. The higher self has to gravitate towards its sun—the universal atman to subdue the lower ego, which may otherwise continue to have upper hand. The first three-and-a-half root races perfected physical form at the cost of spirituality. From this turning point higher ego reigns over animal ego and spirituality is on an ascending path now. Only in human form spiritual ascendance is possible; angels are intransitive, and they too like to descend on earth to take human form for this reason. With the destruction of the last remnants of *Atlantis* some 12,000 years ago, an impenetrable veil of secrecy on truth was created as the ring pass-not. This veil can be broken only by becoming a 'twice born' with the possibility of becoming absolute once again. The fifth race is re-establishing the truth again, with the upsurge of spiritual giants in sixth century BC.

Swami Sri Yukteswar presents his theory of evolution that is based on eight steps of yoga, parallel to the yoga-sutras of the great sage Patanjali of sixth century BC. He points out that seeing of divine light and hearing of divine sound are signposts of graduation from earth, becoming an initiate or 'twice born.' There are seven divisions of the cosmos: *Bhurloka* (gross matter), *Bhuvarloka* (fine matter and electrical impulses), *Swarloka* (magnetic impulses and aura), *Maharloka* (creation of four ideas—word, time, space and atom, where the atom or *jiva* or 'individual soul' is created for the first time. It is the middle plane between three lower or material worlds and three upper or spiritual worlds. For this reason it is called the 'tenth door' or *dasmadwara* which then opens for the initiate to travel to higher spiritual worlds), *Jnanloka* (plane of *jnanis* or wise men, plane of spiritual light or brahman, where the initiate becomes one with Brahman), *Tapoloka* (plane of holy ghost or divine love force, anointed by spirit. The Initiate becomes Christ, the saviour and attains a state of *Jivanmukta Sanyasi*—liberated while living), *Satyaloka* (baptized or absorbed in the holy sound or word or Aum one arrives at the highest region of SAT and becomes one with God, out of the clutches of *maya* or illusion once and for all. This is the state of *Kaivalya*). According to Swami Sri Yukteswar absorption or baptization in *Pranava Shabda* or Word or Aum is the only way to God.

Srimad Bhagavata Mahapurana is the gist of all vedas and upanishads and carries direct instructions from the Lord Himself from time immemorial. *Sattva*, *Rajas* and *Tamas* are the three states of being which direct a man subconsciously for spiritual worldly and no activities, respectively. So a man should indeed neither be praised nor blamed for what he does since it is the three states or *gunas* that are responsible. A self-realized person is above the three *gunas* and remains unaffected by them. Even his worldly enjoyments do not bind him into karma. Enjoyment or suffering is *prarabdha* or destiny, which clears up only by living through it. It is the mind that connects organs of action to the organs of sense, and hence the control or demise of mind will enable divorce the mind to itself from sense objects of the material world. The Lord advises one to shake off identity from *buddhi* or Intellect and its attachment to three states of wakefulness, dream and deep slumber, and get established in the fourth state of *witnessing*. Sankhya is the science of differentiation between spirit and matter, and *yoga* is the science of connecting soul to supersoul. The Lord says that he loves more than anyone else, a devotee who has nothing to call his own, has subdued passion, is free from wants and has fixed his attention on the Lord sitting in his own heart. *Yoga* as taught by the Lord to Brahma and other sages suggests 'withdrawing the mind from everything else and duly and directly establishing in him.' One is advised to sit in a chosen posture, concentrate on breathing and on the sound of Word or Aum, and fix his attention on the Lord's form. Gradually, misconceptions about matter, knowledge and action will be cleared and the practitioner will become one with the Lord.

Ishopanishad, Upanishad of Ishwar or God, elaborates the relation between the first cause/supersoul and the individual soul. Conditioned soul has four deficiencies—mistakes, illusion, philosophy without knowing the truth, and imperfection of senses. Therefore it cannot acquire true knowledge. Knowledge of the Vedas comes directly from the Lord to Brahma to his sons and disciples, then to their disciples. Hence, knowledge comes from discipNic succession, and is therefore authentic. Independent experiments will lead to the same knowledge. There are two classes of transcendentalists—impersonalists and Vaishnavas.

Preface xvii

Impersonalists believe in impersonal Brahman, while Vaishnavas believe in personal features of Godhead having a form. However, both believe Krishna to be the highest authority. Originally, there was only one Veda. People at that time had sharp intellect and strong memory, so they could remember the instructions mentally. Some five thousand years ago, Sage Ved Vyas thought that henceforth men will have weaker intellect and memory and hence he wrote down Vedas in four parts and eighteen Upanishads, and put his disciples in charge of them. In the end he wrote the summary of everything in the Vedanta for the scholarly and philosophical people.

Swami Prabhupad observes that, Upanishads point at the indirect but *Bhagavad Gita* points at the direct attention to primeval Lord Krishna. He is the proprietor of everything animate or inanimate in the creation, and no one else should claim the proprietorship. The Lord has internal, marginal and external potencies. Through external potency inanimate matter is created; through marginal potency demigods, men and animals are created while through internal potency the spiritual sky or atmosphere is created. One-third of the space contains millions of material universes of solar systems like ours, while three-fourths of the space has spiritual sky and millions of spiritual planets in it. The effulgence of the Lord emanates an infinitely powerful light called *brahmajyoti*, which clouds his face and form. Material universes are situated at a corner of the *brahmajyoti* and are enclosed in a coconut-like shell that needs light from various suns. Also the shell acts like a 'ring pass not' because of which the *jivas* or individual souls cannot know the truth unless they become 'twice born' or an initiate. Planets in the spiritual sky are self-lighted because of *brahmajyoti*.

The Lord expands himself to paramatma and Brahman forms to run his creation. The Lord's Brahman feature is the Lord's impersonal form present everywhere while the paramatma feature makes him the controller of all souls as Supersoul and He resides in the hearts of everyone. The Lord resides in his abode, which is highest in the spiritual sky, and yet present in every particle of the space. God realization is a great science. Impersonal transcendentalists come to know about impersonal Brahman as *brahmajyoti* and become one with it. They are known as *jnanis* or wise men, who are said to have realized Brahman. It is said that the knower of Brahman becomes Brahman himself. This is the beginning of the spiritual sky. *Sankhya yogis*, who differentiate between spirit and matter, get the knowledge of the 24 elements that make the material universe, and come to know about the various potencies possessed by the Paramatma feature of the Lord. They are said to have realized Paramatma. A *jnani* and a *yogi* cannot go beyond these stages of realization. If however, the practitioner persists with true *bhakti* or devotion to the Lord then he can pierce the veil of *brahmajyoti* that covers the face of the Lord, and see the Lord face to face. This is the highest form of realization. At this stage one may live in the spiritual sky or on one of the spiritual planets called *vaikunthalokas* or even live on the planet of Lord Krishna. Once an entry is found in the spiritual sky there is no rebirth for the *jiva* or individual soul.

A *karma-kandi* or a worker with actions and their fruits can endeavour and/or meditate and on being successful he can reach the goal of his choice. Thus one who takes delight in eating meat can be born as a tiger, one who likes spiritual activities can be born as a Brahamana, one who loves to be with his demi-god can go to his planet. The highest one can attain in the material universe is the abode of Brahma, called Brahmaloka. These are the achievements in the material universe. Therefore better than a *karma-kandi* is a *jnani* or impersonalist who can cross the Brahmaloka and enter the spiritual sky and become one with *brahmajyoti*. Better than a *jnani* is a *yogi* who realizes the paramatma feature of the Lord sitting in every heart, and best of all is the *bhakta* who goes a step further, pierces the *brahmajyoti*, travels through the spiritual sky and reaches one of the *vaikunthalokas* or spiritual planets, the highest of which is the *Krishnaloka*.

My observation based on my personal experiences is that a practitioner passes through almost all the stages described in any faith or tradition. This means that any prescribed path may be followed and the results ultimately would be the same, depending on what one's aim or goal is. For example, I have experienced the steps prescribed by Swami Sri Yukteswar for a *yogi*, such as, going through the eight-fold path of *yoga*, seeing the divine light and sound and following the Word or Aum to become one with Lord. Srimad Bhagavatam has prescribed the rule of sitting in a posture, withdrawing one's attention from the material world, following the inner sound from root centre to crown centre, and fixing one's attention on the Lord till one finds Him. This also I have gone through. Carl Jung's process of individuation requires the balance between masculine and feminine personalities that is between intellectuality and sentimentality, which leads to the inner marriage and birth of the divine child, which completes the process of self-realization. This too has happened with me. *Sankhya yogis* would separate spirit from matter, undergo the experience of death (of ego) and witness oneself as atma or soul, which completes their goal. My autobiography shows that these were also my experiences. Swami Prabhupad states that one should realize brahmajyoti first, then realize the paramatma feature of the Lord, and finally see the Lord face to face; even this has been the order of my experiences. And finally, Shaktipath, or the passage of energy from Guru to disciple awakens Kundalini and activates it so that it passes through seven *chakras* and meets the Lord in the crown centre. These have been my experiences duly described in my books on Kundalini and published through papers in the Academy of Spiritual and Paranormal Research. Hence any authentic scale of measuring spiritual progress can be used and the results found would be the same.

My recommendation is as follows. Faith and an attitude of surrender to the Lord would be the best starting point. Although this level is attained by people after Karma Yoga or action without an attention on the fruits, and Jnana Yoga or acquiring the knowledge through reading and contemplation, one can start the three simultaneously. Sri Aurobindo talked about Integral Yoga, which amounts to the approach I am suggesting. I have given such a formula explicitly in my book *'Kundalini for Beginners'* by the name Integral Path. Keep an eye open to find a Guru of the Shaktipath cadre who can pass spiritual energy into the disciple and awaken the Kundalini in a short time. Just as a hen can hatch the eggs by sitting on them and passing energy, a fish can develop its offsprings by looking into their eyes and passing energy, and a turtle passes energy to its offsprings still under the ground by its will power, so also a Shaktipath Guru can awaken and activate the Kundalini in the disciple by one of the means. Then answers to questions and direct instructions from the Lord will begin to come in three ways: books and scriptures, meeting someone suddenly and getting the required knowledge, and through dreams and trances. Do not aim at anything in the material universe up to the Brahmaloka, and keep your goal on the highest level of meeting the Lord in person. Remember that first is the realization of self and Brahman, second is the realization of paramatma, and third and final is the personal encounter with none other than the Lord himself.

The last chapter deals in detail with the theory of Shaktipath. Maha Yoga or the great yoga in the theory of Shaktipath, so called because it involves all kinds of yoga in one, has four stages of development that are found in all kinds of yoga. Stage1 (*arambhavastha*) includes *kriyas* or automatic movements following the awakening of Kundalini. This marks the beginning of real *Yoga*. It induces the form of Hathayoga or *yogic* postures that are necessary for the development of the practitioner. *Asanas* or yogic postures give stability to the body, *bandha* or locks and *mudras* or gestures give strength, *pranayama* or breath control gives subtlety, and the purification of nerves gives perfection and balance in everything. Thus the first stage brings automatic perfection in Hathayoga for the practitioner. *Stage 2* (*ghatavastha*) enables the body to be purified, empowers it with *sattvic* (pure and spiritual) qualities; greed and lust get destroyed; God becomes continuous; Hathayoga and Layayoga (yoga of absorption) become easy and smooth. One remains zealous and uncomfortable due to separation from God. The first two stages run together as stage one unifies the body while stage two unifies the mind. Both body and mind become purified and strong. Kundalini finds its path unobstructed and travels easily and smoothly to the crown centre. *Prana* or life energy becomes static and the mind becomes stable at the second stage.

In stage 3 (*parichayavastha*) the Prana is absorbed in the inner sky or *akasha*. Kundalini Shakti on establishing *prana* in the heart centre or *anahata-chakra* gets united with Shiva in the crown centre or *sahasrara*. As long as *prana* remains static, the practitioner's body becomes motionless and gives the appearance of being lifeless, although he is fully alive internally. *The atman gets united with prana* and the practitioner is now called a *siddha* or adept, who attracts power from beyond and acquires unworldly capabilities. *Prana* crosses all the seven *chakras* and rests in the crown. Semen converts into energy and the practitioner finds intuitive knowledge flowing into him. The practitioner on becoming an adept or *siddha* can pass over energy to others and awaken their kundalini. Karma is burnt, all doubts are removed and the knot at the level of the heart is opened by the grace of God Almighty. He is absolved and has the power of absolving others too. Even if such a person appears without morals outwardly, his knowledge cannot be camouflaged by anything whatsoever. Those who criticize him take these sins with them, and those who praise him take these virtues with them. He has seen the way to the realm of brahman and when he leaves this world he will arrive straight into the realm of *satya* or truth. The Lord conveys that such an adept is acquainted with me and now he can show the way to anyone he likes.

In stage 4 (*nishpatti-avastha*) the practitioner-turned-adept or the *Siddha* witnesses himself as the soul or *atman*. He has reached the level of Siva-ness (Kundalini Shakti is absorbed in Shiva), and he is known as *jivan-mukta* or liberated-while-living. He experiences the universe being absorbed in his own atman.

I can say that Shaktipath works very effectively; the only requirement is faith and surrender. In the last three years I have initiated about 20 people and almost all of them have their Kundalini activated, and there is a complete change in their lives. We have developed centres in various parts of the world but the main ashram is in Delhi and Haridwar where all the facilities are available.

Margaret Dempsey
Mind Research Institute, London, U.K.
and
Swami Gopalanand Tirth
Narayan Kuti, Devas, India.

THE AURA OF THE FIRST AUTHOR
(RAVINDRA KUMAR)

An aura contains the colors of the rainbow—VIBGYOR: Violet, Indigo, Blue, Green, Yellow, Orange and Red; representing the seven *chakras*—crown, eyebrow, throat, heart, naval, sacral and root in the descending order. Appearance of white represents the transcendental and spiritual qualities, beyond the seven *chakras* located in the physical body. The violet, followed by white and blue, and a tinge of green, dominates the aura. One can see clearly a *white channel* extending from the crown centre and beyond. The interpretation follows in the next paragraph.

Violet indicates intuition, idealism, magical personality, sensuality, vision, charisma, creativeness and inventive. White stands for transcendence, transformation, healing, calmness, sensitivity, living in higher dimensions and strong spiritual connection. On top of these properties there is a white channel connecting the crown centre with the infinite suggesting that the ideas and knowledge or wisdom come directly from the spiritual realm, and not from the material world. This channel also confirms the text that the soul is taken in tow to the supersoul by the cosmic sound, generated within after the culmination of Yoga. Outskirts of aura have some fading of the white invaded by the blue or indigo; this indicates some loss of energy through discussions with other lineages because of doubt in one's own perfection. The aura reader strongly advised not to lose energy in this way and have firm faith in one's own spiritual power, which is exceptionally good for the guidance of others. However, I was advised to keep grounding my high energy through regular heavy walks and physical exercises to keep the balance. There can be occasional stomach upset due to such an imbalance. The aura reader said that the divine knowledge and calmness suggested by the aura should help many in the world.

Small amount of blue in the aura suggests harmony, loyalty, sensitivity, loving and helping nature while dealing with the people of the world. Indigo stands for calm, turned inward and searching. Little amount of green mixed with white shows socialization and communication with others for spiritual purposes. Tinges of yellow here and there show the nature to be warm, charming and entertaining. Absence of yellow, orange and red colors shows withdrawal from the activities of the world for which these colors are necessary ingredients.

An advice given by the aura reader is to recognize the importance of dreams in my life. Unknown divine talks to you through dreams and trances and this is proportional to the level of consciousness developed in you.

A Part of Initiation

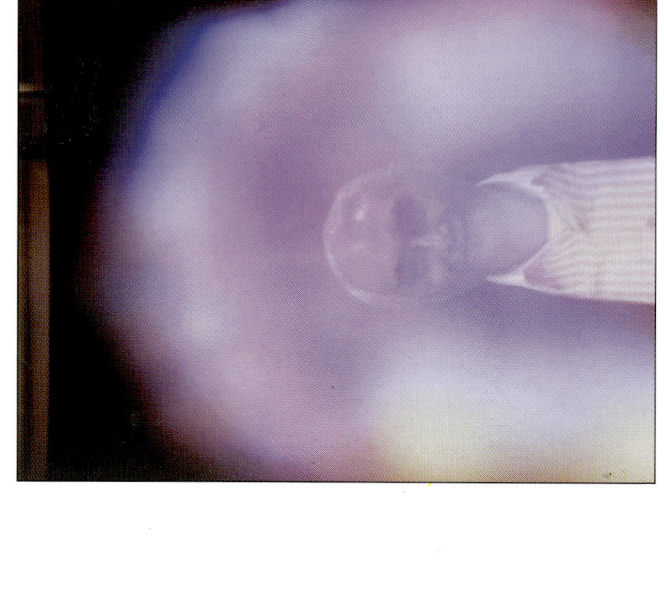

Aura of Ravindra Kumar

Aura of Jytte Kumar Larsen

THE AURA OF THE SECOND AUTHOR
(JYTTE KUMAR LARSEN)

Nearly the same interpretation, with some variations of course, holds good for the second author who has been working closely for several years. Notable difference is that the second author has less white and more indigo. However, the white channel connecting crown centre to beyond is nearly the same in both.

The reading was done on 2 September, 2006 in Copenhagen, Denmark by Lene Kopwski Schack.

Telephone: (45) 28188873,
website: www. leneschack. dk.

The Divine Light, Sound and Touch

Spirit and Nature, the two inseparables, forming our illusory universe, remain in the universe of ideas till it lasts, finally merging back into Parabrahman, the changeless one. 'The Spirit, whose essence is eternal, one and self-existent,' emanates a pure ethereal LIGHT—a dual light not perceptible to the elementary senses—in the *Puranas*, in the *Bible*, in the *Sepher Yetzirah*, the Greek and Latin hymns, in the *Books of Hermes*, in the Chaldean *Book of Numbers*, in the esotericism of Lao-tse, everywhere[1]. In the Vedas, it is BRAHMA. According to Kabala, this light is the Dual Man, Androgyne (sexless) angel, better known as ADAM-KADAMON. They solidify and complete the ethereal form of man, which emanates from the divine, though a far lower being in their comparison.

According to occultism and Kabala, there are three kinds of light. (*a*) The abstract and absolute light, which is darkness; (*b*) the light of the manifested – unmanifested, called by some the logos; and (*c*) the latter light reflected in the *Dhyani-Chohans*, the minor *Logoi* (the Elohim, collectively), who, in their turn, shed it on objective universe[2]. However, in the thirteenth century the Kabalists re-edited and adjusted the Kabala to fit the Christian tenets, where the three lights are described as: (*a*) The clear and penetrating light, that of Jehovah, (*b*) reflected light, and (*c*) light in the abstract.

The Divine Light, Sound and Touch

My hypothesis is that a spiritual practitioner witnesses these three kinds of light in succession, whenever he/she reaches the level of self-realization. This is the objective proof of his/her subjective experiences on the path of evolution. To supplement it with my own experiences over the years, I would submit that the witnessing of the three kinds of light came to me in the reverse order, with an interval of nearly two to three years between them. Thus I first saw the clear and penetrating light in 1984 (Nigeria), then the Logos entered me in 1987 (Zimbabwe), and finally I got connected with the Abstract and Absolute Light-Darkness in 1990 (Malawi). The three experiences have been narrated in detail here.

One day, somewhere in the middle of 1985, while completely engrossed in chanting, I achieved deep concentration. In losing my sense of the world, even the counting of beads was forgotten. In a flash, I heard the sound of lightening, like an electric spark jumping between two poles. Hearing a high pitched sound, my eyes opened. I saw a thick, cool, dazzling spark of pure white light about six inches high and three inches wide, about four feet from my eyes. The spark slowly vibrated as it moved to the left one or two feet, slowly diminished in size, and then vanished completely. I was amazed and I looked around to find the spark's source. I thought it had leaked from a light bulb or some other source of electricity. Slowly, as my amazement subsided, I understood the light had materialized out of nowhere. Now I know it was the physical manifestation of Brahman or God, according to the scriptures, and is called *brahmajyoti*. Carl Jung referred to this 'light' as the high self, and the Polynesians in their Huna code call it the *'aka* body' that manifests as a comforting *amazing white light*. After that day I was filled with inner happiness and my spiritual practice became more regular.

My prayers in the morning from 3 a.m. to 6 a.m. were regular as before during July 1987. One day early morning, I woke up and became aware of the constant sound of someone blowing a conch shell. When I asked others in the morning if they also heard such a sound the answer was 'no.' Plugging my both ears tightly, I found this sound came from inside my head. I went to the ENT specialist at the hospital who said there have been other cases like mine. For some, such sounds vanish after a time while others live with it permanently. This is not due to any ear or nose blockage. This sound, he said, is not a sign of irregularity or insanity. Now I know that it is the sound of Aum or Logos or *Shabda-Brahma* that stays with me till today, having become more pronounced in the course of time.

In the early morning of 15 March 1989, I felt a pressure between my eyebrows. I felt as if a screen was obstructing light and only scattered light could be seen. Slowly the screen started moving to one side and I saw a bright point of white light opposite my third eye. Soon after that, I opened my eyes and got up from the bed.

During December 1989, I was at the University of Malawi, Southern Africa for a week, attending a mathematics conference. I felt relaxed and happy as usual. One night I woke up several times but while dreaming or in trance I felt connected to the infinite void, full of indigo colored darkness, a strange and previously unknown experience. For a few seconds I was afraid, but gradually my fear was replaced by pleasure. And then I suddenly felt dead as my head dropped to one side. Soon I woke up and everything that happened in my dream/trance appeared to have happened in my waking life. I even felt some pain on the side of the neck where my head had dropped. This experience stayed with me for some time.

End Notes:

[1] Blavatsky, H.P. 1979. *The Secret Doctrine Vol. II—Anthropogenesis*. Adyar, Madras: The Theosophical Publishing House, pp 36-37.

[2] —— pp. 37.

Cosmic Consciousness

We are all aware of the five usual senses in life—sight, sound, smell, taste and touch. When awareness of a new sense arises, different from these five, it is not by chance. There are prerequisites for the birth of new sense awareness, extraordinary health (physical, mental, emotional and spiritual), charismatic, and sweet disposition. It happens with the extinction of lower faculties, such as love of materialism and worldly possessions, sense of sin and fear of death. A purely subjective phenomenon becomes objective; in fact for an individual with the new sense there is nothing subjective or objective. For the new man (or woman for that matter) the old world of matter continues to exist, yet, the old world has been transcended and made new; *he/she is in the world but not of the world*. Events are no longer seen through the eyes of the 'lower self', but through eyes becoming more and more clear as this new reality is 'realized.' Bliss, attunement with nature, absolute oneness, and intuitive knowledge of a universal flow, is now realized with the dawning of this new sense. A self-realized individual will be conscious of three things: existence (we are infinite, we were never born and can never die), intuitive knowledge (understanding of the perfection of the universe) and bliss (ever-existing inner happiness). The new sense awareness reshapes the individual. *'Existence-Knowing-Bliss'*, the innate nature of the conscious universe, is reawakened.

The newly awakened man or woman is not immediately established in a permanent state of understanding. They are like newborn children alternating between the old self and the new. The new awareness becomes prominent from time to time, in varying degrees and stages, until one day it becomes the individual's permanent, dominant feature. Exhibiting this new sense awareness has been defined in different ways by different faiths and traditions. Hindus, through the Vedas and other scriptures, called it 'Mukti' meaning 'Liberation from limiting conditions or freedom from *Maya* or illusion" and creating a new individual with a new self. For Buddhists, it is 'Nirvana', the achievement of the state of highest good. Because of the peace and happiness belonging to it, Jesus called it the 'Kingdom of Heaven' or the 'Kingdom of God'. Jesus came to be known as Christ after the awakening of this new sense. Mohammed identified with this new sense as the separate individual living in him and talking to him, and called it 'Gabriel'. Dante identified the new sense with the happiness it brings and named it 'Beatrice'. Balzac identified the new sense as a specialization and called the new individual 'Specialist'. Whitman identified it as the permanent feature within a person and called it 'My Soul'. Richard Maurice Bucke called it 'Cosmic Consciousness', and this became a permanent label for this new sense or type of awareness in psychological study.

INTRODUCTION

In recent years there have been two books in the market that caught my attention: *How to Know God* (Dr Deepak Chopra), and *How to Find God* (Sri Herald Klemp), the Eckankar leader at Minnesota. These books prompted me to realize the three steps in nature: first to know God by inference through *jnana* (knowledge), then to find God through experience of *yoga*, and then become God through *bhakti* or devotion. These ideas matured in the research paper 'We Are All Gods in the Making,' appearing this year in *'The Journal of Spirituality and Paranormal Studies,'* Connecticut. The knower of Brahman becomes Brahman—is the central message of this book, which further elaborates concrete steps to achieve this inevitable goal.

Complete realization of the self takes place in three stages: first is the realization of the impersonal Brahman, as *brahmajyoti* or effulgence from the Lord that lights all the material and spiritual worlds and is omnipresent, and that is the identification of atman with Brahman. Many seekers stop at this stage, considering it to be the final goal. Of course, the chain of repeated births is broken and one finds an abode in the spiritual sky that is lighted with *brahmajyoti*, in contrast with innumerable material universes, each of them having their own sun for light and energy. Buddha too talked about the 'Light of the Void' as the final realization. The second stage involves the realization of the paramatman aspect of the Lord in the form of his powers as yogis talk of siddhis, and his presence in each heart as the supersoul looking after every soul or atman in an individual. The soul and supersoul are realized as a simultaneous presence in the heart, for example, through automatic *sphurna* or a special ecstatic vibration emanating from the heart. When one continues further and is able to pierce the *brahmajyoti* that is extremely bright and dazzling, covering the face of the Lord, he has a face-to-face pleasant encounter with the Lord. This is the third and final realization of the self. One then lives on one of the spiritual planets called *vaikunthalokas* in the spiritual sky.

I have presented my autobiography as the first chapter, corroborating my experiences with various faiths and traditions, and giving details of various milestones that a practitioner passes through in his spiritual journey to Godhood. I have been unknowingly following the eight-fold path of yoga, and every time I got an experience it was explained by some agency in one way or the other. Teaching and researching in mathematics for more than 30 years in various countries I never knew about Kundalini until it was awakened in me through sustained yoga practices. Dreams and visions have invariably been my friends telling me of things that have happened or are about to happen. My first encounter was with my inner Guru, my Higher Self, and then although I did not need a worldly Guru, I took initiations from some Masters for my own satisfaction. The whole journey is described in full detail, including the various factors that assist in the process, and I hope it will help some seekers on the path.

A fact worthy of attention is that scriptures and holy books are not understood in their right perspective unless one becomes an *initiate* or "twice-born." This is the reason why the followers of different religions are fighting with each other in the name of God, who is one and the same for everyone, by whatever name you may call Him. The "truth" has been concealed from mundane readers some 12,000 years ago with the submersion of the great Atlantis, as the angels or devas did not want the facts to go in the hands of unworthy

Introduction xxxiii

people. For example, astronomy is reduced only to the science of stars without the knowledge of the spiritual entities and their activities associated with it. Hence one's first aim should be to become a "twice-born" and that requires a "crisis"—moral, scientific, physical or religious, which is not under one's control. However, yoga and meditation, and other metaphysical practices can bring a calculated "crisis," which is in a way under one's control.

In subsequent Chapters I have elaborated the fact that we are all Gods in the making, which is inevitable and predestined. However, the difference is that some will have this realization in present life, some in a future life and yet some in future manvantaras, depending on the level of interest and persuasion they have. Madam Blavatsky's *The Secret Doctrine* has been very enlightening and informative, and I have tried to present her collected ideas in a simple form for the benefit of the readers. Starting with the method shown by Blavatsky for the "journey back to the Lord," I have presented the method of Swami Yukteswar that I have been following unknowingly. And then the way shown by the Lord Himself in *Srimad Bhagavatam,* and *Sri Ishopanishad* commented upon by Swami Prabhupad is presented in brief. Finally I have elaborated the method of Shaktipat that I learnt and practised on many prepared practitioners successfully, raising their Kundalini in shorter time as compared to the time taken by classical methods of self-efforts.

It is amazing to note whatever method of Self-realization may be chosen; the experiences are verified by each one of them. The reason is that various faiths and traditions lay stress on certain selected aspects of realization only, according to their bringing up with the method, but spiritual development is universally the same process. For example, hearing the Cosmic Sound internally is the sure sign of spiritual awakening mentioned in all religions. Hindus call it Shabda-Brahma or Aum, Jews and Christians call it the Word or Logos, Muslims call it Kalm-I-Ilahi, Pythagoras called it the Music-of Spheres, Eckankar call it the Divine-Sound, and some others call it Amen. Similar names can be found elsewhere too. Seeing the Lord as a "divine child" at the culmination of the spiritual process is detailed not only in Hindu scriptures but in other traditions too. Thus, the most famous philosopher and psychologist of the West—Dr. Carl Gustav Jung writes about the birth of the "psychic child" after the inner marriage between masculine and feminine aspects of personality has taken place, and as a proof of the "process of individuation" being completed. The Chinese, Zoroastrians and Egyptians have also talked about the birth of such a child in very clear terms. Very interesting details of this fact can be read in their famous *Book of the Golden Flower* in Chinese.

I have also given my recommendations and suggestions to the seekers, based on my own experiences. The best way is to begin with *bhakti-yoga* or the path of devotion to the Lord in some way, which of course is not the only way. However, if one does so, then the *jnana-yoga* or the path of knowledge and *karma-yoga* or the path of selfless action become easy and also the help comes from nature in a good way. This develops an all-round approach to Self-realization that should be aided by an *initiation* from a Guru of the Shaktipat order. The advantage of *initiation* is that one gets spiritual energy through the Guru, which could otherwise take a long time through self-efforts. Success can be achieved in a comparatively shorter time and certainly in a single lifetime.

Academy of Kundalini Yoga and Quantum Soul **Ravindra Kumar**
Ganga Laksha House, (Now Swami Ravindranand)
58-61, Vashisht Park, Pankha Road, Founder/Director
New Delhi-110046, India.
Tel: 9891467723, 65956688.
Email: kumarravi@mail.com
Website: www.quantumsoulaware.com
Europe: Sofus Francks vaenge 6,6;
2000, Frederiksberg, Denmark.
Tel: (45) 36169250
Email: jytteravi.kumar@mail.tele.dk

CHAPTER 1
THE AUTOBIOGRAPHY—MY JOURNEY TO GODHOOD

Introduction

Credibility is the first major point in the mind of the reader when such a book based on personal spiritual experiences is in hand. It is for this reason that I decided to first write down the steps in the process of self-realization, as followed by some well-known faiths and traditions, and then corroborate my own experiences as a natural growth compared with those steps. This is like laying down the theory first and then doing the practical on specified lines. Having been a scientist perhaps this was natural for me to do so—theory and practical. However, I had the experiences first, as if some unknown force was guiding me all along, and then I found that they have been according to the theory although I did not have that in mind. I have found the common line through some of the famous spiritual traditions, and I am glad to say that my growth has been parallel to the directions shown by those traditions. This corroboration serves two purposes – (*a*) for my own satisfaction that I have been on the right path and the results achieved by me are genuine. I know where I have reached and what I have to do in future, and (*b*) true seekers of truth may find some help going through the series of my experiences and get some guidance in their own spiritual progress.

To be specific, I have been unknowingly following the eight-fold path of Patanjali Yoga: *yama* (morality or self-control: non-injury to others, truthfulness, non-stealing, continence and non-covetousness), *niyama* (religious rules: purity of body and mind, contentment under all situations and obedience to the guru), *asana* (a steady and pleasant posture of the body), *pranayama* (control over the *prana* or life force), *pratyahara* (withdrawal of the senses from external objects), *dharna* (concentration), *dhyana* (meditation) and *samadhi* (final absorption). My whole autobiography will be seen to have run on these lines, although I never knew about it while involved in those practices. It is after achieving a result that somehow I will come to know about it, either through someone telling me, or reading a book or some written literature about that experience. These two ways of knowing things seem to be appointed by nature or God, since they used to happen in a sudden and unexpected manner. After the experience I would be looking for its explanation eagerly for some days and in that I would meet a person who will explain it to me. Most of the times I will suddenly come across a book by chance (there is nothing that happens by chance), will unknowingly open on a particular page, and lo! the answer to the query I had in mind would be there. Sometimes I will have an inner urge to go to a particular place, either in the town or to another city, sometimes even to another country, and will suddenly find the answer or clarification I had been looking for.

Inner turmoil, death (of ego) and resurrection—are the three stages through which the seeker has to pass. And these three stages span over one's life (for some it could be several lives), till self-realization is achieved. This is what I can sum up my life with. From birth till the year 1987 it was inner turmoil; the year 1987 was the awakening of the hitherto dormant spiritual energy – Kundalini and repeated experiences of death (of ego); and thereafter the continual resurrection with series of inner experiences. The turmoil that included metaphysical efforts and yogic practices of various kinds, and the atomic reactions of the awakening of Kundalini that shook the mind and body many times— all came to a final rest. Peace, inner happiness, contentment, unconcern for the affairs of and relations in the world, loss of interest in any kind of power and position was then my permanent property. Travel to inner worlds or higher realms and knowing the working of the universe became a regular feature.

In September 1994, sitting in the lobby of the house in San Francisco, I resigned from my post as professor of mathematics, after teaching mathematics in ten countries for about 35 years. My interest shifted from mathematics to religion and psychology. The Academy of Religion and Psychical Research, New York published my spiritual experiences in a series of more than 15 papers. The book on Kundalini, based on these papers, published in 1999 has now appeared in seven languages of the world. Eighteen books about Kundalini, life after death, and self-realization have come out of my pen effortlessly, as if some external power has been working through me.

The turning points in the spiritual journey can be briefly described here, while the full details will appear in the text to follow. The first major and perhaps the most important event occurred in the year 1984 while I was in Nigeria. I looked at something that fascinated me the most and began to meditate with the chanting of mantras. In course of time I was deeply engrossed and had no waking consciousness at all. Suddenly I heard an unusually high sound and got my eyes opened. I saw a column of unusually white, dazzling and cool light appear before me. It stayed there for about 15 to 20 seconds and then began to move to the left and disappeared. I was extremely happy and blissful from that moment. I came to know later that this was the manifestation of Brahman before his loving devotee, the first manifestation in form. This was the 'first milestone'.

There is a kind of crisis—scientific, moral or religious—that brings the unusual out of the man or the profound experience or the grace of God. Experience of death (of ego) was the 'second milestone'. For the last seven years I used to get up around 2.30 a.m. and from 3 a.m. to 6 a.m. I would meditate chanting mantras. During July 1987 I was fully engrossed in meditation. In the third hour of meditation that is between 5 a.m. and 6 a.m., I was feeling extremely helpless, alone, without a Guru, and desperate for divine help. I was crying with tears rolling out of my eyes and praying to God for help. I was repeating that there is no one to help me except God himself in this hour, as no result is coming out of my long years of meditation. I do not know whom to turn to at this time. I was sobbing and repeatedly striking my head on the feet of Lord Krishna. Suddenly I saw my dead body being carried out on the shoulders of four men, who were repeatedly saying that, 'Ravindra Kumar is dead'. There was a crowd following behind and saying words of different kinds. I saw my own funeral. And the next moment I was out of the distress, feeling very relaxed and peaceful and the whole atmosphere around me appeared to be very happy. In a little while my eyes got opened and I was smiling with unusual happiness. This experience of death (of ego) repeated three times in as many months.

After about two months, I was about to take my evening tea. Suddenly it appeared that my body is going to twist like a snake and my backbone may break. Also my head was getting so hot that I was not able to tolerate. Some thing struck my thoughts and I ran out of my house and kept running for about a kilometer and ran back home. I then cycled the sport cycle for about 20 minutes. Then I took a cold bottle of coca cola and drank it up and lied down on bed. Slowly I began to recover and was near normal. However, my thoughts would not concentrate for preparing the lecture and I had to take leave from the University for two weeks. The doctor advised me that if I was not maintaining an unusually good health I could have suffered with brain haemorrhage. He advised me to abstain from teaching for two weeks and stop meditation henceforth. This was the awakening of the *dormant spiritual energy*, known as Kundalini in the East, and the 'third milestone'. For details on Kundalini please refer to my book *Kundalini for Beginners* (Kumar, 2000).

The rising of Kundalini is felt in many different ways. Some feel it as an ant crawling on the spine, some as a frog jumping on the spine, some feel that a creeper is crawling on the spine, and yet some feel like a small and fine snake rising on the spine. I felt it like a sharp snake shaking and rising in the spinal column.

After a few days when I got up early morning at 2 a.m., I found that I was hearing an unusual sound as if some aeroplanes were flying over our house. I asked everyone if they also heard such sounds but they all replied in the negative. The ENT specialist doctor at the University examined me next day. He said there was nothing wrong with my system and said that he had heard about such cases in which people hear some unusual sounds which may continue or subside after some time. That sound I am hearing till date. It was the cosmic sound or the Word or Aum that manifested and I was hearing it through the inner ears. This was the 'fourth milestone'.

It was during those days that once I suddenly saw Mother Goddess in my vision. She was wearing a red sari (Indian dress) and many beautiful bangles on her wrist. I (*jiva* or individual soul) in white clothes was sitting and bowing down before the red-sari clad Mother (cosmic energy of super soul or god), and with folded hands I was prostrating before her, with love and respect. She was blessing me with her right hand just above my head. She was unusually beautiful and bore a lovely smile on her face. This vision appeared about three times in as many months. This was seeing Mother

Kundalini in physical form. It happens for the satisfaction of the devotee indicating that he is moving on the right path. This was the 'fifth milestone'.

I have seen Kundalini in four different and well-defined forms: snake, mother, beloved and daughter. As a snake she has appeared in my dreams and visions innumerable times, as would be seen in the text of the book to follow. Seeing as a mother has been described above. Then I have seen her as the most beautiful lady, dancing and smiling and looking at me in seducing manners. Once I felt her kissing me on my lips and the blissful state that followed lasted for several hours. And finally I have seen her as a loving daughter trying to give me love and care in different ways.

After about three months I was in a house in London with my relatives. Here I experienced the opening of Third Eye and having the visions of Lord Krishna two times in less than 12 hours. On the night of 31 December 1987, I was half asleep and half awake, which is called the twilight zone by parapsychologists. Suddenly Lord Krishna appeared in front of me as an extremely beautiful child/boy. He was looking at me with love and bore a beautiful smile on his face. He turned around himself but continued to look into my eyes. When the vision gradually disappeared I fell asleep. Again on the morning of 1 January 1988 when I was still half awake and half asleep, suddenly the vision of Lord Krishna appeared before me. As a most handsome child/boy he was smiling and looking at me. He turned a little bit but continued to look into my eyes. The vision lasted for some time and gradually I came to my normal waking state. However, for a long time I was in a half awaken state and in unusual blissfulness. This was the 'sixth milestone'.

Seeing God is a very important event. On successful culmination of meditation through a 'seed mantra', the deity of the mantra appears before the disciple. This is how I saw Lord Krishna as God. However, this is still a state of duality or *dvaita* involving *jiva* or individual soul and the Lord as the super-soul. Awakened Kundalini automatically takes from here and leads the devotee to a non-dual or *advaita* state of self-realization. In this state the devotee realizes the formless state of Lord God and becomes one with it. After passing through the palace of Brahma, I was guided by my Inner Guru to proceed further. I crossed over a wide blue river of deep waters in a formless state, as if travelling on a bridge made of hair-like material. Crossing the river I arrived at a group of mountains and returned to my physical body. After a few days, I crossed the mountains and entered a 'huge cotton or snow-like body' in my minute form and felt extremely blissful and happy. I came out of that huge body and looked at It and then looked at myself as a tiny part of it and made of the same material. Realization came to me that I have always been a part of it will always be so. This can be termed as the 'drop losing its identity in the ocean and yet retaining it'. This was realization of the formless state of Brahman and becoming one with it, which is *final self-realization*. This is paramapada of Blavatsky, *Kaivalya* of Swami Sri Yukteswar (1984, 43) and 'sitting on the throne with Lord Jesus. This was the 'seventh and final milestone'. Knowing the final truth I feel liberated with the grace of God and help of Mother Kundalini. This is possible only through love and devotion to God Supreme. After liberation one enters *Vaikuntha Lokas* or spiritual planets.

According to *Srimad Bhagavatam* and *Bhagavad Gita*, which is the essence of all Upanishads and the Vedas, realization of Truth comes in three stages: impersonal Brahman, represented by *brahmajyoti*; parabrahma or paramatma, the supersoul, sitting in everybody's heart as the working form of the Lord; and finally, the Lord himself appearing as Krishna. Brahman and paramatma are planetary expansions of the Lord. The order of experiences may sometimes appear as reshuffled but the *jiva* or individual soul has to pass through all the three states of realization before entering the *Vaikunths Lokas* or spiritual planets. Details of this nature will appear in Chapter 4.

The 'son of man' (ego) becomes the 'son of God' (self), and it is an irreversible process. Once man attains the position of the son of God, which is final self-realization, he always remains in that state, even if living in the world and involved in the works of the world. He is in the world but not of the world. He has realized the three fundamental properties of Brahman—*Sat* (existence), *Chit* (consciousness) and *Ananda* (bliss), and in this he is one with Brahman, the Ultimate Reality or God, the Father. Man as son of God knows that his 'existence' is permanent (he was, he is, he always will be), he is 'conscious' of the truth about Universe and its working, and he is full of 'bliss' or *ananda*. There is nothing more to be achieved. However, he may be assigned with some duties to help the creation, by God, the Father, or he may take them voluntarily.

There are two important milestones mentioned here. The first is the experience of death (of ego) and second is the opening of the Third Eye. The causal body of man dissolves gradually at the experience of death and the mental body comes into formation. With the continuation of the spiritual progress a time comes when the Third Eye opens. At this time the mental body gets dissolved and the spiritual or cosmic body comes into formation with which the soul becomes one with the super soul. This cosmic body is called *Bramha-sharira* (body of Bramha); and the individual is said to become identical with Brahma (in quality) or the knower of Brahma, called *Brahma-Jnani*.

This, of course, is the destiny of each one of us. We are all gods in the making. In the words of Sri Sathya Sai Baba, "...I say I am God. I also say that you are also God. The only difference is that I know it and you do not know it." According to John (10:34) and Psalm (82:6):

Jesus answered them, is it not written in your law, I said Ye are gods.

I have said, Ye are gods; and all of you are children of the most High.

Sooner or later, everyone is going to find out that he is God or Angel or *Devata*. This means both atma (*jiva* or individual soul) and paramatma (God Supreme) are inside every creation and they are interrelated. It is a different thing that some will take less time, some will take more time and some may take a very long time, involving several lives. Effective spiritual practices and grace of God Supreme, the Guru, are the catalytic agents that expedite the search for reality and make one proclaim that he is God or angel or *Devata*.

A word about my Guru would be appropriate here. As would be seen in the autobiography, I have been involved in the meditative practices right from early childhood. I met Siddheshwar Baba, formerly Dr. B. S. Goel (1995), author of *Third Eye and Kundalini* at his ashram near Delhi in the year 1988. After extensive talks with me he told me that I had my Kundalini awakened already, and no physical Guru is required any more. Mother Kundalini is my Guru, he said. Then in the year 2002 I met Swami Devendra Vigyani at Rishikesh, India. He, after holding detailed talks with me, said that I was a Guru myself, who has been successfully initiating the disciples and raising their Kundalini. He also said that I do not have to ask anybody to give the power of the Guru, which has already been given to me by the Guru of all, that is, Mother Kundalini. Yet, however, on my request Siddheshwar Baba gave me initiation in 1988. Later in the year 2002, Swami Dr Krishnananda Saraswati of Uttarkashi, himself the disciple of Swami Narayan Tirth of Varanasi, India gave me the power of Guru to initiate others. Guru Deepak Yogi demonstrated to me the way of 'Shaktipath' (direct transmission of energy from Guru to disciple) and later initiated me to *Guru-pada* (position of Guru), which was already given to me by Swami Krishnananda. I got blessings of the highly respected Guru of the Tirth lineage, Swami Shivom Tirth, who kindly read the manuscript of my book *Secrets of Shaktipat* and wrote the foreword for it.

The experience of death (of ego) is the big milestone after which the personality of the individual begins to change. This event is importantly described by most religions as 'rebirth' after which the devotee is called a *Dwij* (born again). Lord Jesus also said, "unless a man be 'born again', he cannot enter the Kingdom of God." The old nervous system that served the body since birth gets gradually destructed and a new system takes over. I noted many times the nerves cracking down, especially in the head. Because of inner experiences setting in, one begins to come out of the belief, 'I am this body and mind' and establish the new faith 'I am something permanent as soul.' Mother Kundalini, who was the guide/guru until now, of course under the supervision of God, is taken over by God himself as the Guru. If this was not so, many would break down at this important change and go to a lunatic asylum. In the language of psychology this energy (Kundalini) is called cosmic libido, which turns the devotee or disciple into a guru with God-like nature, if it is attracted towards God. Otherwise, the individual suffers with incurable delusions, pains and sufferings. Working in the positive direction, Kundalini as Guru is now taken over by God himself as the inner guru. This is what I noticed clearly in my case.

Guidance from God as the inner Guru has been coming to me from time to time. Once he appeared before me in my dream. I was in San Francisco in the year 1995. I dreamt of a big hall full of people with normal body sizes. Suddenly, an unusually tall and handsome person appeared in the middle of the scene. He looked at me with a smile and blessed me. The word BAPU was written on his chest. He began to move in one direction swiftly but looking constantly into my eyes. After several years when I was standing in front of the palace of Brahma on a higher platform, I was above the ground in a formless state. Three people were standing on the ground in formless state too. They appeared to be talking about me. Suddenly one of them, presumably the inner guru, asked

The Autobiography—My Journey to Godhood 11

me telepathically to move on. I started to move through the green meadows, crossed the blue and deep river and arrived at the group of mountains. I was given the idea that it is 'Kailash Mountain', the abode of Lord Siva. Before entering the place of Paramapada one has to pass through this place, which may allow only the deserving people to go through. This could be the ring 'Pass Not' mentioned by Blavatsky (1979/1888, 90). All along I felt the presence and guidance of the inner Guru around me.

'For reasons which are not easy for the outsider to divine, the possessors of occult knowledge are specially reluctant to give out facts to Cosmogony, though it is hard for uninitiated to understand why they should be withheld' (Blavatsky, 1979/1888, 170). However, after the experience of death (of ego) when man is called 'twice born' (*dwij*) and is said to have become an 'initiate', occult knowledge and facts about Cosmogony begin to unfold before him gradually and in a sequential manner.

Many cases have been reported in which the individual experiences some internal uplifting and pleasures, and thinks that it is the awakening of Kundalini. My humble suggestion is that a genuine awakening will involve the kind of experiences listed above, e.g., visions and dreams of snakes, manifestations of the divine light and sound, experience of death (of ego), and opening of the third eye and vision of God. After a genuine awakening, contentment, peace and cheerfulness follows. On the other hand, after a fake awakening depression follows, and help of a Guru should be sought in such cases. For symptoms of awakening please refer to Krishna (1967, 1975), Goel (1985), Woodroffe (1981), Sivananda (1991) and Tirtha (1993).

Only 'seven major milestones' have been mentioned in my spiritual journey. However, there are many other in-between milestones or events or signals which need clarification. This chapter on my autobiography is going to be the longest of all, dwelling in details about the proceedings of my life as narratives of happenings. Describing the details of day-to-day living, particular spiritual experiences, and opening of the 'knots in the causal body' or crossing of the ring 'pass not' before the especially profound experiences would take place, are narrated in a fully explanatory manner. Various circumstances that led to a particular experience have been described in detail. I hope the reader would like the text and I would feel my efforts worthwhile if the reader finds some kind of help or guidance from the same in his spiritual quest and realization of the truth.

Historical Background

I was born in an average Hindu family living in the northern part of India. I had a religious background at home. Living in a large joint family with many uncles, aunts and cousins I saw most of them praying or worshipping God in different ways. A common activity was to sing devotional songs to God in the evenings and I used to be a part of it. Lord Shiva was our 'family deity'. We used to sing a particular devotional song for Shiva called *aarti*. Gradually I found that I was most devoted to *aarti* and would not miss it at any cost as far as possible. For example, one evening I was in the garden away from home and playing some games with fellow boys. Suddenly I realized that it was time for *aarti* and I had a strong urge to be at home. I left everything and ran home as fast as I could. Reaching home I found no other person was doing *aarti* for some reason or the other. I immediately prepared the plate for prayer, lit the cotton wand dipped in ghee (cultured butter) and recited the *aarti* alone in full sway. On completing the ritual I felt great satisfaction and happiness. This became my habit and I got involved in devotional songs, wherever I was, whether at home or outside or even in another city.

I was good in studies and games. I had a group of three friends and we stayed together in whatever activity we were involved.

I was a bit naughty in the classroom and used to tease the teachers in different ways. For example, I would make some funny sounds sitting at the backbench and enjoy watching the students enjoy when the teacher was irritated. Some classmates and I would go to neighboring fields and steal some fruits and/or vegetables and use the same during interval in which some food was served to us. Once or twice we were caught by the farmers and got a beating. Once the farmers stripped us off our knickers and on reaching home we had to face the dire consequences. Most of the games popular at that age and time were played by me, for example, playing with glass balls on the mud-ground, flying kites in the sky, and football. We would prepare special thread to fly the kites, coating them with grounded glass, prepare many kinds of colored waters during Holi, the festival of colors, take part in fire-works during the festival of lights, and play different kinds of games like hide and seek in the streets.

To sum up I was a person who took equal interest in all activities, be it studies, throwing up pranks, playing games, or conducting religious prayers. These habits continued from school to college and I achieved good results in each field. I was captain of gymnasts' first eleven while in graduation and won several cups in long jump and other ground activities. I was the vice-president of the mathematical society at the college and got prizes in debates. I invariably took part in plays and dramas at the college and won many awards. The longest drama I played was Gautam Buddha for eight hours, in which I played the leading role of Buddha and won several awards. I used to sing too and entertain others and myself at home or in gatherings. A few years later I learned ballroom dancing and was good at it in India. Several years later when I went to England for post-doctorate research in mathematics, I became very good in these dances as these activities were normal at all colleges of residence in UK. I was also fond of photography and made several albums while travelling in different parts of UK.

I can now think that interest and achievements in all the various fields of activities or the possession of various talents could be due to the awakening of Kundalini to some extent at an early age or as a continuation from previous life. An awakened Kundalini provides excellence in whatever field one takes interest. However, I did not have the inkling of any kind of this knowledge at that age. Even after proper and full awakening of Kundalini in the year 1987 I did not have the knowledge of Kundalini at all. As I mentioned in the 'Introduction', knowledge of everything was received by me after something had happened to me.

My father was not highly educated and had an ordinary job. My mother travelled to another town for her education so that they both could earn a good income someday. She lived in a hostel and would come home on weekends. My grandmother looked after me from that age until I first left for England in November 1972 and she was my only companion. I missed my parents and felt very lonely. She died in 1973 when I was in England. Right from the early age I have mostly lived alone, as if nature conspired to throw me into loneliness. When I reached the middle years of my life, I felt lonely and homesick. Later this loneliness became an integral part of my experience, even if I was in a gathering or party.

My grandmother acted as my guardian during my schooling, while my father was transferred from one place to another as a military officer. He moved every three to four years and my parents thought it better to keep me with my grandmother in our hometown. Many times I felt homesick beyond my control and I would run away to my parents' place without telling my grandmother or other relatives, and would later be warned not to repeat this and was then punished by my parents. So I had to live away from my parents. Later, I lived in hostels away from home as I furthered my education, and again when I served in eight different countries teaching mathematics. I was mostly by myself. Gradually 'disturbed loneliness' evolved into *'healthy solitude'*, although I missed the company of people at times. Most of my spiritual development and experiences took place when I was alone. Yet, however, I would like to be with people, especially in the evenings. This habit eventually got the regular shape of a 'satsang', that is, talking about spiritual matters related to God and self-realization. I would be pleased to discuss and remove doubts from the minds of the people in such matters.

Another important factor I have noticed since my childhood was my disinterest in material possessions and relations out in the world. I did not show interest in buying toys like balloons and whistles when I went out to a fair with my parents. My mother tells me that I would simply keep looking at things without asking to have them and would quietly follow my mother or father while holding their finger. When I graduated from college I was good in gymnastics and hoped to get the award as best gymnast or captain of the first eleven. When I received the captain's 'color' and put it on the pocket of my jacket, I did not feel anything special about it and even lost interest in wearing it. Before our examinations we would talk about getting good results. However, when the results would come out and I was placed in the first division with distinction in some subjects, I did not feel anything special. Around the same time, my younger brother aged 15 drowned in a swimming pool in Delhi, and I lit the fire under his dead body at the crematorium. Everybody in our family was crying but I was simply doing things and watching his body burn to ashes. During a recent burial in India, when we were at the crematorium, I read an inscription on the wall, which said, 'Who says that I have died, I was on the journey outside and have now returned home'. This thing was subconsciously always in my mind, and perhaps intuitively, I knew that we have not departed forever. And hence, I was not perturbed by such happenings, like the death of a relative.

Thus loneliness and disinterestedness in the affairs of the world were noticeable in my nature, right from the early life. As I think now, my ideas and thoughts were probably a continuation from my previous life's experiences and spiritual development.

Love of the unknown and the mysterious things have also been some of my major interests. I would always be excited about going to a new place, whether it was in student life or professional. And then I would like to explore the unknown roads and localities of the new town. I would like to stroll in new parks and gardens, visit new cinema halls and even go to neighboring towns and villages to see what speciality lies there. For sometime I was also interested in 'ouija board' and I talked successfully to some people, for example my deceased grandmother, whom I loved very much. I found that she continued to have the same beliefs, interests and feelings as the ones while she was living on earth, for example, some people/things she liked and some she disliked, and this continued to be so after her death. She warned me not to entertain some relatives who were going to visit my place in near future, because she hated them for certain happenings. Later I talked to my deceased father a couple of times through a medium, while I was in America, an experience to be described later. Repeated conversations with my grandmother and my father convinced me of the belief in the *continuation of personality after death* and the fact that one's personality remains unchanged after physical death.

Dreams have played an important part in my life. Since early childhood I foresaw major events coming into my life through dreams. For example, I would get a bunch of fruits or flowers in dreams, a day or two before I received a letter of appointment. To be specific, I was teaching as a temporary lecturer at the central polytechnic, Chandigarh, India in the year 1961. The letter of confirmation was in the waiting that made me feel insecure at times. One of the nights I dreamt of receiving a bunch of ripe grapes from somewhere. And the next morning when I reached my office I received the letter of confirmation of my job by mail. I would see myself naked whenever some kind of humiliation was to come upon me. In the year 1980 I was serving as an assistant professor at the University in Delhi. In an examination fraud a group of teachers were under enquiry and everyone was worried about the result of the enquiry, whether one was guilty or not. One of the nights I dreamt of seeing myself naked. After a day or two I came to know that I was one of the teachers who was going to be suspended for some time. The letter of suspension came a few days after the dream. This was a matter of big humiliation. It is another matter that after some time I was acquitted of the charge and was reinstated in the job.

I would be chased by dogs and even bitten a few days before I was to face defeat in some family matter or be insulted by someone. In a matter of division of the property amongst us six brothers and one sister—a row was going on for quite some time. I being the eldest of the brothers, shared much of the responsibilities of my parents, and in most matters my parents consulted me. Some of my brothers thought that I was advising them against them. One evening one of the brothers came home heavily drunk. He had an empty and broken glass bottle in hand, ready to attack me if required. In this position, he challenged me and called me many bad names using dirty words one would not use under normal circumstances. It was a disgracing affair for the family in which my brother openly insulted me in the presence of even neighbors. Seeing the sensitivity of the situation nobody took an action for fear of fatal happenings. Although the misunderstandings were later removed and things became normal, it was a great insulting evening for me. And, it was a night or two before this happening that I dreamt of dogs chasing me in the street and even trying to bite me.

I would dream of receiving a letter, money or precious stones a day or two before I would get some important payment from somewhere. Just this morning, 8 March,

2002, as I am writing this paragraph, I dreamt of 'escaping from confinement', which meant, 'rise in the commercial world'. Around 11 p.m. I got an e-mail from Llewellyn Worldwide Ltd., USA saying that they are going to post my article on Shaktipath on their website, and within 30 days I am going to be paid for it. What a timely and accurate prediction through the dream!

You can make your own dream journal and find that recurring dreams will tell you about the life you are going to have in the future so that you can be prepared for it.[1] For example, I have seen parallel lines in dreams indicating that discipline is required in the daily affairs. This would happen whenever irregularities would come into my routine. Seeing crowds or being in crowds is a sign of advancement in one's position or realization of one's ambition. Dreams of crowds recurred to me in 1999 when I got my Kundalini book accepted for publication by Llewellyn publishers, Minnesota. Recurring dreams of having fun with people are an indication of rapid success of our hopes. I would see such dreams before I got invited for an important presentation or before I got a manuscript accepted for publication. Dreams of a pair of things, such as a pair of corns, bananas or pens would recur whenever I was or going to be in a state of indecision, caught between two alternatives. I always got a warning of this kind before the situation came into being. This would reduce my tension and help me in taking decision in favor of one of the alternatives.

Dreaming of happy people, elderly males and people in high offices indicates reputation in society, fortune, honor and dignity. Several times after seeing such dreams I have received invitations for giving talks on yoga, meditation and spirituality. Once I dreamt of a carriage with two cisterns full of milk to the brim. This predicts improvement in financial matters and unexpected fortune. After such dreams recurring a couple of times during May 2000, we got our application accepted for the financial grant by the

The Autobiography—My Journey to Godhood

government to run the yoga centre to treat people for diseases without medicine. My publisher in India gave me a cheque for Rs. 20,000 towards the publication of four mini books on occult sciences. Also a proposal was given to me for writing another eight mini books of that kind. One of my brothers with whom I had differences for a long time suddenly came to me and asked for settling the differences and be good friends. Weeping with or without grief means great pleasures in life and I have always found this to be so in my life. On the other hand laughing too much indicates sorrowful events to come and this too I have experienced to be true. For long I had been seeing dreams of high buildings, recurring to me which meant long life of plenty, travel and exploration of distant countries. Such dreams were normally followed by my travels to foreign countries. For several decades, I have been seeing such dreams and have lived in ten countries in this period. Falling on the ground without injury or sustaining a fall means victory in struggles, and this I experienced many times. Dreaming people eating food indicates rapid success of hopes. Shopping centres, store or market has always brought good fortune following efforts. Seeing stores full of goods in dreams indicate prosperity and advancement, a ring in some way or the other has indicated advancement in a relationship, and dreaming nice hotels has normally brought success of hopes.

Seeing myself in strange places and meeting strange people has always been part of my dreams. Recurrence of such dreams took place when I inherited property from my parents. Seeing wide and long roads has always brought good results in pursuits. Being in a car driven by someone else indicated that someone else controls your affairs. On the other hand, if you are driving the car yourself it means you are the master of your affairs. I have seen such dreams many times in life and the results indicated were found true. Seeing a judge indicated a legal settlement of certain matters in life. Many times I have dreamt of getting ready for a trip before receiving some financial gains. Missing a train or losing shoes always came in dreams before serious differences with my wife, which took a long time to settle. There could have been a divorce if things would not have worked out. Dreaming of being happy has been an indication of realization of ambitions many a time. Kissing someone on the face has been an indication of coming success. Dreaming of birds has always indicated improvement of circumstances and family reunions in some way. Climbing stairs has always been an indication of happiness and prosperity. On the other hand stepping down or falling on the steps has been an indication of failure or dishonor. Such dreams have always occurred in my life before an event of importance took place.

Dreams of flying in the sky have always been a part of my life. Dreaming of a wayfarer on the path and flying in the air are indications of congenial work and good news. On 17 September, 2000 I dreamt of a wayfarer, and the next day I received two messages from my literary agent in America; one, Llewellyn publishers, who had have sent proofs of first book on Kundalini, and two, the publishers who wanted the revision of the second book and then to be resubmitted. Certainly, the dream indicated congenial work and good news at the very right time. I have many times seen long queues and sometimes seen myself standing in the queue. This is an important dream, which has appeared many times in my life successfully predicting either a reestablished friendship or a very important beneficial event. Many times I have dreamt of being left alone in a house. Loneliness in dreams has always been an assurance of happiness. At times I have dreamt of a beautiful big library nicely kept with books on shelves and this has always been an indication of rapid progress in work. All my life I have been seeing children in different forms. Children at play are an indication of abundance in life. I have been dreaming of climbing a wall at times, which I considered to be a indication of overcoming obstacles in the matters I was involved at that time. Dreaming of a house has been an indication of financial security.

Travelling in a car, train or carriage foretells good fortune, family love and happiness. Having loving and passionate moments with the opposite sex is also an indication of happy times. Being bitten by a snake may foretell problems in love affairs including a possible break. Dreaming of disappointment in certain matters means success in the same matter, that is, indicating an opposite effect. This has happened with me many times and I can say for sure that this is true. Dreaming of a dog indicates loyalty by those involved with you in some way, according to the loyal nature of a dog. Similarly, a dream of a cat indicates treachery in some way by the people involved. Again it is in correspondence with the nature of the cat. Crossing a bridge may imply change of business occupation. Swimming in clear water means success in one's affairs. Dreaming of a pool full of water indicates approaching good fortune. On the contrary, a pool without water is the sign of loss or disappointment. Dreaming of a bunch of keys indicates the key to success, peace and happiness in the future. Dreaming of returning from a trip foretells unexpected joy. To dream of a table preparatory to a meal foretells happy union and prosperous circumstances. Seeing a couple copulating is a sign of abundant means. Once again I may say that all these things I am writing from my dream journal with recordings of my personal experiences of the same kind over and over again.

Once I dreamt of a beautiful shop and after a few hours I received a parcel of four mini books of mine published in India. Dreaming of clear water is a sign of abundance. On the other hand muddy or dirty water indicated loss of some kind. Drinking from a glass of water may indicate prompt relationship with the opposite sex. Once I dreamt of three vacant seats in an aeroplane or a theatre. And the next day I received good news from three friends. It was amazing! Seeing a newborn infant shows pleasant surprises are awaiting. And that day I received two copies of the

Kundalini book published by the publishers in US. Fear of the unknown definitely shows someone is going to take care of you. Such were the dreams that recurred to me several times in June 2005. And it was in the month of July that I met William. Henry Balk at the conference near New Jersey in which he offered me to work with him. It was a happy meeting. It was at his place that I successfully wrote my first book on Kundalini. Henry provided all kinds of help to me at his place.

Once I saw a baby crying, and the next day I had arguments and serious differences with my wife, which lasted for some time. Hence, the crying of a baby may foretell disputes in the family. Being in a hall has not proved to be a good sign. This dream recurred to me a few times during early December 2000. I began to expect something important to happen, good or bad. On 11 December I received the information that our application for funding the 'project of yogic discipline curing patients without the use of medicine' was rejected by the government. Dreaming of a sexual organ in good condition has been a symbol of successful creative activities. Seeing a beautiful landscape, flying high in the sky and seeing lakes or rivers full of clear water have always indicated luck and prosperity. Seeing someone or yourself as a big person in physical form has always preceded the receiving of some honor or financial benefits. Questioning the merit of a thing may be dreamt of in the event of suspecting someone you love of unfaithfulness and there may be fear of speculations. Asking questions in dreams foretells earnest striving for truth and being successful.

Dreaming of an officer or people in high office has always preceded moments of honor and dignity in my life. Once I dreamt of finding a shining needle and the dream occurred once or twice. This has been associated with having appreciative friends and spiritual people around. Being lost in streets has recurred to me for several years. This has been associated with 'joy without profit', meaning inner happiness without any material gains. I had been living an unprofitable life since 1994, when I resigned my position as a professor of mathematics at the University of Dar-Es-Salaam, Tanzania. No salary from anywhere, living moderately with inner happiness and journeys beyond was the life when dreams of getting lost in streets recurred. Other dreams that used to recur in those days were meeting an unknown person or a stranger, and being in a strange place alone, all of them meaning 'joy without profit'. During December 2000, I had dreams of numbers written on papers, travelling in a boat, beautiful landscapes and seeing plates full of food being served, all of them indicating a pleasant happening. And, what I got at that time was the 'permanent residence card' for Denmark from the immigration authorities—a good achievement. Other dreams, which have also been predicting realization of ambitions, are gray or tan horses being tossed in the sky, seeing magnificent buildings and flying in the air.

I have been seeing such dreams all along my life. I used to keep a notebook by the side of my bed and used to write the dream as soon as I woke up. I have a collection of several notebooks being filled this way. Seeing dreams on a regular basis is a sign of consciousness being open to the beyond. I can say that the universe has in some way been programmed to answer your questions in dreams. It may also be said that God talks to you through dreams and/or you receive prior information of the events to come if you train yourself to keep open to the beyond. There are some people who never see dreams and you will find them strong headed or unemotional.

I have had a religious bend of mind from early childhood. The normal religious activities performed by my elders further strengthened this interest. I was devoted to Lord Shiva, and every evening I prayed around 6.30. In the morning, after my bath, I would read the *Shiv-Chalisa* (religious text about Lord Shiva) regularly. I always had great respect for my elders and spiritual persons. Faith and surrender to such people was part of my nature. I would easily believe everyone. People thought of me as simple and I was not clever in matters of the world. My simple nature was exploited and taken advantage of by both my friends and relatives. They would misuse me in many ways until I would revolt. I got married in 1960 to my Indian wife and most of my time was spent with my family, parents, five brothers and a sister. The relatives misused my simplicity as I was not mature at that time. The marriage was not successful although I got a son and a daughter from this wedlock.

I worked at various universities in different parts of the world, India (1959–1972), UK (1972–1974), Iraq (1976–1978), Nigeria (1981–1986), Zimbabwe (1986–1988), Ethiopia (1989–1991), Fiji (1991–1993), Tanzania (1993–1994), USA (1994– 1996) and Denmark from 1997 to date. My spiritual interests never diminished. On the contrary, mixing with different kinds of people increased my love for humanity and the world appeared like a big family. Through palmistry and numerology I could see that human beings in general suffered with similar weaknesses or enjoyed similar feelings, no matter which part of the world they belonged to. My interest has always been to know what kind of belief people have about God and what means they adopt in knowing him. Almost every two years I have been changing the country after serving the contract of teaching at the university. This has taught me the big lesson of not getting attached to the people you meet in life, although behaving well with them always pays dividends. This has also taught me non-attachment with places I lived and to any kind of particular circumstances. Being open to the new circumstances has always been my habit and adjustment with different kinds of people has never created any problem to me. In fact, it is this habit that has led me to the quest of unknown spiritual truths and bringing successful ends to them.

An important thing to mention here is the fact that I never occupied a 'managing position' in my profession for the whole life. I never took up as 'head of the department' in about 35 years of teaching at about ten universities of the world. Even the smaller positions such as the timetable in- charge were never given to me due to internal politics. Sometimes I used to feel that nature was not giving me a good deal, but later I understood that it was the design of the nature to keep me free from poor worldly positions, which would have only raised my ego. Sri Herald Klemp, spiritual leader of Eckankar at Minnesota, has written, 'Little goals are dry runs'. This thing has perfectly translated in my whole life. It served a twofold purpose: first, I was saved of the ego of the power and attachment to the position, second, it saved a lot of time that would have been wasted in the execution of duties related to those positions. It also saved me from the situation that you can never satisfy everyone as head of something, since a section of people would always be dissatisfied, however best you may try to please everyone. Someone has rightly said, 'I cannot tell you the formula of success but I can tell you the formula of failure, that is—try to please everyone.' I could wholeheartedly concentrate on my spiritual activities. What a design of God Almighty! I thank him from the core of my heart. It seems he has always been pulling me towards himself, without being lost into petty attractions. How lucky I have been?

I was always interested in the occult in one way or another. Besides teaching and researching in mathematics, I devoted a few hours to the study of palmistry every day during the 1970s. I studied the work of many renowned authors such as Cheiro, Benham and Saint Germain, and helped others by guiding them in their pursuits. In November 1972 the Indian Institute of Technology sent me to the UK for post-doctoral research in mathematics on a British Council scholarship. One day, after seeing the British Museums near Tottenham Court Road in London, I went through bookshops that had a good collection of old books. I bought a book on numerology, *Romance in Your Name* by

Dr Juno Jordan of California. I was so fascinated by it that I studied it minutely and repeatedly and started practising numerology by making charts for friends and relatives and giving them their life reading. Then I bought several books on numerology from different parts of the world and worked to master the subject. It became my favorite hobby and I practised it in all the countries where I lived. Eventually I wrote the book *Secrets of Numerology*[2] that was later translated and published in several languages of the world.

Looking at my life and achievements in general so far I could say that the following properties were embedded in me—loneliness, disinterestedness in the affairs of the world, love of the occult, openness to dreams such that they occurred almost every night to me successfully foretelling about the coming events. Religious bent of mind, prayers and worships, reading of religious books and biography of saints, chanting of mantras, doing Yoga-asana or yogic postures, pranayama or breath control, games and sports, swimming and walking four to five miles every day were very regular in my life. It seems that my consciousness was already open to the beyond and it was waiting to be triggered for higher spiritual experiences. With this background, I will now describe my life in greater details since it was now the beginning of significant spiritual developments.

Life in Africa

In August 1981, I left India and came to Nigeria. I had collected several books from all the places in the world I had been, written by yogis who got their serpent power aroused and had penned down their experiences. These books served as guidelines to me and provided incentives. To mention in this context are the works of Swami Muktananda, Swami Yogananda, Pandit Gopi Krishna, Acharya Rajneesh, Swami Sivananda, Swami Satyananda Saraswati, Dr B.S.Goel, Sir John Woodroffe, Richard Alpert and Richard Maurice Buck. All these realized persons wrote their first-hand experiences in the course of the arousal of their Kundalini.

From 1981 to 1986, I was in Nigeria, teaching at the University of Port Harcourt. Until June 1982 I was happy since I had the family in the house. From then onwards I was never mentally settled because I was alone in the house with the exception of my house girl Elizabeth. It was now that I was driven to regular *mantra-jaap* or the chanting of mantras. On an average I was concentrating for about two hours a day. At the same time my tantric activities were quite frequent resulting in periods of ecstacy. There was a beautiful Krishna temple run by the ISKCON (International Society for Krishna Consciousness) in Port Harcourt where they had regular services and discourses. I attended quite regularly and generally I was engrossed in devotional songs and many a time I would go into ecstasy with tears flowing from my eyes. I became a life member of ISKCON in 1984, although I never confined myself to any single faith or tradition. My chanting of mantras became more regular and longer from the middle of 1983. Many times I sat to chant between 9 and 11 in the morning. I knew there were techniques to get quick concentration. Either keep looking at the image of your chosen deity or at the physical representation of the Tibetan mantra 'Om Mani Padme Hum', meaning 'the jewel is in the lotus', which is a phallus (male principle) deep set in the yoni (vagina). I would get concentration any time I would chant.

After a few months of joining the university I came to India on vacations. One day I was walking on the roads of Connaught Place in New Delhi. I just walked to the bookshop on the path and began to look at books. A book on mantras, *Mantra Rahasya* by Dr Narayan Datt Srimali caught my attention. I bought it and carried back to Nigeria. This happened without any preparation as if someone subconsciously guided me to do so. I began to devote two-to-three hours, on an average, to the chanting of mantras.

I selected mantras that appealed to me and started chanting. The first mantra I selected was for Lord Ganesh, who is the bestower of success in anything one does. Second, I selected a mantra for Lord Siva, who provides protection from accidents, ill health and gives long life. Third, I selected a mantra for Lord Krishna, who bestows both worldly happiness (*bhukti*) and spiritual liberation (*mukti*). According to the book on mantras, the mantra for Lord Ganesh was to be chanted during afternoon only, so I used to do it between 12 noon and 2 p.m. for two hours. The other two mantras I would chant in the early hours of the morning. Something would goad me up between 2.30 and 3 a.m. and after washing, I would sit down to meditate. After around 6 a.m. I would go for a long walk and on my return I would perform asanas or yoga postures for about 45 minutes. As far as asanas are concerned, I recall doing them since the mid 70s. I have been an athlete all my life with a serious interest in table tennis and swimming. During the 80s my intimate family life was regular, rather it increased in frequency during those years. Periods of meditation and ecstasy in intimate family life both seemed to bring my consciousness to an unusual concentration and happiness in general. I had collected several books by yogis and self-realized people from different parts of the world and read them for a few hours each day. These books served as guidelines and provided incentives. Feelings of loneliness, which used to be with me very much in the past, diminished. Mantras became my companion. Unconsciously I would be chanting some or the other mantra all the time.

One day, somewhere in the middle of 1985, I looked at something that attracted me much and began to meditate between 9 and 11 a.m. While completely engrossed in chanting, I achieved deep concentration. The counting of beads was forgotten but the chanting of the mantra continued. After a while I lost my sense of the world completely. In a flash, I heard the sound of lightning, like an electric spark jumping between two poles. Hearing a high pitched sound, my eyes opened. I saw a thick, cool, dazzling spark of pure white light about six inches high and three inches wide, about four feet from my eyes. I was looking at the spark till it remained in manifestation with full concentration. The spark slowly vibrated as it moved to the left one or two feet, slowly diminished in size, and then vanished completely. I was amazed and I looked around to find the spark's source. I thought it had leaked from a bulb or some other source of electricity. Slowly, as my amazement subsided, I understood the light had materialized out of nowhere. Now I know it was the physical manifestation of Brahman or God, called *brahmajyoti*, according to the scriptures. Carl Jung referred to this 'light' as the High Self, and the Polynesians in their Huna code call it the 'aka body' that manifests as a comforting *amazing white light*. After that day I was filled with inner happiness and my spiritual practice became more regular.

In the evening I met Professor S.D. Bajpai, head of the department of mathematics at the technical university at Port Harcourt, who was himself a very religious person. He gave me the book, *Chitshaktivilas* by Swami Muktananda to read and understand what had happened to me in the morning that day. I read the whole book in a few days and could see that the signal of the light was the first sign of the unfolding of Kundalini as manifestation of the *Chitshakti* or Cosmic Energy.

After about a year in the month of May/June 1986, I was standing in the verandah of my house in Port Harcourt around 8 in the morning. It was a clear sky and there was sunshine on the road in front of me about 15 feet away. Suddenly, I saw a black cobra, about three feet long, driving the hens around him who were trying to attack him with their beaks. He simply moved his head with a hissing sound towards them and soon they all left him. My house girl Elizabeth was looking at the cobra and she was naturally afraid. She shouted loudly to call the gardener or any other man to come with a stick and either kill or drive the snake away, but no one came. After getting rid of the hens the snake turned towards me and stood at the edge of the road with his hood fully open, about four inches wide six to nine inches high on the ground. Elizabeth was still afraid and shouting but my feelings were different. A feeling of love and respect got aroused in me and I said *namaskar* (salutation) to him in my heart. I was now reciting a mantra of Lord Shiva and there was no sign of fear at all. The snake remained in that position before me for about four to five minutes and both of us were constantly looking into the eyes of each other. After about five minutes he lowered his head, turned back to the direction it came from and vanished into the long grass.

The incidents gave me a good feeling of love for God. I started thinking that there is someone in nature who is aware of me and perhaps keeping a watch on me. I cannot say in worldly terms whether it was really a spiritual signal or just an incidence of those kinds. Could this be the manifestation of Mother Kundalini (energy from the causal plane) into physical form of a snake to show to me 'her oneness with me' or 'her awakening inside me'? It is quite possible and I am waiting for some expert to comment on this incident. On searching my heart I find that now I do not fear any poisonous animal and I never like to kill it in general.

In fact, before this instance I had been seeing an unclear vision of a snake in coiled form subconsciously and in my dreams. Sometimes while driving the car I had a feeling that a coiled snake sat near the gearbox and my hand might fall on him instead of the gear lever. Sometimes I felt that there was a snake sitting in the glove box or dickey of my car. Another feeling I had sometimes was of my body becoming straight and long. Sometimes there was a momentary feeling that I am one of the very tall people, more than 20 feet tall, walking in the jungle. My prayers/meditation continued between 3 a.m. and 6 a.m.

In July 1986 I left Nigeria and joined the University of Zimbabwe. If someone asks which of the ten countries I have lived in was the best, I would say it was Zimbabwe. Being there for two years, I led a complete physical and spiritual life while enjoying teaching mathematics. The university campus was massive with a beautiful swimming pool, tennis and table tennis courts, where I enjoyed a regular swimming and sports program. My three-hour practise of *yogic asanas* (postures), reading scriptures and chanting mantras became very regular along with my numerology practice. I helped people with life readings and suggested remedies to their problems using spiritual practices. People often spoke of feeling strangely happy on entering my home, not wanting to leave after their reading was over. I met a variety of people in Zimbabwe this way, mostly British and American. I learnt a lot about life, with five to six people coming to see me on an average every day. I began writing on occult subjects and my interest in mathematics began to diminish.

It was on 3 October 1986 that I began to write my spiritual diary in Zimbabwe, of which the present book is the outcome.

As for concentration, my mind would wander sometimes, especially during the first half of my prayers, but short intervals of concentration would come now and then. A strange feeling of happiness and a thrill ran through my body, especially during the latter half of my prayers. My prayers to the Lord were almost regular.

Visions of snakes in different forms always continued. Sometimes I felt a snake crawling along the wall parallel to me. I never felt fear. Rather, I found the word *Mata* (mother) coming from my mouth with an ecstatic feeling of bowing to her with namaste.

Detailed here are more of my experiences during this time. (1) I used to get a faint vision in mind that very tall people are quietly walking in a strange garden. This happened many times. (2) A faint vision of a vast space around me with several bright stars twinkling at different places. (3) Once in the morning around 6.30 to 7 a.m. when I got up from my second sleep, I had a clear feeling of *tingling* of a sharp and short snake like an electric current rising up from the base of my spine, reaching my naval region in my back. (4) Many times, as I got up from the sitting position, on completing my morning prayer, I felt a sweet but heavy pain below the root of my spine with the feeling that my neck was stiff and had straightened up. (5) I felt a marked inner strength and power of retaining the semen.[6] Once, as I completed my prayers and lay sleeping on the sofa around 6.30 a.m., I was suddenly awakened by the feeling of a reptile trying to crawl up the back of the sofa, its two front legs reaching the edge of the sofa's back. I looked everywhere and found nothing. I felt this was the effect of an inner happening.[7] For five or six days my left eyelid constantly vibrated and I had the feeling of some bad news on the way. Then, in a dream, I saw a close relative with his head and forehead covered with blood and a cut on his left cheek. His face and eyes were pale and withered. Two days later the message came from India that he was passing through extreme mental agony with a highly pessimistic feeling about life, including a weak desire to commit suicide.[8] On 9 April Dr Kirri of the University of Zimbabwe examined me thoroughly and found me in very good health. He stared at me in surprise, saying that my blood pressure, haemoglobin and other things were even better than the young students at the university. He said that he had seen such a good health after a very long time. I told him about my regular meditative and yogic schedule. Yet, he was amazed.[9] There was a considerable reduction in my appetite. I needed to eat very little to keep going, being as strong and fit as ever.[10] After prayer, I normally took rest or a little sleep between 6 a.m. and 7 a.m. During this time I had a distant feeling, like a sealed bottle wanting to open up. Sometimes I got the faint vision of a toilet seat being twisted and crushed and the hand gear of a car being twisted and crushed.

While absorbed in meditation once I heard the roaring of a lion and the sound of a waterfall coming from somewhere inside me for a few seconds and then disappearing.

On 16 May 1987, I was busy with prayer around 5 a.m. Suddenly, I wept bitterly, unable to stop myself. Thereafter I put my head on the table and said to the Mother Goddess, 'I have no Guru, please protect me my Mother, only you are my Guru.' After some time I found stability in my heart and chanted the mantra for Lord Shiva and then for Lord Krishna until around 7 a.m. afterward, I lost complete identity of myself. In those moments of absorption I saw a scene from the film Devdas where his dead body is taken from the train and carried on the shoulders of four men to the cremation ground. I saw dead body being carried and heard a voice coming from inside me saying, 'Ravindra Kumar is dead. He died just today.' Soon after that I came out of my absorption feeling relaxed and happy. Everything appeared beautiful.

This was the experience of death (of ego). The death of ego appears as a physical death in trance, vision or dream. Most of the yogis pass through this experience after which they are called *dwij* or 'twice born' or an 'initiate', in the language of Blavatsky. This opens the Kingdom of Heaven for the 'initiate', as Lord Jesus said, 'Only the twice-born can enter the Kingdom of Heaven.' Dr Elizabeth Kubler Ross described her experience of death (of ego), going through the pain of all her patients. She suffered for quite sometime and asked for a shoulder to rest her head on, which she was denied through an inner voice. However, after the suffering was over, a pleasant resurrection took place. St. Paul said, 'I die daily,' which was associated with his inner journeys to higher realms. This is what exactly happened to me after the experience of death (of ego).

Almost every night I would find myself on some inner realm with strange but pleasant experiences. These journeys to higher realms are referred to by Jesus Christ as, 'entering the Kingdom of God or Heaven'.

As mentioned earlier in the introduction to this chapter, it is a sort of crisis—moral, religious, scientific or physical—which brings the unusual out of the individual. For example, St. Paul was struck by an unusually bright light on way to Damascus that blinded him for sometime. When he came to his senses the conditioning on his thinking against the Christians had been removed. This was a 'sudden revelation', following a 'moral crisis'. Sir Fred Hoyle passed through a 'scientific crisis' that resulted in 'sudden revelation' that 'the particles in the atmosphere have decision-making faculty'. British actress Sarah Miles had her 'first revelation' after the loneliness and agony of *masturbation* in front of men triggered a spiritual experience in her. Britain's best-known mountaineer, Doug Scot got 'sudden revelation' while, being catapulted down head over heels, heading towards a long drop. The experience lifted him up to a new way of looking at the whole business of being alive. A female parachutist could not get her parachute to open, in spite of her best efforts. Seeing imminent death, she came out of her body and found that she had forgotten to press the correct button. Quickly, she reentered her body, pressed the required button, and landed safely. Her 'heightened perception' while out of her body changed her entire view of life; she was never the same person again. For complete details and other cases of this kind please refer to my book, *The Kundalini Book of Living and Dying* (2004).

It is this 'crisis' that makes the individual pass the great circle of 'Pass Not' called *Dhyanipasa* or the 'rope of Angels' guarded by the Dhyani Chohans (*Devas* or gods), which separates the phenomenal from the noumenal Kosmos, so that it does not fall within the range of our present objective consciousness. An 'impassable barrier' is created around the manifested world by the *lipikas* or Recorders of the Karmic Ledger because of which the occult knowledge does not pass on to the practitioner until he becomes an 'initiate' after passing through the crisis. It is hard for the uninitiated to understand why the knowledge should be withheld from him. I can say with my own experience that reading the holy scriptures such as *Bhagavad Gita* did not convey the meaning of the statements made therein before I became a 'twice born'. And afterwards, the facts presented were very clear and comprehensive. You really feel that you are a new person with some new faculties, which were not possessed earlier. Many things which we tried to believe earlier because Lord Krishna has said them, were now clear and understandable such as the permanence and indivisibility of Atman or Soul, since you experience yourself being so after becoming a 'twice born' or an 'initiate'.

Thus a sudden crisis brings a 'sudden revelation', but you cannot have a control over such a situation and make it happen for you. However, a 'religious crisis' is created through yoga, meditation and prayers one day that brings the unusual out of you and gives a 'sudden revelation'. An experience of death (of ego) by the yogis is the result of such a 'religious crisis', which is self-created or is the result of self-efforts.

This 'self-created crisis' can be brought about in a single lifetime if certain principles are followed carefully. I got the result in exactly seven years. I give a simple example at this stage. If we have to boil water in a container and we put a candle underneath it, the water will never boil. But, if we put a strong burner underneath, the water will boil very fast and convert into steam. In the same way, if the applied spiritual practices are strong enough that can bring a spiritual boiling point within, you become God just as water becomes steam. Usual spiritual practices in any religion are not stronger than a candle and hence the conversion does not take place. Some rare ones are able to bring the spiritual boiling point within and become God and then they exclaim,

'I am God.' Let me explain the easy way this can be achieved.

The main problem is created by the mind that keeps us connected to the past and future, and not to the present. Brooding about the past and speculating about the future, neither of them can serve any purpose. If we can stay in the present and get connected to the 'energy within', then we can listen to the silence, achieve stillness and know and become God in an easy way. We do not have to change our lifestyle, keep doing what we like to do, and have the best of both the worlds. Vedic and ancient findings by the yogis lay stress on four paths: (*a*) yogic asanas or exercises of Hatha Yoga, (*b*) Karma Yoga or path of selfless action, (*c*) Jnana Yoga or path of knowledge, and (*d*) Bhakti Yoga or path of devotion. One can incorporate these factors easily in one's life. Half an hour to 40 minutes of selected yogic postures, Pranayama or breath-control and morning walks can keep you physically fit, free from diseases and ready to attain higher spiritual goals. Make a habit to do things or take an action according to the situation, without attaching personal benefits with it; thinking it to be one's duty assigned by nature or God, preferably. Make a habit to read regularly spiritual literature about self-realized people and scriptures. If possible, select a mantra and chant it regularly for an hour or so; and/or offer prayers to God by sitting in an easy posture, closing the eyes and concentrating on third eye, which is the space between the eyebrows. If the thoughts about the world and its problems trouble you, concentrate on breathing in and out of the nostrils; feeling the sensation of breath rubbing against the nostrils both ways. After some time you will see that the mind has become still and you can connect to it from within.

Sitting in a cross-legged position close the eyes and focus on the third eye. Now chant aum for 15 to 20 minutes starting the first part from *mooladhara chakra* or root centre; carry the sound along the spine and then pass it out of the third eye till it subsides. Take a full breath and repeat the process. This will bring concentration on the third eye. Keep your eyes closed. Feel that you are dipped in the ocean of white light and the same white light is entering your body through *sahasrara* or the crown centre. Feel that this liquid white light is fully conscious and is carrying God-energy with it. Feel it flow through every part of your body, starting with head, neck, shoulders, arms (feel that the arms have become heavier and longer than before), chest, spine, stomach, pelvic region, legs and toes. Feel that every part has been energized and is becoming disease-free. Now you will be losing consciousness of the outer world, attaining concentration on the third eye, going within and getting connected to the Unmanifested First Cause. Peace, stillness and blissfulness are with you now. This is what I did for about seven years and experienced death (of ego) one fine morning.

It is quite appropriate to mention here *The Power of Now* by Eckhart Tolle (1999, 224) regarding 'the quieting of mind' that leads to the realization of the highest one:

"Since resistance is inseparable from the mind, relinquishment of resistance—surrender—is the end of the mind as your master, the imposter pretending to be 'you,' the false god. All judgements and all negativity dissolve. The realm of Being, which had been obscured by the mind, then opens up. Suddenly a great stillness arises within you, and unfathomable sense of peace. And within that peace, there is great joy. And within that joy, there is love. And at the innermost core, there is the sacred, the immeasurable, That which cannot be named." Thus the whole thing is about quietening the mind, either by direct method, which is not easy, or by yogic methods discussed earlier. The old way to enlightenment was the 'way of the cross', which should not be dismissed or underestimated, since it still works. According to it the worst thing in your life, turns into the best things that ever happened to you, by forcing you into surrender, into 'death', forcing you to become as nothing, to become as God—because God, too, is nothing. This 'death' has to take place either by natural happenings, on which there is no human control, or it should be created through yogic practices.

The way of the cross is *enlightenment* through suffering, that is, pain and problems forcing one into the kingdom of heaven. One finally surrenders when pain is not bearable any more. However, the pain and suffering may continue for a long time before it happens. Living in the present and not in the past or future, and saying yes to what 'is' brings an end to the pain. In this way one has to decide oneself when to end the pain and suffering. By living in present and connecting to the power of 'now' one gets connected to the source of everything, the highest one.

One day, between 15-20 June, during my usual morning prayer, I suddenly saw myself fly over the Ngorongoro Crater and the neighboring hills in Tanzania that housed the hotel I stayed in. I felt I was about to rise above the chair I was sitting on. This happens when the astral body wants to separate from the physical body. In another vision, I sensed a snake rising from the ground and then the Mother Goddess dressed in pure white clothes appeared before me and I bowed to her, putting my forehead on her feet. Many times I saw my own figure very clearly, praying and chanting mantras. Once I had a strong feeling of someone watching me with two sparkling eyes, and sometimes with one eye. A voice inside me said I was being watched.

A few days later, in a flash, I saw clearly in my mind's eye the Mother Goddess's extremely beautiful face with a red vermilion spot on her forehead, clad in a red sari (Indian dress). Wearing white clothes I bowed down to her, touching my head to her feet. I saw her hand, adorned with bangles, touch the top of my head as she gave me blessings with a smile on her face. This was the manifestation of Kundalini energy in human form for my satisfaction confirming that I was on the right path and that I had her blessings and support.

My prayers in the morning from 3 a.m. to 6 a.m. were regular as before during July 1987. On the night of 7 July I was having a very happy time with my family and had a very satisfying experience. I practised distraction from my sensual pleasure and focused on my thoughts of God all along. I slept the next four hours. Around 2 a.m. I got up to answer nature's call and became aware of the constant sound of someone blowing a conch shell. Asking others in the morning if they also heard such a sound they all answered 'no'. Plugging both my ears tightly, I found that this sound came from inside my head. I went to the ENT specialist at the hospital who said that there have been other cases like mine. For some, such sounds vanish after a time while others live with it permanently. This is not due to any ear or nose blockage, nor is it a sign of irregularity or insanity.

About marital relations, which are in fact useful and act as catalytic agents in spiritual path for many, Swami Satyananda Saraswati has to say the following:

> 'A person who has controlled his lower impulses, a yogi who is practicing higher sadhana, doesn't have to give up his or her partner and the marital relationship. If you think to be a yogi you must give up sex, why don't you also give up eating and sleeping? Yoga has nothing to do with giving up these things; it is only concerned with transforming their purpose and meaning.'
>
> Saraswati: 150.

In fact, one does not care for opposite sex or the satisfaction of passion, one is only concerned with awakening an experience and sublimating it. That is the way to open the higher centres. Also, through the sexual act, a female can awaken *mooladhara* and *swadhisthana* chakras if her partner is a yogi (*ibid:* 0149).

This was a very important happening in which the cosmic sound or the Word or Aum had manifested inside me. This primeval sound takes the *jiva* (individual soul) in tow to paramatma (universal soul). This is the beginning of automatic meditation all the time. This sound has been mentioned in all faiths and traditions. In Islam it is known as Kalma-I-Ilahi. Pythagoras called it the 'music of spheres'. In Eckankar it is known as the 'divine sound'. Many religious leaders, for example Saint Kabir, have advised the practitioners to concentrate on this sound, which will take the *Jiva* (individual soul) to all spiritual stages of perfection. Saint Sheel Nath, respectfully mentioned by Swami Vishnu Tirth, had this sound awakened since childhood, which should have been the effect of his past life. He used to sit for hours together and listen to this sound, which brought all kinds of spiritual experiences to him for which he is well known in the lineage (*Sadhan Shikhar* by Swami Shivom Tirth). Much has been said already about the cosmic sound in earlier chapters.

The manifestation of the cosmic sound indicates the opening of the heart centre or *anahata chakra*. The second of the Ten Commandments says, 'Thou shalt love thy neighbor.' When you ask any Christian, more often than not he will say that this is not possible. After the opening of the heart centre 'loving they neighbor becomes automatically possible'. In fact, one cannot help but do it. Heart becomes so full of love that there is no place for hate. One begins to love even one's enemy because he has seen the truth beyond physical existence. He now knows that every animate or inanimate existence in the universe has the same element of God common to all. One reaches the state of balance in which there is neither love nor hate and he wishes good of all. He is full of bliss all the time; contentment and equanimity become part of his nature.

One evening, 2 or 3 days later, I suddenly felt my whole body twisting like a snake with a very heavy pressure on the top of my head, threatening to blow my head off. I quickly ran out of the house with heavy hand and leg motions for a kilometer. On returning home, I worked out on my exercise bicycle for 15 minutes and then continued exercising vigorously, finally regaining some feeling of control over my situation. Next day the doctor again examined me thoroughly and said that if I were not in such good health I could experience paralysis or a brain haemorrhage. He warned me and asked me to suspend all meditation and heavy mental activities, which I did from then on. The next week my head was blocked with heat and I could not think or read. I did not deliver lectures at the university for two weeks. Slowly things returned to normal.

I met Dr B. S. Goel, the saint in Delhi, on returning from my tour of the US in August 1987. He told me that the Kundalini shakti had aroused in me and there was no further need of mantra chanting. He also advised me to suspend all physical and mental activities that put pressure on my head and further said that now Shakti will take me to the final destination herself, and I should lead a simple *satwik* (pure) life and pull myself away from all materialism. *Satsang* (being with people on path of God) and *kirtan* (singing religious songs) would be helpful, he said. Dr Goel took retirement after his Kundalini awakening and set up an ashram near Delhi. His book *Kundalini and Third Eye* (1995) was very well received and appreciated round the world. Many people stayed in his ashram from all over the world and took initiation. He wanted me to give up going abroad and stay with him in the ashram permanently, which I could not do. I still wanted to remain free and gather experience round the world. Unfortunately, he expired before I decided to settle in India.

On 27 October 1987, I played an hour of table tennis from 6 p.m. to 7 p.m. What I found interesting was that towards the end I still felt very energetic, making some powerful shots. Suddenly I felt a sensation of concentration between my eyebrows and a very strong desire to sit down and pray. I left the game and sat on a chair facing the corner for a few minutes. I then got up, as I wanted to reach home as quickly as possible. While driving, my desire to pray increased, and internally I felt a sort of death experience. The old internal voice was repeating the words that Ravindra Kumar is dead. On reaching home, I closed myself in the prayer room and happily prayed for 15 to 20 minutes. Slowly and rhythmically, I chanted the Krishna mantra. The feeling of death and inner happiness was constant throughout. Tears flowed from my eyes and my throat felt choked. My tranquil mood prevailed until I went to sleep between 10.30 and 11 p.m. Before going to sleep I had a very satisfactory time with my wife, after which my tranquil state increased. As I closed my eyes to sleep I saw a large garden with tall green trees and magnificent white buildings. Then, on the grass I saw fairy-like beautiful women materializing from everywhere and assembling at one place. The next night I saw a garden full of small trees bearing fruits of various kinds. The scene was very pleasing and satisfying.

I was teaching at the university and living peacefully in Zimbabwe in (1986 – 88). I could concentrate on Lord Shiva during periods of ecstasy as I did in July, but I was afraid of some unhappy results damaging my brain. Therefore, I observed the precautions suggested by my doctor and Dr B. S. Goel, and avoided meditation. However, pictures of Lord Shiva and Mother Goddess (most likely Mother Kundalini) were constantly in my mind. I sat gazing at a picture of the Mother's lovely face for minutes at a time. It felt so satisfying. I reduced my alcohol consumption to a minimum, restricting myself to such indulgences only at parties or special occasions. I simply lost my taste for alcohol.

Many times a picture of my son Atul appeared in my imagination and would enlarge infinitely so the whole sky and the universe were engulfed. Sometimes I felt my own figure enlarge infinitely as well. Many times, in my imagination, I felt a snake encircling my neck and on contracting itself, cut my head off. Sometimes I felt my head floating separately from my body. An inner voice saying, 'Ravindra Kumar is dead,' would accompany me at times. Sometimes scenes from my life appeared one after another in a backward time progression, that is, from present to the past, to the events of early childhood. It was very much like a life review. This used to happen to me quite often during 1956 – 57 in Meerut while I was a student of B.Sc. Like this it has happened to me many times in my life. Those days I was concentrating on three things that Dr Goel had advised me to do: (*a*) living a *satwik* (pure) life, (*b*) controlling and reducing of sexual thoughts and activities, and (*c*) controlling and killing *ahankar* (ego) or pride. I used to pray constantly inwardly and request 'Shakti Maa' to help me in achieving the results.

For the last few weeks of December 1987, I saw through my imagination inverted snakes. I petted their 'smooth white surface' again and again. I remember that I always had a strong liking for clothes of flame color or the saffron; most of my suits were almost of that color. Consciously or subconsciously my eyes would always fall on such colors. Once in the evening I was walking on the road and looking at a very high building belonging to the State Trading Corporation. Suddenly my body jerked with something unusual and I nearly lost my balance. Somewhere in the passage from the centre between the eyebrows to the back of the skull, the point where Hindus keep a tuft of hair, I had a clear feeling of two nerves breaking down with a sound like the cracking of fine dry sticks. In a flash, I saw a big rectangular rock before me, the size of a house, with sunlight spreading from its top.

This was an important happening indicating the change in the physiology and chemistry of the body. The old nervous system breaking down and the new are being formed to facilitate the process of enlightenment. It was clear by the fact that light was seen coming from the top of a building soon after the breaking of the nerves. This showed the enhancement of *Chit* or consciousness about the understanding of the working of the universe.

My journeys to different countries were quite regular for one reason or the other. On 1 January 1988 I was staying in the house of a relative in London. Around 11 p.m. I was about to sleep with a clear and peaceful state of mind.

Suddenly I saw an open eyed, beautiful child with a blissful smile looking back at me. I cannot say whether it was a vision or I was seeing through my mind's eyes. On the morning of 2 January around 6 a.m. when my sleep was half broken, I clearly saw the same child facing in a different direction. What tranquility, what peace and what happiness! Later, Dr B.S.Goel told me this was the childhood form of Lord Krishna, which I saw as the final result of my *sadhana* or yogic practices. The deity of the seed mantra I used to chant had appeared before me.

Sir John Woodroffe in his famous book *The Serpent Power* (p. 120) observed that the worshippers of Lord Shiva see him in child form. Dr Carl Jung in his book *Man and His Symbols* said when the process of individuation is complete, the practitioner would see the 'psychic child' born as a result of the inner marriage between the male and female principles. When one is united with the 'other side' of one's own psyche, the 'inner child' appears as a symbol of wholeness, as the birth of a new individuality. If the energy flows outward, it creates in the outer world, while if it is checked and flows inwards, it creates within the individual. Chinese teachings have also elaborated on the birth of a 'holy child'; see for example, *The Secrets of Golden Flower* by Richard Wilhelm. Lord Jesus at one point has said, "an 'inner marriage' will give rise to the 'inner child' whose birth brings release from the power of death."[4]

It was a very happy day for me to reach this milestone. I was convinced that Lord Siva and Mother Kundalini were taking full care of me. Most of the time I found myself singing religious songs internally. Even when I was not conscious of it, a song sang itself inside me. I would like to sing or listen to only religious songs and no other.

During January 1988 I had flying dreams. I first saw myself flying through a big hall closed on all sides. I could not find the way out of the hall and a feeling of confinement remained for some time. After surveying the walls I suddenly hit and broke out through one wall and flew free over the land. I flew over a crowded area and saw a woman on the ground. I descended to talk to her and then flew up again. Next, I flew over a clear blue ocean, then green meadows lined with trees and surrounded by mountains. I would accelerate and decelerate at will to land softly and then fly up again.

Another night I dreamt of a wide canal of beautiful clear blue water with concrete banks on both sides. People were moving around. There were large buildings everywhere. Flying from one bank to the other, I noticed people on the ground pointing towards me. With other people I entered my house where I found long, thin snakes everywhere. Even my clothes were turning into skinny snakes. My hair too appeared to be like bunches of thin and very fine snakes hanging out of my skull. I came out of the house and flew off again with a joyful heart.

Once, I had a special kind of dream in which I felt supernatural powers were bestowed on me and I was testing those powers. I saw something like an electric pole at a distance. I moved and rotated my fingers, pointed toward the pole and the pole twisted. I could stop a moving vehicle through my will power and I could throw a big stone from one place to another simply by finger gestures. Flying was as normal in my dreams as walking is in my waking state. In this dream, though a short one, I felt myself being superhuman although with humble and polite nature. I could travel anywhere and do anything by the power of thought and hand gestures. This probably was the indication that I can acquire and use paranormal powers if I want, which are normal tools on higher realms. At the same time I had the intuitive feeling that I should never try to develop and use such powers, which could be a hindrance in my spiritual development.

It is important to point out here briefly that the *jiva* or individual soul first passes through the stage of a *jnani* or the path of knowledge that gives you the realization of the elements responsible for the creation of the universe. One comes to know about the five sheaths covering the atman or soul. Next he passes through the stage of a *yogi* who realizes the powers of *yoga* without getting entangled into them. If one entangles there he is caught up there and begins to use or show his powers. He feels like a special person and the ego stops his spiritual progress. That is why the practitioners are warned against it. Nature showed me the truth about *yogic powers* and helped me in progressing further on the path of spiritual perfection. The next and highest stage that comes is of *bhakti* or devotion to the Lord, which takes the *jiva* closer to the Lord. Those who have *bhakti* or devotion from the very beginning they cross the stages of *jnani* and *yogi* quickly and without any entanglement. Lord Krishna told his disciple Arjuna in Bhagavad-Gita that one who remembers him all the time is the best of all *jnanis* and *yogis* and he comes back to him finally and lives in his own spiritual abode never to be born again.

While praying I felt I was about to rise from my chair and float in the air. For a moment I worried about the lightness of my body. This happened to me more than once. I also saw myself sitting and praying at a distance. This was an experience where my astral body separated from my physical body and I saw my own double. On another occasion I dreamt of cars coming towards me with very bright headlights that normal eyes could not tolerate. I felt a spark of lightening in my head. Suddenly, a bright and very fine snake passed through it. Visions and dreams of snakes were quite common in those days. This was a clear indication of the awakening and the active working of Kundalini, which has the form of the snake.

According to Swami Satyananda Saraswati, 'When *Mooladhara* (root-centre) awakens, a number of phenomena occur. The first thing many practitioners experience is levitation of the astral body. One has the sensation of floating upward in space, leaving the physical body behind. This is due to the energy of Kundalini whose ascending momentum causes the astral body to dissociate from the physical and move upward. This phenomenon is limited to the astral and possibly mental dimensions, and this differs from what is normally called levitation—the actual displacement of the physical body.'[5]

Engrossed in short prayers of 10 to 20 minutes, I would achieve concentration with a sensation between my eyebrows. I felt like a new eye wanted to open up. I also felt someone watching me with one clear eye at the centre of his forehead.

On the morning of 29 May 1988, I was lying in the bed around 6 a.m. I clearly saw a 'blue star' with my eyes closed. Sometimes it appeared as a diffused deep blue light. Since then whenever I close my eyes and look between my eyebrows, I invariably see the blue light, either as a star or as a diffused form. I felt a new happiness and sense of security at an invisible being around me, guiding me. It was around this time that I came in contact with the people from Eckankar in Zimbabwe. Paul Twitchell of Eckankar in his book *The Spiritual Notebook* has written that one should concentrate on the blue star and let oneself follow it to the other worlds.

I am going to describe here either a vision or a lucid dream I had in mid 1988. In fact, it was a unique soul travel experience. Blue shining water extended over a vast area, a strange mountainous region with green trees on both sides, I was conscious of myself flying. Looking at myself I found I was without hands or feet or any body at all. I was ecstatic. People with the lower half of their bodies missing were entering through a gate into a translucent mini fortress and others were coming out of another gate. The two gates were on either side of a small canal flowing from under the fortress. I was up in the sky and three lower bodiless entities were standing on the ground, talking to each other. One of them asked me telepathically to move. I moved through the beautiful green glowing area until I reached the bank of a wide canal flowing with crystal clear light blue water.

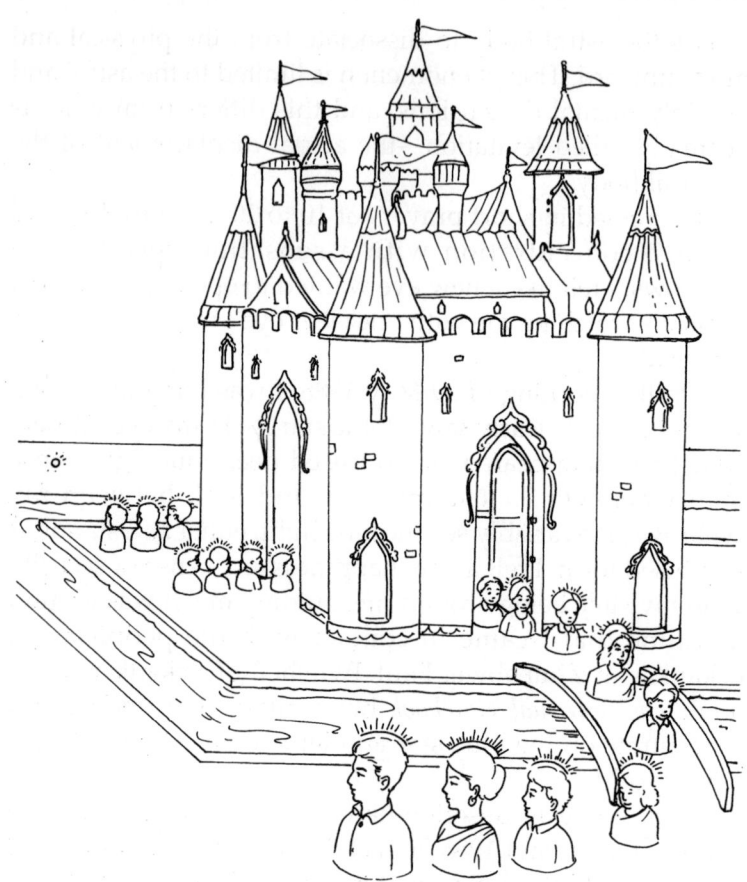

Souls entering and leaving the palace of Brahma

I began to cross as if I was moving on a fragile bridge made of hair. I looked into the deep clear blue water. Sometime later, I arrived on the other side of the canal and found myself in the midst of a wide range of hills. I kept moving until I was close to one of the hills. I suddenly found myself back in my body on earth. My sleep, now broken, was replaced with a new peace and happiness.

In Harare, Zimbabwe I began to write the book *Destiny, Science and Spiritual Awakening* that was eventually published in 1997.

The Autobiography—My Journey to Godhood

On 4 August 1988 around 5 p.m., I was walking with a friend on the Janpath in Delhi. We came across the very tall State Trading Centre building. I turned my head up to stare at its highest point to look for something. Suddenly

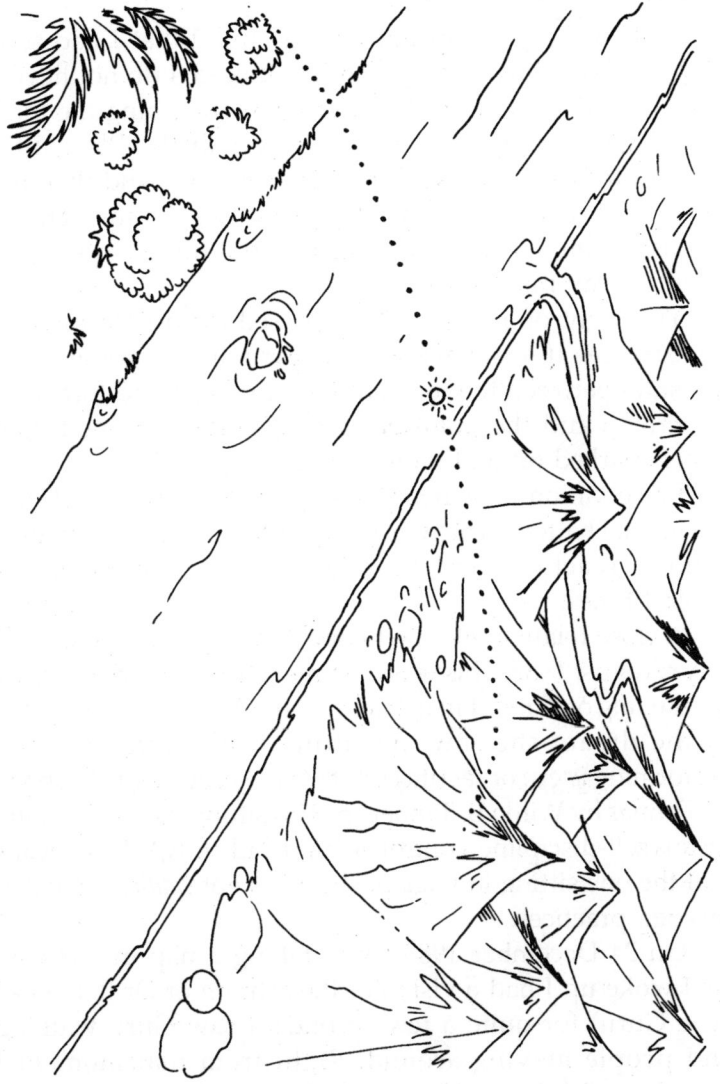

The author's soul crossing the ocean of divinity

something struck the bottom of my crown centre from the inside of my skull. I felt nerves cracking like fine sticks being snapped. There was a slight imbalance in my body so I stood quietly for a few seconds stabilizing myself. It felt like a mild earthquake.

A dream began repeating in my mind that I had seen 25 years ago. Slowly ascending to a hilltop, I do not have a form or body but am in full awareness. Reaching the top I saw a very bright temple of white marble. Pleasantly amazed to see it, I looked at it for some time and then my sleep was broken. I got out of bed with the pleasant memory of this dream, most likely an actual soul travel experience, haunting my mind for days.

The night of 4 August 1988 passed almost sleepless. It appeared as if some action and reaction was going on in my skull between the top centre of my head and forehead, the crown and the point between eyebrows. Some bright lights sparked off and on in my visions.

Preservation of semen plays an important role. Clearly the mental battery is heavily charged and triggers with these actions, reactions and experiences. I have noticed this several times.

A close relative told me I appeared in her dream during July/August 1987. This was the time when I experienced my awakening of Kundalini in Harare. The dreamer was in Delhi. In the dream she saw me sitting in the lotus posture performing *yagya* or sacrifices with fire. According to the book on *Dreams* by Wilda B. Tanner (p. 355) sitting in yoga posture means self-discipline, control of mind and body, which means that the one sitting in yoga posture has got *siddhi* or success in yoga practices.

On 24 December 1988 I was taking a nap in our van. As I woke up I had a vision of the ashram of Dr B. S. Goel (The Guru) for quite a few seconds. I saw Guru walking and people moving around. Right from that moment I experienced bliss for five to six hours. The pleasure was similar to what one would experience at the culmination of coition, but was so unique and real, as if I was absorbed in a ceaseless act of copulation and continuous ejaculation with a constant pleasure/bliss of equal intensity. The situation lasted for about six hours and it was constant ecstasy.

I joined the University of Addis Ababa, Ethiopia in January 1989. I got a small but good accommodation to live at the campus and began to meditate regularly. During the whole month I constantly felt a white snake twisting and turning in my thoughts/visions. A feeling of constant ejaculation of some fluid in a vertical direction upward through an invisible capillary was there all the time. Many times it was accompanied with ecstatic states of happiness. During the last one week I was having visions of a 'magnified capillary tube' surrounded with flesh, through which constant upward ejaculation of some fluid was taking place. It was accompanied with very pleasant feelings and was there all the time in my thoughts/visions.

On 10 February 1989 the whole night I had dreams of snakes of various kinds around me. Some unknown person gave one snake each to two or three people like me. I held the snake around myself. It was taking out its long and sharp tongue again and again and was looking at me all the time. I was holding him in a friendly way without any trace of fear at all. The next night many pigeons and bat like birds were looking at me. Their bodies were tied with some extra loads and they were trying to fly but were unable to do so efficiently. A bat was successful in flying across from one point to another though his body was tied with some weights, and he was looking at me. The dream could mean that my spiritual progress was being hindered by some worldly involvements, and it was a suggestion by my high self to give a practical shape to detachment and renunciation for having full-blown spiritual experiences.

In the early morning of 15 March 1989 I felt a pressure between my eyebrows. I felt a screen obstructing the light and only scattered light could be seen. Slowly the screen started moving to one side and I saw a bright point of white light opposite my third eye. Soon after that, I opened my physical eyes and got up from the bed. A few days later, in the early morning hours, I was dreaming about big buildings and construction on some meadows and then I was watching a show with some others on a platform. I had to move to one side to see around a pillar in front of me. And then I clearly saw the lighted program before me. I found myself talking to my mother and saw Chandra Vishwain in three different forms at three corners of the room at the same time. She was dancing with a smile just in front of me. She was moving slowly to my right and talking to someone. And from another angle I saw her standing quietly and looking at us with a smile. I saw her very clearly in three different places in three different forms simultaneously. During those days I saw an 'unusually beautiful child' in my visions in the early mornings. This happened on a few occasions and was similar to the experiences I had in London in January 1988. This unusually beautiful child was none other than the Lord Himself, and it implied that the *jiva* or individual soul had qualified to reside in the spiritual planet of the Lord and there was no further births. The meaning should be the same whether the practitioner is a Chinese, a Western philosopher of Jung's group, a Hindu or one belonging to any other part of the world.

I was reading a spiritual book from 2 a.m. to 5 a.m. and then slept for an hour between 5 a.m. and 6 a.m. During this hour I had a soul travel experience with a dimensionless form seen consciously. I was moving in a big valley with waterfalls flowing from the top of a mountain. I moved to a cavity very close to the falling water and enjoyed the scenario for quite some time. I enjoyed going in and out of the waters many times and moving freely around the waters and enjoying the mountaintop and the atmosphere around. The waters did not wet me and there was no fear of falling down on the ground. This was a wonderful experience in

The Autobiography—My Journey to Godhood

formless state, which proved that the soul couldn't be wet by water or hurt by any other physical means, as stated by Lord Krishna in the *Bhagavad Gita*. This is how the *jiva* or individual soul on becoming a *twice born* gets the proof of statements in scriptures, which can now be understood by him. This is why Blavatsky wrote unless one becoming an *initiate* or *twice born* crosses the ring "pass-not" the scriptures are not understood. Scholars may read and research on scriptures and get a doctorate, yet they do not understand the *truth* and they are not changed internally.

During July 1989, I noticed that for the last more than a year I was having some strange phenomenon going inside my testicles. It felt like something is overhauling, adjusting and readjusting, the testicles squeezing and sticking to the body, never hanging down in the loose way. Casting the seed or ejaculation became too much delayed and it seemed that it does not want to take place even after a long duration of lovemaking. Even the desire for lovemaking was reducing every day and the attention would mostly remain focused towards the thoughts of God.

One day I was sitting in meditation for a short while around 5 a.m. Suddenly a flash came in my vision and I saw saint Kabir sitting on a chair with white beard and hair. He was looking at me affectionately. The vision lasted only a few seconds.

In the early hours of the morning on 12 June 1989 I dreamt of an extremely beautiful, white complexioned, perfectly built woman dancing in a jungle from one point to another. She was constantly looking at me with big alluring eyes giving seductive looks. She was wearing a sari and blouse (Indian dress); most of her marble smooth body was naked. The dream went on for about 15 minutes. The feeling in me arose sexually but it sublimated in a motherly attitude towards her. Certainly it was the manifestation of mother Kundalini. Perhaps it indicated the transformation of sexual love into divine love within. One of the books on Kundalini says that Kundalini in the beginning acts like

Mother; but when the practitioner masters the process, it acts like a beloved. Another interpretation says that nature tests the practitioner whether he would be lured into sex or not.

A night in November, 1989 was a restless one for the conflicts, arguments and uneasiness in me. I went to sleep late, around 2 a.m. and slept till 7 a.m. In this dreamtime I saw my penis separate from my body like a ripe fruit, easily leaving the tree. I looked at it for a while and then placed it on a shelf. I readjusted my body and moved around. When I woke up in the morning I was unusually happy. All anguish forgotten, I was calm, peaceful and smiling as I went to my department at the University in a happy mood. I was happy the whole day. I believe the erotic sense rising in the body is converted into love and understanding, a step towards the transcendence of sex.

On 4 November 1989 I dreamt that my penis was very big and standing erect. Suddenly it enlarged further and became big enough to enter my naval. For a minute it entered my naval opening and remained stuck there. I had little sexual desire in those days and the inner sound became more pronounced. Perhaps a sublimation of sexual and erotic desire had taken place. I had the urge to meditate most of the time, although I was still observing the doctor's direction not to meditate. According to Swami Satyananda Saraswati in *Kundalini Tantra*, these were the symptoms of Kundalini successfully passing through my second centre, called the sacral or Swadhishthan chakra.

During December 1989 I was at the University of Malawi, Southern Africa for a week, attending a mathematics conference. I felt relaxed and happy as usual. One night I woke up several times. While dreaming or in trance I felt connected to the Infinite Void (*shoonyata*), a strange and previously unknown feeling and a very pleasant one. For a few seconds I was afraid, but gradually my fear was replaced by pleasure. And then I suddenly felt dead as my head dropped to one side. Soon I woke up and everything that happened in my dream appeared to have happened in my waking life. I even felt some pain on the side of the neck where my head had dropped. This experience stayed with me for some time. According to scriptures void or *shoonyata* is nothing or God, wherefrom everything originates. This experience is also a milestone on the path of spiritual knowledge.

On 2 January 1990 in a dream there was a way leading to the top of a mountain and someone in white clothes was going up. He asked me if I wanted to follow him. I was with many people. I left them and followed the man. After reaching the top we entered a big house surrounded by water. A few seconds later, a friendly man perhaps moving on crutches, came out. He smiled and greeted us.

Around this time I had several meetings with Mr. Olson, leader of the Eckankar group in Harare, Zimbabwe. My discussions with Mr. Olson were very enlightening. He said going slow on the path acquaints you with all the details of the journey and is not risky. Going fast can lead to a hasty arousal of Kundalini and can cause problems. In the early morning hours I would usually have flying dreams with both hands stretched like wings over populated areas. I felt happy but some heat in my head made me uncomfortable. Reading the Eckankar book *The Far Country* I discovered my Soul travels in January 1988 were to the Brahma Lok[6]. Standing in front of the fortress of Brahma is recommended since it burns karma away and makes the practitioner pure. Many leaders take their disciples there for this purpose. After crossing the sea/canal I reached a group of mountains and then I returned into my body on earth. Perhaps you need the help of a guide to cross the mountains and reach the sacred area of Sach Khand.

I noticed that my interest in sex had almost been lost. Whenever I would engage in lovemaking I would lose interest in the middle of the act. I would withdraw and go to sleep. I would not have ejaculation for a long time. My mind was always focused on thoughts of God, in one way or the other. My sexual partner would normally get her orgasm before I withdrew. The frequency of lovemaking went down considerably and my partner would grumble at times for this reason. However, it was never a total stop and things continued somehow.

Observations
Here is a list of relevant dreams:
February 18, 1990 I dreamed of flying over tall modern buildings. In a crowded park, a woman flew from one corner to another. I flew past that place. After flying by many times I was asked by a policeman to come down and stop at gun point. Dr. Michael Newton has researched and found there are other worlds in which flying is the normal mode of living. In our dreams we may sometimes be actually visiting such worlds ([7, 8]).

One night I dreamed of losing the ring from my right hand in a swimming pool. I dove down and was amazed to find there was no wetness to the water and the floor shone with light. I found the ring and picked it up.

In the early hours of March 15, 1990 in Addis Ababa I dreamed that my brother, Rajendra, and some friends and relatives were standing on the terrace of a high building on the shore of a vast sea. I asked Rajendra to look after my body, as I left it behind to go out over the sea in Soul form. As he said okay I used my imagination to gently force myself out over the water. I flew for quite sometime and then collected some water in my cupped palms for those standing and waiting in the building. Before doing that I looked at the rest of my body, which was there as normal. I pinched my left hand but there was no sensation. I flew back to the top of the building. Before this dream I had other flying dreams to strange places. On March 19 I dreamed of flying over vast blue seas, and from the bottom of a tall building up to the top.

On March 20 I dreamed of water below ground seen through a clear glass wall. Small animals; a rabbit, a green tortoise, a black snake with one big spot like a single eye at the centre of its hood in the back, a few white mammals and so on, all in dazzling white light seen through the glass.

On 5 April 1990 I was in London. In the early morning hours I woke up with a very strong erotic feeling lasting for a minute. I held on to it simply observing what was happening. During the process my organ was hard erect and quivered with strong sexual desire for more than half-a-minute. Suddenly the wave passed and then slowly my sexual tension lessened, replaced by love, tranquility, peace and inner happiness. The experience was very similar to the one described by Swami Muktananda[9]. A natural state of "celibacy" was arriving without being forced down. A forced state of celibacy has the potential of erupting back any time, as in the case of several spiritual heads of churches reported in recent years.

In April I bought the book *Taoist Yoga* by Lu Kuan from a London shop. It was a pleasant surprise to read on page 106 the following statement on page 106: "If you so train you will certainly produce the immortal seed which, however, before it matures, tends to arouse and shake the penis without prior warning."

In the last few years I have received explanations for unknown events through books. Soon after the event I came across a book explaining what had happened within me. Many people who saw me on the 7th of April said I had a special glow on my face as if some energy was radiating from me. I felt very strong physically and calm mentally.

For 10 days I saw dead snakes hanging from their heads with their white undersides facing me. This happened at night in dreams and in visionary flashes during the day. This could indicate the taming of Kundalini.

Two important things I noted in Taoist Yoga are: (1) On maturity there is an experience of death and then resurrection, (2) When the seed of vitality is fully ripe it appears in the form of a "golden bright light" seen between and behind the eyes when you close them. This morning after my regular yogic exercise and bath, I concentrated on and found a "golden light" the size of a large pea with light shining around it. I have seen "sky blue light" for several years but I saw this golden light for the first time. This circle of golden light varies between 1 and 2 cm in diameter and is surrounded by either golden or sky blue light. I continued to see this light regularly while praying. Sometimes the light would have a copper-red color and would spread all over. According to Swami Satyananda Saraswati in *Kundalini Tantra*, practitioners may see a flaming lamp, like the morning sun, when the Ajna or eyebrow centre opens.

On April 28, 1990 I saw two important dreams. In the first one I was sailing on a boat over clear water extending over a vast land. Shining white light illuminated everything on the ground, visible through the water. In the second dream I heard the voice of Chandra Vishvain coming from a *bodiless form* around me. I could tell where the voice emanated from as it spoke and moved around me.

During May 1990 I felt Kundalini symptoms hitting the crown of my head. There was an interaction going on between my eyebrow centre and crown centre. My entire head heated up and I found it difficult to concentrate. On the 8th of May between 3 and 5 in the evening I had the feeling that something was hitting me very hard on the back of the head, which was very hot and painful. It felt like blood was sucked out of me and my face went pale like in 1987 and I was nauseous. I sat in a friend's house and drank two cokes. I felt a sort of emotional climax inside me. And then the experience subsided, giving me a complete feeling of emptiness. I felt as if the tank full of water inside me had been emptied. I relaxed and closed my eyes. Then I felt very hungry and I ate two bananas, which was unusual under normal circumstances. The next day my mind and body were back to normal and I did my usual paperwork.

A deep sky blue color on one hand and a deep golden-red on the other were always seen when I closed my eyes. Normally the golden color would first appear as a spot, expanding slowly, and then blue would come and then the two would mix, a beautiful combination producing violet at my *Ajna* or eyebrow center. Sometimes I had visions of the corpses in the British Museum, sometimes a plane taking off from the ground and going into the sky, and sometimes visions of towers and meadows moving below me. These dreams signified the death of ego and spiritual progress, and some of them were actual soul travel experiences.

During July 1990 I noticed that my tongue was sticking to my palate and my spit just would not slide down my throat, rather it collected until sizable and then I would forcibly gulp it down. This had been happening for many years. However I became conscious of it only after reading about it in the book *Taoist Yoga*. This stated it was necessary for the formation of the vital seed. Even today I notice the tongue sticking to the palate and spit gathering and going down the throat in a gulp.

On October 24th 1990, in a flash, I saw a white lotus. On focusing on my third eye and listening to the high sound of Logos, I felt the sound moving towards my left ear. Sometimes there was pain in the left side of my head. Sky blue light and burning copper light would appear together producing a purple color. A feeling that I can enter solid matters and fly anywhere prevails. A feeling of being dissolved in the infinite universe and losing myself surfaced many times.

Most of my flying dreams were actually out-of-body experiences of soul travel. Eckankar travellers, in their books, have described many places I had also visited. For example, the beautiful city described on page 111 of Terrill Wilson's book *How I Learned Soul Travel* was visited by me, and I remember many of the same details. Narrow, pebble paved streets, sidewalks, colorful buildings built close to each other and crowds moving around. I flew over the whole street and peeped into many windows from the top. Once

I landed on the ground and asked a question to a beautiful young woman walking there. She answered with a smile and then I took off and flew again. While flying I saw my full body, which was made of a cloudy white material, and with arms stretched, I flew like a glider. I have been flying like this for several years. My visit to the Brahma Lok in 1988 and seeing everything exactly as described on page 18 of the book *The Far Country* by Paul Twitchell confirms my actual Soul travel to that plane. Many times I have flown over unknown places, over very high buildings, sitting on top of them, flying over wide jungles of strange trees and flowers. However, Terrill Wilson, while stating that Soul travel is one means of expanding consciousness, suggests the aim should be to achieve spiritual perfection rather than fascination with out-of-body experiences. Paul Twitchell has rightly said that one should aim for the Highest plane of God Absolute and the lower planes would follow automatically according to the necessity and the will of God. One's aim should never be less than Self-realization.

I completed my two-year assignment with the University of Addis Ababa, Ethiopia in January 1991 and I did not agree with the Head of the Department to renew it for another two years since my father wanted me to be in Delhi to build the second site of our property there. Most of the year 1991 I was in Delhi and with my brothers built the four storey building on five hundred square yards, where at present we have the head offices of our Academy of Kundalini Yoga and Quantum Soul. One of the precious gifts of my stay in Zimbabwe and Ethiopia for four years was my turning to write on occult sciences. I wrote the book, *Secrets of Numerology* (1992) there. The book has now been translated and published in Malaysian and Indonesian languages. Another book I began to write at that time was *Destiny, Science and Spiritual Awakening* (1997). I began to write research papers based on my personal experiences that were published by *The Journal of Religion and Psychical*

The Autobiography—My Journey to Godhood

Research, Connecticut from time to time. Eventually I joined the Academy of Religion and Psychical Research, Connecticut, and I am now one of the "trustees" and member of the "publication committee" for the about last five years, at the time of writing this book in July 2002.

On 13 April 1991 in Delhi I listened to the high whistle in my head and contemplated this for 30 to 45 minutes before falling asleep. In my dream I found myself in a large temple building. With leg and arm motions I started flying up over a vast jungle landscape. I saw a huge palatial building in the distance. On waking I felt happy and peaceful. Next morning I dreamt of an elderly woman, and after putting my head on her feet I flew from a big building into the distance over green trees. After sometime I flew over a Shangri-La valley full of beautiful and strange trees. Flying around, admiring the beauty of the place, suddenly I saw a lion roaring at the jungle's edge. I was about to land at this point; instead I flew on and returned later.

During November 1991 while staying at the Hotel Grand Pacific in Suva, Fiji, in order to join the University of South Pacific on my new three-year assignment, I had an immense sexual desire with an erection lasting about half-a-minute, just as I experienced in London about one-and-a-half years earlier. After the feeling subsided there was tranquility, peace, happiness and love. State of "celibacy" coming in a natural way.

One morning I had visions of unusually colored flowers and then the colors of VIBGYOR as in the rainbow, such as I have never seen on earth. Once I dreamt of flying from the bottom to the top of a very tall building and on reaching the top founding statues of snakes with open hoods. One day in June 1992, in Suva, Fiji Islands, I felt connected to the Infinite Void for a moment, dark and vast, a bit horrifying in the beginning but with a feeling of love. It was similar to the experience I had in Malawi during December 1989—connection to *shoonyata* being repeated.

On 7 September 1992, in Suva, I sat for meditation around 6.30 p.m. For one whole hour I had such a wonderful concentration that I was in peaceful *samadhi*. I could have continued much longer if I was not disturbed and asked to come for dinner. I was amazed because this was a rare instance of going so deeply into samadhi. Later that night I came to know that it was exactly the time my father died in Delhi, India. His Soul was released and might have been in tune with me, his peaceful state of non-physical was shared with me. Both of us loved each other very much and he missed my not being with him when he passed away.

During December 1992 I had visions and semi-dream states in which I felt snakes rising from the ground and saw someone throwing rope rings over them to catch them. The snakes were caught and tamed. This was an indication of Kundalini being under control and in its benevolent form represented by Goddess Durga in India. Freshly aroused Kundalini is in its violent form and very difficult to control; at that stage it is represented by Goddess Kali. From this stage onwards one has very pleasant experiences with Kundalini; its form changing from *mother* to *beloved* and to *daughter* at times. I have experienced all the three form at different times.

On 7 January, 1993 I had a Soul travel experience. In my dream state I found myself hovering around a large white marble statue of Lord Shiva, with many small, thin snakes around his neck. While travelling round his neck I was astounded when I saw myself passing close to a snake. But soon my fear was replaced with a feeling of strange peace and love. I felt the snake was representing Mother Kundalini. Certainly it was a visit to some higher realm and I was in my Soul form without a body but with awareness. I felt tranquility, love and peace of mind.

I joined the University of Dar-es-Salaam, Tanzania in February 1993, after resigning the job in Fiji. On 5 March 1993 I dreamt of flying high over oceans and mountains, tall buildings shining clearly in bright shining light and descending to the ground and again rising up. I was looking for a way or destination but there was confusion and no clear way was seen. Nevertheless, a feeling of peace and happiness prevailed. On the 9th of April I dreamt of being dropped from a very high altitude into a wonderland with tall thin objects like statues. It was a land full of light, peace and tranquility.

I was at the Mt. Madonna Yoga Centre in California from June 18 to 22, 1992, as one of the invited speakers at the First International Conference of Kundalini Research Network. A young American woman came and asked to speak with me. I replied that we could talk later. A refined middle-aged woman, who was an author and speaker, sitting close to me, started talking to me; and, although I was talking to her but my attention was somewhere else. Another woman who was quite attractive and smiling all the time was also very interested in talking to me. Yet again I did not show much interest in talking to her. I noticed that I was not interested in a physical relationship with a woman; otherwise it was a good opportunity for me to develop a friendship there.

During October 1993 two mantras emerged inside me. One was "Om Namoh Bhagavate Vasudevaya," which was also suggested to me by the Tantric guru and author Dr. B. Bhattacharya in Delhi. The other was, "Mahanta Sri Harold Klemp, The Living Eckmaster." Both these mantras, with repetition, would generate power and heat inside me. Another mantra, suggested to me by Bhrigu Rishi was "Om Hrim Shrim Govindaya Namah." However, with a lengthy repetition I would feel too much heat in my head and I would stop it. There were other mantras that I also knew. The mahamantra "Hare Krishna, Hare Krishna, Krishna Krishna Hare Hare, Hare Ram Hare Ram Ram Ram Hare Hare," produced a pleasant cooling effect. According to Swami Radha[10] practitioners in the latter stages would find mantras coming to them and could repeat and enjoy one of them. The point is—*all power is one*. You need to stick to one of them and enjoy chanting with the one that pleases your inner self. This is the stage where one has gone beyond dependence on mantra chanting.

Transcendence of the lower and disturbing forms of sex shows the successful passage of Kundalini through the *Mooladhara* and *Swadhishthan chakras*. This is also certified with the experience of "rising of the body from the ground," which signifies the separation of the astral body from the physical. Self-expression through writing spiritual papers and through Soul travel to higher realms shows the crossing of the *Manipura chakra*. Opening of the Anahata chakra is suggested by hearing the Cosmic AUM and seeing the blue lotus star. Vishuddhi chakra is certified by good health, freedom from diseases, rejuvenation, power of speaking influentially and writing spiritual texts. The Ajna chakra or eyebrow centre is opened with a "golden light" at the center, the opening of the third eye through which astral travel and clairvoyant experiences are held. This is also certified through the knowledge of paranormal powers, though in dreams, such as uprooting a pole, stopping a vehicle, hearing a relative who has no body, and seeing a relative at three places at the same time. Activation of the Bindu chakra is signified by a connection with the *Shoonyata* or Great Void, and the properties of Vishuddhi chakra, since the two are connected internally. Sahasrara is seen as a white dazzling lotus with many leaves. Death experiences and snakes signify death and resurrection, which again signifies the opening of ajna or eyebrow centre on one hand and control with an awakened Kundalini on the other.

Over the months I felt my experiences had stopped, for example, flying dreams or visits to other realms. Sexual desire does not occur at all although I enjoy female company. A feeling of quiet, calm, happiness, satisfaction, compassion, detachment, lack of jealousy and lack of hatred always remain. The cosmic sound of AUM and the blue and golden lights are always there. I am writing spiritual papers constantly. The indications are that a stable stage has been reached and there will be no more paranormal experience distractions.

During a nap on 28 February 1994 I saw a large tree laden with beautiful unearthly colored flowers, falling constantly to the ground, which was already covered with them. This scene repeated two to three times within a few moments. I had seen similar colors in January 1992. Certainly it was a clairvoyant viewing of some higher plane. On both occasions I had a feeling of long lasting happiness.

The night between the 6th and 7th of March 1994 was notable for an unusual experience. In the early morning hours I suddenly felt severe pain in my first chakra—mooladhara. I ran to the toilet expecting to pass a stool but that was not to be. The pain became unbearable and I was about to scream. Suddenly I concentrated on my third eye and saw a dazzling white star surrounded by bright blue light. As I stared at it the pain subsided and was finally gone. The star was shining off the central line. It was bright and pointed. As I looked at it directly it vanished. It was different from the blue light that normally spreads on my mental screen. Swami Shivananda in his book *Sadhana* mentioned that seeing the shining blue star means nearing the culmination of yoga practice, the star being oneself as Soul, seen internally. It is the sign of liberation from *Maya* or illusion, since you see yourself in your true form, and then attachment to the body and mind is completely gone. You will be placed in a suitable higher realm after physical death. According to Sri Herald Klemp, spiritual leader of Eckankar, the star shows a high state of consciousness and involvement of the inner Master with the Soul. Around 11 p.m. on the previous night I had a long satisfactory and pleasant time with my wife and then I slept well for about four hours. Around 3 a.m. this ensuing pain and ensuing experience with the star took place. I recollect the night in 1987 when I had a similar relaxed and good time before going to bed and after a sleep of about four hours the *cosmic sound* appeared within me. Yet again in 1984 it was after concentrating on the picture of a couple from the Tantric text that I went into samadhi and eventually the *brahmajyoti* appeared before me.

It is the recognition of the sex drive, which brings about spiritual developments in fastest possible way, if handled with knowledge and care or under the guidance of a Master. It is the sexual lever, which is called the "philosopher's stone" in *alchemy*, which is responsible for converting *normal consciousness* into *Higher Consciousness*, known as conversion of iron into gold by the stone. It is one of the sure ways to bring the "crisis" and have the quantum jump into divinity. However, one should be reminded that continuous devotion to the Lord is a necessary safeguard against the things going wrong. This is a prerequisite.

In the previous year I felt energy and my vital fluids being sucked up from my pelvic region into my head. I had not lived family life for several months. There was a big change in my metabolism. The book on *Sexual Secrets* (p. 233) talks about Chandamaharosana, a set of 13 positions of "kama sutra" where we find, "entering yoni without knowledge results in countless rebirths; entering yoni with knowledge results in distillation of sexual energy in the head center, producing subtle hormonal changes and opening of intuitive wisdom." This according to Hindu thoughts means conversion of *virya* or semen into *ojas*, which is the prime factor for *enlightenment*. A very important fact is presented here for those who would care to know about it. In his book, *Living with Kundalini*, Gopi Krishna writes, "The incessant and rapid natural suction of the reproductive secretions that occurs at this time is the only way open to Nature to save the brain from damage and to contrive the enhanced activity of the vital organs. Energy is drawn from every part of the body through the nerves lining the genital organs to meet the highly increased demand without interruption. If interruption occurs, the consequences can be dangerous. The newly activated chamber in the brain must be constantly fed by what is described by the ancient masters as a stream of ambrosia (p. 132)."

I am happy I did not feel like having female company anymore, instead, longed for a more profound intimacy with God. During September 1994 I was feeling quite lonely, cut off from social life and missing female company. On one of those days in the early morning hours in Delhi I received a "divine female kiss" on my lips and the sensation lasted for the whole day. It was intoxicating and divine. As Vimal Ananda said in the book *Aghora*, the kiss could be from Shakti-Kundalini, who assumes the form of a beloved at times, after the process has been completed. The Mother, before awakening and activation, becomes the Beloved after meeting with her master Shiva in the crown centre.

The fall of 1994 was a period of major changes in my life once again. During September 29 to October 2, 1994 I was involved in the International Conference of Kundalini Research Network (KRN) near San Francisco. My paper was very much liked by the members of KRN, who advised me that it was time for me to settle in America. Soon after the conference I made the decision to resign my professorship of mathematics in Tanzania. I sent the letter of resignation by mail. This was a good-bye to mathematics for the rest of my life. The second big thing that happened to me was that I decided to end my marriage with my English wife, which was not based on spirituality and was proving to be an obstacle in my further progress. I got the divorce in about a year's time. Third important thing that happened at that time was that I applied for permanent residence in United States of America and I got my green card in less than a year. I rented an apartment in San Francisco and started to live there with my mother, who is also very spiritual and devoted. Our prayers and religious songs, and going to the temple in San Francisco, which was run by American devotees, became very regular. I felt I was making good spiritual progress there. I began writing the book on Kundalini at that time which was eventually published in India in 1999.

A strange thing happened around the 9th of November 1994. I was feeling a bit sexy when suddenly a pleasant sensation came to my pelvic region and around the reproductive organ and I had mental orgasms. There was no ejaculation. The pleasant sensation lasted a long time and I had a good sleep afterwards.

At 8.55 a.m. on November 25, 1994 I had a vision of a crowd cornering a man and stabbing him to death. He was lying peaceful and smiling on the ground with a knife in his heart. When I looked at the face of the man, it was none else than myself. I also heard someone internally saying, "Ravindra Kumar is dead," similar to the event in 1987. During prayers that morning I felt a divine child kissing me all over. I could feel or visualize that it was a female baby, benevolent Mother Kundalini coming this time as a daughter. Sometime back she came as a beloved and kissed me, as mentioned earlier. I was thrilled with happiness. I had an insatiable desire for love, which perhaps could not be satisfied by any human. It was the third time that year that I received divine kisses.

During December 1994 I read the book *Aghora* by Svoboda, containing the teachings of Vimalananda[11]. I noted two things there. (1) The fire of tongue burns what you speak through it—bad things as well as good things including spiritual achievements. This was a warning given to me by a relative in Delhi also, sometime ago, and also by Ray Olsen of Eckankar in Zimbabwe. I have been talking to people about my spiritual attainments, losing thereby some good effects perhaps, if not all. Bad karma repeatedly confessed likewise burns it off, which should be done. (2) Penance and tapas or austerities cause the heating up of your head. If you indulge in anger or lust, you burn the accumulated Shakti. Controlling the temper enhances the process towards enlightenment. Vimalananda used to put ice on the top of his head. I needed these two lessons very badly.

In the morning of January 23, 1995 I saw in my vision two slim white shining snakes moving fast. According to some writers this meant intuitive knowledge coming through the perfection of the Kundalini process.

On January 31, 1995 I got a sort of realization through the book *Aghora* by Svoboda. In 1987 the divine appeared to me as the Mother Goddess three times. In 1994 she kissed me as my beloved consort at least on three occasions. And many times I have seen her as a female child. So Shakti has appeared before me as a mother, as a beloved/consort and as a daughter/child. I have seen the beautiful child many times in male form too.

On February 4, 1995 I started a 41-day program of chanting a particular mantra of Lord Krishna, two hours a day. In the second hour I would sometimes experience firework explosions of divine colors, not to be seen on earth. On February 10 I saw, in my vision, a young child, around one year of age, laughing and looking all around inside me. He appeared to be full of happiness and innocent love. On March 10 I saw lady saint Anandmayi Ma coming close to me and looking at me. A child would appear in my visions every now and then. During the month of March I would go into states of trance from time to time while meditating. Once I saw myself as a dimensionless Soul fast approaching a temple, entering it and then striking at the closed door, perhaps wanting to open it. On another occasion I saw beautiful female figures, and had sudden orgasms without ejaculation, very satisfying and transforming. A divine presence would be felt now and then but I could not recognize any figure. But I was happy and blissful. On my inner screen I was a bright yellow color along with the purple one.

In the middle of the year 1995 I had a very important dream. I was in a hall with many other people involved in various activities. I was looking at them. Suddenly I saw a man about one foot taller than everybody else, very attractive and graceful. His radiant form set him apart from an ordinary man. He passed from one corner to another as if he was standing on a moving platform. He looked constantly at me with a smile and beautiful big eyes. He had the word BAPU written on his chest, the word in India is used for one's grandfather or such an elderly person. His look at me produced an ocean of love and happiness inside me. Some authors on dreams have written that higher personalities can enter the dreams of others for specific purposes, see for example Guiley[12]. I believe it was either my High Self or Guru/God who initiated me into higher spirituality.

April 30, 1995 I had severe pain at the base of my spine, the place of first chakra, for a short while. My body wanted to become straight; chest drawn outwards and there was a pressure in my third eye, also my anus muscles were contracted.

During the month of November 1995 I was in Philadelphia for the Kundalini Research Network's annual conference. In the middle of the night I again had a terribly hard erection with extreme feelings of sexual desire for about one minute. As usual, it gradually subsided, leaving no trace of sexual desire. Bliss followed. I was in the company of American women, but there was never a desire for sex. We had a pure, loving and platonic relationship.

Some life-changing events took place in the year 1995. In summer we normally had the annual conference of the Academy of Religion and Psychical Research (ARPR), and during fall we had the annual conference of the Kundalini Research Network (KRN) every year. During ARPR conference I met William Henry Belk, a big businessman from the East coast. Boyce Batey, our secretary general of ARPR, informed me that some people had come from Charlotte to meet me especially. After hearing my talk Mr. Belk told me that he had been reading my articles in the journal of ARPR for quite sometime and he had also heard my talk now. He offered me to work with him and do whatever I was doing from his table. On his insistence I accompanied him in his home-car to Charlotte and stayed there for about three days. He had more than 4000 books at his Belk Research Institute and a nice atmosphere to work. He offered me a monthly allowance and all other facilities to work as the "professor of comparative religion." I accepted the offer and returned to San Francisco. In the first week of July I arrived in Charlotte with my mother. I had a wonderful time in Charlotte with Henry Belk. My book on Kundalini was completed there in about six months time. It was first published in India in 1999 by Sterling Publishers and later in USA in 2000 as *Kundalini for Beginners* by Llewellyn Worldwide Ltd. The book has now been translated and published in seven languages of the world, including Russian and Japanese.

In September 1995, three years after my father's death, a clairvoyant friend in North Carolina assisted me in making contact with my deceased father. A spirit spoke through him saying that Ganga Singh (my father) was not strong enough to talk to me directly. However, as caretaker of the place where my father was recovering, he offered to converse with me and relay whatever my father said, while my father would hear me directly. Through this helpful spirit my father described a hospital setting where large number of people were recovering. After a long rest and feeling very relaxed, his broken leg was mending and soon he would be transferred to a region of brighter light. He wanted me to remove his possessions from the house so that his attention would not be distracted, and requested to be emotionally released by all of his relatives. I asked if he had met my grandmother (his mother) yet, and he replied that she is in a higher region where he can see her but cannot go there directly. He wanted me to tell his wife (my mother) he is very well and no one should worry about him; we then spoke about other family matters. I expressed my sorrow at not being at his side when he left this world. He was also sorry, missed being with me and wanted to embrace me. He suggested we could meet in a dream thirty days later, if I agreed. Naturally, I said yes, and exactly thirty days later, we were walking and talking together in my dream or probably in a real soul travel experience.

The next opportunity to visit my father came in June 2000, at the home of my friend in North Carolina. In this vision, having recovered his strength, my father spoke to me directly, greeting me with folded hands. I experienced much joy, since now my father was talking to me directly, as compared to the last time, when some one was speaking on his behalf. Immediately, I lowered myself in prostration to touch his feet-a traditional Indian gesture of respect and reverence. Saying we were no longer father and son, but now two fellow souls, he expressed his pride at my progress and offered to guide me in my further quest for spiritual knowledge. When asked if he remembered his wife, he replied, "which one?" Other souls had partnered him in other lifetimes. He confided in revealing his new type of existence. In this existence, he sometimes felt like a cloud. He could take form if he wished, however, he felt no need. In this place, eating or drinking was no longer necessary. It was a realm of unearthly colors, as he had never seen. The entire atmosphere was so lovely it was beyond earthly language's capacity to express. Going to meet friends or relatives required only a thought, but usually they would come to see him in groups. Several radiant and serene teachers came from time to time to offer lessons.

Curiously, I enquired about his next incarnation. He said that the choice had not come up yet. The concept of time did not exist and he was happy learning and enjoying his new life. Needing to go, he assured me that I could visit him whenever I wished. When I asked him if my visit had caused him any trouble, he reassuringly said, "no, not at all."

My medium friend suggested that I could talk to his "spirit guide," known as Guru Kirpal, who had translated from earth a few years ago. Guru Kirpal was the same spirit who helped me communicate with my father when my father was *indisposed*. On another occasion, I had an hour's conversation with Guru Kripal. Guru Kirpal told me that he resided only on the mental plane. He explained that souls on the mental plane, on a still higher level, have very subtle bodies, sometimes visualized only as a flash of light. They engage in spiritual pursuits and there are teachers who visit whenever assistance is required.

That fall, during the KRN conference, a group of women from Denmark attended a talk I presented. The leader of this group, Ms. Jytte Larsen, asked several questions, and then asked about the possibility of contacting me later. I gave her my address and received her first letter while I was in India for a short visit. We exchanged more letters. In December 1995 I received an invitation from Tampa, Florida to give a talk on Numerology and Kundalini, which I accepted. Around that time I met several people in Florida, including Dr. Khandelwal, Dean of Hindu University, Tarpon Springs, Florida. He invited me to work with him as "professor of yoga philosophy and meditation." I joined Hindu University in April 1996. In June Jytte Larsen paid a two-week visit to the University and we became quite close. In July I visited Denmark for a few days on my way to India. We both decided I would return and stay in Denmark after my short visit to India. Since the fall of 1996 I have been living and writing in Copenhagen, Denmark. At the time of writing this book in 2002, I completed the book *Secrets of Kundalini Awakening*, coauthored with Jytte Larsen, which was published that year in New Delhi.

September 11, 1996 in Delhi I dreamt of a thin, long and brightly colored coiled snake. Facing up, its tongue came out again and again. Suddenly it began rising and uncoiled. It changed into a full-grown snake with several pairs of feet on both sides. Bright and strong, it moved up, and soon disappeared. It was a symbolic representation, in my consciousness, of my inner process of awakening and activation of Kundalini. Disappearance of the snake/

Kundalini could also mean my disappearance as *jiva* or individual soul from the face of the earth at the end of present incarnation. Having graduated from earth I may not return and settle permanently in the spiritual sky. This was the reading of *Bhrigu Rishi* in his *Bhrigu-samhita*, which is a record of all souls on earth. However, my attention may be diverted by something towards the end of this incarnation, and for this reason I may have to incarnate once more, which should be my final appearance on earth.

On January 28, 1997 I was in Copenhagen, Denmark. I dreamt of being in a large new building with many furnished rooms filled with people working. A dead body lay on the ground floor covered with a white sheet. I looked at it and then climbed up from one room to another. I reached the top floor, which had a beautiful and big balcony with many green plants. An elderly man came out and sat down on a chair. He pointed towards another chair where I sat down. Two nights later I dreamt of an elderly man again, I felt he was my father. He could be my Higher Self too. He was holding packets of money and gave me one note. Then he told me about the new room I was going to live in. Then he gave me a soothing massage on both arms. Coming to interpretation, a dead body represented, once again, the death of my ego, and my consciousness rising from one level to another, as the rooms represent consciousness. An elderly man represents the inner Guru/God, my High Self, who is always taking care of me, symbolized by his giving a massage to my arms.

For a few days, being worried about family and property matters in Delhi, my sleep was disturbed. I was in Denmark at this time. I constantly remembered asking God to help me. Around 5 a.m. I felt a sudden "rush of love" in my heart. I forgot my grief. Around 6 a.m. there was a telephone call from my son in India giving me information about things being well in Delhi. I do not know how he got an inspiration to call me. My sensitivity became sharply magnified. I felt small things in a big way. I analyzed my behavior over the past few years and held myself responsible for causing unhappiness to my brothers in the matter of property distribution by my father. I thought I could have given a better deal to my younger brothers, even if it was at my own expense. I decided to go more fully into my spiritual process. Around that time one of my brothers encroached upon a part of my property and this made me unhappy. The police and courts were involved. To add to my misery the publisher in America rejected my book for publication. And yet again there was another misunderstanding with a family member causing unhappiness. All this happened at the same time. Everything seemed to go wrong when I decided to go fully on my spiritual path. I brought up my energy reserves and reminded myself that I am the Soul who should not be affected by these happenings. In a few days I returned to normal. One morning I saw unusually beautiful unearthly colors that gave me divine happiness.

On 11 January 1998 Jytte had an experience similar to the one I had in March 1994. Around 6 p.m. that day she felt severe pain after sexual feelings, as if stool was to be passed but nothing happened. However, she felt rush of energy upward and itching in 5th and 6th centres. A feeling of vomit and effect of indigestion was felt in the throat. Blue light was seen but not the star. However, the process appeared to be advanced.

On 28 January, 1998 between 7 and 8 p.m. I was typing the chapter on Jnanayoga. Suddenly I found brittle ash on my fingertips, especially on right hand, materializing spontaneously. I had to do away with it before I could type again, but a part of it remained that I showed to Jytte. A similar thing had happened in Nigeria in 1994 when lot of ash remained on my table of prayer for few days and Professor Bajpai and his wife came to see it.

During January/February of 1998 I decided to go fully on the spiritual path under the influence of the planet Ketu. Just those days I received a phone call from India that one of my brothers was acquiring my property in our family house. I intuitively felt a difficult time was coming. On March 4 I landed in Delhi. Whole of March and April was full of problems I had never seen before. Police, court, lawyer, friends, relatives were all deeply involved because of the property occupation. Another "bolt from the blue" was received when my publisher from Florida returned my book and showed her inability to publish the book. Third serious problem came when Jytte told me on phone that she is going to break relations with me and I should not come to Copenhagen anymore. Everything seemed to be going wrong when I wanted to dip myself fully in spirituality like Sri Aurobindo.

The third week of October 1998 I was in Philadelphia. A Reiki healer gave my body a complete massage. Before starting, she moved a pendulum over my seven chakras one by one. The pendulum rotated slowly at my root centre, its rotational speed increased from chakra to chakra, and rotated with full speed at my crown center—perfect, said the healer. She was amazed at the complete development/opening of the chakras in the correct ascending order.

Between December 1998 and January 1999 I carefully noted the kinds of sound going on inside me. There were three types of them at one time—buzzing of bees, a single note from flute and woodwinds music. Buzzing of bees was constant since its onset in 1987. The other sound I commonly hear these days is the music of the woodwinds. Two other sounds appearing from time to time are "high tension wire" or "humming" and a single flute note.

I began to write the next book on Kundalini but I got little time to work on it since I was doing first course in Danish language since November 30, 1998. Test for it was passed on January 21. The second course began on February 1, 1999. In one-week holiday I planned to type my paper for the Ashby Memorial Competition run by the Academy of Religion and Psychical Research on afterlife. Much of my time went on what my brother had done in Delhi about property acquirement. I had become too sensitive to relationships. The more I wanted to bring the whole family together, the more it felt apart. The same person whom I bestowed the power and position was responsible to oust me from the business. These thoughts occupied much of my time, which I considered a complete waste. I wanted to have a yoga centre at a remote place where such happenings did not disturb me, but it was not happening. I was sorry for this.

While studying in Copenhagen during March 1999 I noticed two "kinks" in my life or personality—first, my understanding of technical/worldly things was slow, second, getting angry with someone and showing my resentment or annoyance does not pay, it creates a break in the relationship. On the other hand, my intuitive understanding was on the increase, and unconditional love (no resentment) is the key. The desire for sex had almost vanished from my system and a natural celibacy evolved. Sometimes there were thoughts of sex but my body and emotions no longer responded to it. Shashanka asana, a yoga posture, proved very useful for going into states of samadhi. Time virtually suspended in the Shashanka asana, that is, I felt two or three minutes pass, while about 20 or 30 minutes had gone by. This asana proved very useful for turning inward.

During May 1999 I decided to give up drinking and smoking. After a week of this I noticed my dreams becoming clearer.

It was around that time that I decided to form the Academy of Kundalini Yoga and Quantum Soul (AKYQS) with its Head Office in our own building in Delhi and centres in Copenhagen, Bradenton-Florida and London-UK. The academy provides training in an all-round development of personality: physical, mental, emotional and spiritual. Eventually one is guided into the practices for Self/God realization. The academy was soon recognized by the Government of India and registered in 1999 as a non-profit body. We started the publication of a quarterly bulletin from the beginning of 2000 and the academy has now members all over the world. I began to write small books on different kinds of yoga and occult sciences. So far 12 books have been published by Sterling Publishers, Delhi in their "All You Wanted to Know" series. They are on the topics: hatha yoga, kundalini yoga, kriya yoga, chakras and nadis, dreams, aura, psychic development, mantras, bhakti yoga, jnana yoga, karma yoga and tantra yoga in that order, at the time of writing this book in July 2002 (13-24).

I felt that I was judgmental towards my brother who had taken my power, position and money from the school. The reason could be that a decision was taken before incarnating to have this lesson of loss, since in past life I had redirected the funds for poor people towards my personal use. I was told of this sin committed by me in the thumb impression reading in Delhi. My feeling was that I had to learn this balancing lesson in this lifetime.

On 12 January, 2001 I had a wonderful dream, an actual Soul travel experience. It came after a two-year lapse. I flew high over a clear blue ocean, and reached the other side, there were buildings and people. I moved around the area and talked to people working there. It was a very happy experience. Later, whenever I concentrated on the dream, my heart became full of a strange happiness. In my book, *Secrets of Kundalini Awakening* I have written that my Soul travel experiences are always full of happiness, because I am free of my body's confinement. I devoted an entire chapter to this experience.

I have visited spiritual planets that are self-lighted; possess vast green lands, beautiful trees laden with fruits and lovely ponds and canals of clear blue water. People live there in the form of different lights but bodily manifestations take place at times. Most important thing to remember was the moment I entered such a planet I was full of strange inner happiness and feeling of bliss. May be some Souls would choose to live on such a planet while others may like to merge with the Great Void. There may be other alternatives too for the liberated ones. Also I cannot say whether it was one's own choice or it was an automatic placement. Swami Prabhupad, founder of International Society for Krishna Consciousness has said at one place that three-fourth of the universe is inhabited with spiritual planets while one-fourth has other planets and solar systems like ours. I cannot express my authority at this point although I have been visiting spiritual planets from time to time.

An important observation that is worth a mention here is about the extra-sensitivity I have always had physically, mentally and emotionally. In physical terms I have noticed that I could never wear a shirt without an under vest in summer, even though I saw most of my classmates doing so at the college. If I wore a shirt without a vest I would soon start sneezing and have a headache. As soon as I entered the swimming pool I would sneeze many times. If I would sit under a fan with bare arms I would start sneezing, consequently, I would normally wear full sleeve shirts. Going to Kashmir to stay with my parents during summer vacations, I would soon start sneezing unless I covered my head and body well, although others would still not do so. I remember while walking on the streets of Rome in Italy during the summer of 1973, I would start sneezing through the sweat and would need to cool down myself for being normal. Thus, whether it was extra cold or hot, I needed protection for my extra sensitive body. Coming to the mental part of sensitivity I would never rest unless I had worked out all details of the daily life and had sorted out the associated problems to my maximum capacity. Those who knew me would advise that I should have a habit of forgetting many details that are comparatively not so important, but I would not.

More important was the area of emotions concerning sensitivity. With the advancement of age I became more and more sensitive. Especially after the experience of

Kundalini in 1987, my emotional sensitivity became very strong. Although I had the habit of sitting and analyzing my actions and events of the years gone by from time to time, this habit became more acute and pressing after 1987. There are two types of feelings: you being hurt or insulted by others, and you hurting or insulting others. Before 1987 I would not forgive others in the first case, and the hurt would keep me pinching until I had retaliated in some way or had taken some kind of balancing action. After 1987 I found that I would not give so much importance on being hurt by others and gradually I began to forgive the offenders. Now I do not take a notice if some one tries to hurt me, I would laugh and get out of the situation in one way or the other. In the second case where I had caused a hurt to the other I would not forgive myself, more so after the 1987 event. I would keep myself analyzing and find the cause of my action. Then I would try to compensate the damage done to the other person, in one way or the other, and would not feel peaceful until the compensation had been met with. I would also curse myself and punish myself in some appropriate way. Over the years of course I have learnt and have advocated the art of forgiving others as well as yourself, knowing that there is never a single reason or cause for an event to take place. It is the whole machinery around us in the nature that causes an event to take place. Now I do forgive others and myself and do not take a notice of either honors or insults. Letting go everything—every possession and every relation, in the symbolic sense—is the motto.

I was a good sportsman, who achieved honors in gymnastics and table tennis, although I was interested in other extra mural activities too. I always felt that the right side of my body was weaker than the left. My strong teeth and jaws on the left, and stronger left arm and leg, and stronger left shoulder. Lifting weights I would put it on the left shoulder. At night I could sleep on the left side as long as I wanted, but when I wanted to sleep on the right side I soon got tired and had to change to the left. My left eye has always been strong; the glasses I used for reading now have stronger correcting factor on the right side than on the left. I always wondered about these observations but in spite of my conscious efforts I could not reconcile the difference between the two sides. After meeting Margaret Dempsey over the e-mail through my book *Kundalini for Beginners* (Llewellyn, 2000) and having discussions with her I was pleasantly surprised to find the answer to my long-standing query about the reason why the left side of my body was stronger. It was because I had a more dominant right brain.

From childhood I was equally interested in mathematics and spiritual activities. I achieved first class marks in mathematics and science as a student from primary to post-graduation. I completed the requirements for the doctorate degree in three years and then did some post-doctorate research at English universities in UK. As a teacher I was acclaimed as one of the best in eight countries during my career. I could remember long mathematical equations and could learn off by heart the lecture I would deliver to the classroom. I was the author of several books on engineering mathematics and had more than 30 research papers in mathematics published in various journals throughout the world. At the same time I devoted much time to yoga, meditation, chanting of mantras and reading of scriptures. Until then I was as good in mathematics as before.

Soon after the experience of Kundalini I was advised by the doctor to stop all meditative practices, and not to take classes for two weeks at the university. After two weeks when I started to prepare the lecture in mathematics I would not find either the same interest or the same capacity to do so. It was an effort to remember small equations in mathematics, while prior to the Kundalini awakening I could remember even the most complicated ones. I then began writing articles in religion and psychology for the first time. My interest in mathematics diminished constantly until in 1994 I found it too painful to continue. I have written more than a dozen papers that have been published in the Journal of Religion and Psychical Research, USA, and 18 books on various branches of occult sciences. By drawing on all this experience I concluded that my capacity for mental work was not reduced but transferred from mathematics to religion and psychology. Now I find that I have no interest in calculations of any kind big or small. Even receipts and bills concerning daily life do not interest me. Since the episode in July 1987, I believed that my consciousness is operating mostly through the right side of the brain.

With Kundalini rising the Soul is in charge and it uses Kundalini to stimulate new areas in the brain. Kundalini-Soul energy passes up the central column of the spinal cord through the seven chakras and into the right side of the brain where it causes millions of more neurons to fire. This results in a reorientation of energy, which manifests as physiological and psychological renewal and rebirth, and thoughts.

Before Kundalini rises the activity of the Soul is minimal. It is largely working through the inner voice to assist the mind in gaining control over the senses through disciplining the ego. Once the mind has this control then the Soul works through it. The greater the control of the mind over the senses the more Soul energy can imprint on the brain. Energy from the Soul forms the etheric body, which is an energy layer containing the body. Kundalini rises when the mind has control over all emotions through the effect of newly directed energy on the body's nervous system. From here the Soul controls the flow of energy into the brain through the opened chakras and newly stimulated areas in the brain. At this point there is no separation between mind and soul, they have become one.

The month of November 2001 was quite important for my spiritual progress. I had a keen desire to meet with "higher order yogis" with whom I could advance further on the spiritual path. I made an appointment with the popular female saint Guruma, whose discourses are on Indian TV every morning for half-an-hour. Jytte, my brother, my mother and I booked our stay by phone and stayed at her ashram on the night of the 12th of November 2001. She had a lavish lifestyle living in a modern building set on seven acres, some 80 km west of Delhi. There were 30 rooms, with attached bathrooms, for visitors. Around 5 p.m. she comes out and sits on a swing to grant audience to visitors. During a private, one-hour conversation I asked many questions, wanting to know her views on "shaktipat." I could see her skill at motivating people to pursue their spiritual path, but was frustrated at her avoidance of commenting directly on the act of shaktipat. After repeated questions she finally replied that shaktipat is possible if the practitioner is ready. Looking directly at me, she asked specifically, was I ready, to which I answered, "yes." She immediately closed her eyes and for two minutes I felt something happening around my heart centre, an upsurge of love, peace and quiet. However, she did not ask me to meet again and I could see that she did not belong to an order of Shaktipat Gurus. After returning home I soon met another holy man near Sonepat, north of Delhi. He talked about nice things but he admitted that for him the power of shaktipat comes only occasionally, after meditation. This made him look pretty shallow from Shaktipat point of view. I was disappointed for not having met a Shaktipat Guru yet, in spite of my intensive search.

A few days later, one of my numerology students brought me a book written by Deepak Yogi. I quickly finished reading his book and decided to meet him at the earliest moment possible. Jytte and I made an appointment and spent four days at his center. We discovered He is a Shaktipat yogi of the lineage of the well-known Swami Vishnu Tirth and is the first person to convince me with his silent power. We chose to become his disciples and receive his initiation. I experienced a passage of power from him into me as he touched me and I went into "vibratory meditation" under his supervision for 45 minutes, and then I had to lie on the ground in a state of yogic trance. My concentration was beautiful. I felt I might leave my body when some figures appeared, in addition to the indigo color on my mental screen. The Yogi observed me for three days and said he was very satisfied with my performance. He said he was looking for a person to whom he could give the powers of "guru" and now he recognized the possibility in me. It was a day of extreme satisfaction for me also. I asked him why I needed further initiation as I had already experienced the awakening of Kundalini, resulting in the manifestation of Divine Light and Sound, and Soul travel to subtler realms. He said Kundalini needs further modifying for its full activation. Also, it is better to be a "shaktipat yogi" of a "lineage of the tradition of saints," than to be an independent one, in order to be effective and of service to others. Being in the lineage attracts the power of all other saints in the lineage, even after they leave for higher realms.

    I had two specific experiences after receiving this Guru's initiation. One, my back grew very hot, with strong itching sensations behind my spinal column for a few days. I rubbed my back against the wall for relief. Two, I had a recurring dream of a huge chimney with smoke pouring from it. According to Wilda B. Tanner this dream meant, "Place to safely vent or let off steam, smoke, fire. Could represent the flow of Kundalini, agni (fire) yoga, the fire of purification and burning away of the dross...."[25] (p. 157). It could mean the clearing of the veins through which the Kundalini is passing. The dream appeared to rightly explain my burning sensation in the back with the passage of Kundalini. I also dreamt of horses running in all directions. Brhadaranyka Upanishad-I says that horses are related to cosmic meaning. Wilda Tanner writes that "four horses refer to four lower chakras and seven horses indicate seven centres, the whole chakra system. Horses running free could represent loss of control or can be a wonderful freedom." (p. 99-100). I have been seeing blue to violet colors both in dreams and on the internal screen. For colors blue-violet Wilda Tanner writes "High spiritual qualities, devoted, inspired, rich in spiritual truth, trustworthy, honorable; often a spiritual leader of some kind in a quiet, unobtrusive way." (p. 173). To the gold color that I have been seeing these days she writes "Spiritual rewards, refinements, attainment, God's love and approval; also the enhancement of whatever it surrounds." (p. 174). Dreams have come as friends over the years, conveying the information in a subtle and regular way.

For some time I experienced breath-control after inhalation and sometimes after exhalation during my one-hour practice; these are the inner and outer "kummbhak." Sometimes my breath would be violent, signifying "bhastrika pranayama." On a few occasions I found " uddiyan bandha" or naval lock taking place by itself. One day when I was in bed, preparing to sleep, I felt something crawling up my back, from the base of my spine, up the length of my back, in repeating wavelike motions. In trance, I would sometimes see birds taking off from the ground, heading towards the sky. Sometimes I flew in the sky. During that time I felt bliss and a connection with the Infinite Void. During the day I felt happiest with closed eyes, not wanting to open them and reconnect to the outside world.

I continued with my one-hour daily practice of *kriyas* or automatic movements, suggested to me by the Guru. This gave pleasant experiences and results. After two months there were no more disturbing side effects of any nature.

I constantly see blue-violet colors and friendly snakes have been in my dreams for half of the life. Many times I have been seeing things in golden color. These colors have been interpreted a little while ago. Serpent is taken as the "symbol of mind power, wisdom, the creative force, mysticism, or Kundalini when dream feelings are positive (p. 104). Tiger represents go-getter, great strength and power of overcoming. I had a telephonic talk with Guru Deepak Yogi who was happy with my sadhana and asked me to increase time from 45 minutes to one hour and twice daily, which I immediately complied with.

February 3, 2002 we were in an exhibition in Copenhagen, where our auras were photographed. It had mostly blue and indigo colors meaning strong intuition and seeing subtle things within. Then there were four antennas-channels connecting to higher realms; which the expert photographer explained to me that "four superior beings are there to help me in evolution. Some brown color meant I have to drink much water and remain grounded for a balanced growth."

More than once I have dreamt of a big chimney with smoke coming out of it. The chimney signifies the clearing of the passage for Kundalini, as explained earlier. Dreaming of an open door and a high stool offered to me to sit implied, "higher point of view, and a more spiritual outlook. Can be high point of exaltation (high position), may depict being closer to God. Open door meant available, ready for you, wide open opportunity, way to go, or can be openness to receive." I dreamt of drinking clean water from a glass that is full. This symbolizes quenching your spiritual thirst, drinking in spiritual truth, or your need to do so.

During trance I saw a beautiful white swan flying in the sky. Once I felt being in the lap of the mother and drinking milk from her breast. Once I saw a garden with beautiful flower plants of unearthly colors. At another occasion some scripture in Sanskrit opened before me. I read the first line. Next I saw a clear shining thin and long road going into the sky, on which I am walking slowly upwards. Pranayama (breath-control) and kumbhak (retaining the breath) were going on automatically those days.

On June 4, 2003 I saw during my nap a saucer full of articles. As soon as I poured it on something the articles vanished.

On December 12, 2003 I read the message from the book by Sri Raman Maharishi: Get rid of the thought that 'I have no realization.' God, Soul are all concepts. Consciousness is the only reality. This realization came practically many times during the year 1987, when I experienced the awakening of Kundalini.

a. I saw myself as consciousness moving along a waterfall and enjoying it, going in water and coming out, and moving along.
b. As consciousness I stood before a translucent fortress, then moved along an ocean like river as if on a hair-like bridge.
c. The place had no sun or moon but was lighted bluish-green; I saw people as circles or points of light.
d. I entered momentarily in a space of a planet or something where I felt extreme bliss—perhaps a realm of anandmayalok or an infinite flame of light. Since then it has happened many a time.
e. In subtle body I have had innumerable ventures into subtle realms.

On December 30, 2003 in a nap I saw big-fly flying freely and happily here and there, sitting at different flowers for some time, tasting and taking the honey and then flying freely again. This could represent my inner state of being at the time. Then I dreamt of a white tiger as my personal escort on whose back I am riding for a long time, as people do on a horse. Suddenly I began to fly up above the land. Returning home I find the tiger and the child who was with me waiting for me with a loving and serving attitude. Once I saw a lion majestically sitting in front of me. Slowly it walked towards the room where some others and I were sitting. I was not afraid but others were. I told them to close the latch of the door and sit quietly without fear. Another time I saw a beautiful lake of clear water in which some swans were swimming majestically, their neck being green. On another occasion I saw a clear lake of water with blue leaves of lotus spread everywhere. I dreamt of flying over many locations, low and high, with clear water in the pool.

A committee wanted to take me as president of the society, which I first refused but accepted later. I dreamt of a pot full of honey and standing on stairs, slowly going upwards. Wilda Tanner's remarks on these dreams are, "Moving closer to God, meditation, prayer, communion, moving on up on the world, raising your consciousness, moving to higher levels of mind, a step up, or taking steps in right direction."

August 5, 2005 was a night in Copenhagen wherein I dreamt of Jytte weeping bitterly, tears coming out from both eyes on the cheeks and I am consoling her. According to Wilda Tanner's dream book (p. 353) this is a sign of your High-Self (God-Self) being distressed over your past actions or the decisions you are making. A warning that you need to reevaluate what you have done or are about to do. Then I saw my father telling me or advising me about the do's and don'ts and beg pardon for mistakes. Father depicts authority, responsibility, discipline, may be punishment, leader, man of the house or other qualities you associate with fathers in general or your father in particular (p. 273). I thought over the whole situation and took appropriate decisions. Dreams are the language in which God talks to us. My advice to sincere readers is to maintain a journal of dreams, keeping a pen and diary on the bedside and pendown the dream the moment you wake up, otherwise we forget many details and even the dream itself. You can always know what God wants to tell you.

August 29, 2005 I was in Copenhagen. I meditated in the morning for one hour-and-a-quarter and got connected to the palace of Brahma, seen during 1987. In trance I felt that I am entering the palace and it is disappearing, the two of us dissolving in each other. The mantra Om Hrim Shrim Govindaya Namah brought peace, bliss and attraction to that palace. Then I exercised heavily for about 40 minutes. The whole day I was feeling pain in the *mooladhara chakra* or the root centre. There was some kind of aching in the spinal column and head, and I felt like I was having temperature. In the evening between 6.30 p.m.

and 7 p.m. I suddenly started shivering with cold, so much that I put on many clothes and finally entered in bed with a quilt on, still I was shivering. Jytte gave me a drink but I could not hold the glass, the hand was shaking too much. After about 45 minutes I suddenly began to feel very hot; my whole body and forehead were too hot. I threw off all clothes except kurta-pyjama and was comfortable. Slowly I came to normalcy. It seems some knot had been hit and broken open by Kundalini or otherwise. Inwardly I felt happy and blissful. As soon as I concentrated I got the sight of that palace.

December 24, 2005: Early in the morning around 5 a.m. when my sleep was broken I saw Lord Ganesh in vision. The day went very successful with bank matters and loan application, pleasure in the day and good going in the evening.

January 1, 2006: During *sadhana* or spiritual exercise today I saw a newspaper where the following message was written in bold letters, "Ravindra Kumar is Dead." I had a very good inner feeling with peace and happiness. Connection with Bliss Mountain or Infinite Divine Flame—*brahmajyoti* was made as usual.

April 29, 2006: I have been living a good and regular life for the last one week. Last night I dreamt of a beautiful bird sitting with her back towards me. Suddenly it turned its face towards me and looked into my eyes. At another time I saw a very elderly *sadhu* or spiritual man with long white beard, getting ready to take food. I asked him if I could make tea for him? He said that he would make it himself. I felt very happy talking to him and had an inner satisfaction. This should signify my own state of inner being.

August 4, 2006: Yesterday there were long discussions with our spiritual friend Kalgi, who says that he is an *avatar*, who tried to force me to chanting 16 rounds of Mahamantra. He asked me to give up family life completely and finally, like he has done. I have been seeking answers from the Centre of command or *ajna chakra*, to be answered by the

Guru. This morning I had a successful chanting and meditation for about two hours. Towards the end I was in trance as usual, wherein I saw some shining and clear symbols which seem to answer my queries. First number '2' appeared before me, then it was number '3', and then a ripe fruit which I tried to pluck. Wilda Tanner's book on dreams has the following explanations. *Number 2*: Double weakness or double strength, division, Soul, receptivity, subconscious mind. It could mean interest and achievements both in worldly and spiritual matters. *Number 3*: Trinity, great strength, completion, creativity, or your ability to create. It may represent the physical, mental and spiritual combination, and achievement of the goal. *Fruit:* Representative of the fruits of your labors in particular, and your talents and good deeds. Guru's answer indicates success both in worldly and spiritual fields and the completion of the spiritual goal. I need not change my ways of living and continued to help the humanity as usual.

My life was now divided between India, the U.S. and Denmark. More than half of the year I spend in Denmark, where I lived peacefully and had perfect conditions for meditation and writing. I received permanent residence status in Denmark in December 2000. We have been planning to establish a yoga centre outside Delhi, in addition to the one we had in Delhi, where free and specialized training in Shaktipat was given to a few but genuine practitioners, who wish to raise their Kundalini quickly and safely[26].

Based on my personal experiences the theory and working of evolution can be summarized in the following observations:

(1) Being of a religious bent of mind and/or faith in God was a good start for me. On this basis my spiritual evolution was expedited by regular yogic asanas or postures, building a body strong enough for other catalyzing factors, such as chanting of mantras, reading scriptures and regulated family life. This regulated family life worked as my final and strongest catalytic agent.

(2) My evolution was aided by reading scriptures and the personal stories of evolved persons around the world. This helped in this way—my thoughts were always turned towards God, because of this any activity performed by me went in the direction of my spiritual evolution. Regulated family life at this stage took my energy upwards and the vital fluids were redirected towards my brain to make it rich enough to receive enlightenment, as the seed was ripe.

(3) Having developed such a background systematically, my mental withdrawal from the activities of the material world became smooth and automatic. Disinterest in material possessions developed in a natural way. The reason was that I came in touch with a "higher pleasure" that naturally withdrew me from worldly pleasures. This is called *sahaj-yoga* or natural yoga. Yoga means the joining of the Soul with the Supersoul or joining man with God in common language.

(4) I used a combination of Hatha Yoga (performing yogic asanas or postures), Karma Yoga (working without attachment to the result), Bhakti Yoga (devotional practices), Jnana Yoga (studying scriptures and the personal stories of yogis and saints and meditating on them). My practise of Tantra Yoga was to focus my attention on God during all worldly activities, including intimate moments with my wife. This is the way to transcend sex and become *celibate* in a natural way. Just as a thorn removes the thorn from the body, even so *tantric sex* or intimacy with constant attention on God is the right way to pass this hurdle of sex once and for all. One talking against sex in the open and having it in the private is a forced *celibate*, who can never get close to God or Truth. Regulated family life in this way gives a form of switch to the individual—whenever the switch is put on, one can have intimacy, and otherwise nothing can force him to do so. It is a wonderful situation to be ex-

perienced by practice, it cannot be explained otherwise. This is the control of senses and mind possessed by most yogis. Also I find it unfortunate that the so-called spiritual covering in a country like India takes away the chances of knowing the "philosopher's stone" of alchemists, which could convert iron (*normal consciousness*) into gold (*spiritual consciousness*) permanently and in a very short time. I carefully refrain myself from talking about it in my lectures, lest I may be misunderstood and criticized for the same.

(5) My spiritual awakening and Kundalini activation symbolized itself through seeing snakes in dreams and visions. Part of the reason is that Kundalini resides in the root-centre in a form similar to a snake sitting in three-and-a-half coils, and on awakening the energy rises up similar to the movements of a snake. Another reason is cultural identification. I grew up steeped in the Indian religious and cultural lore surrounding Kundalini. I saw Lord Shiva wearing garlands of snakes around his neck, symbols that unconsciously and consciously connect with Kundalini, and transcendence of sex. Naturally these symbols come to me in the same way as a Tibetan sees Buddha, westerners may see Jesus or Mary, and Arabs may see Mohammad. Our beliefs and conditioning determine our experience. Those with the most expanded beliefs seem to have the widest variety of experiences. Possibly formless energy, seen as light or colors, is the most universal symbol of **cosmic consciousness**. All representations are valid; we simply envision what is most dear to us.

(6) Shakti-Kundalini is the female counterpart of male God-Absolute, and consequently this energy appears in different female forms in my consciousness. When it was awakened it appeared as the benevolent and respectful mother, giving blessings and bestowing peace. Later it has appeared as a beloved and as a daughter at times.

(7) Indications of the completeness of the process come from time to time. Vital sexual fluids are sucked up from the region of the cervix (females) or from the testicles (males) and are pumped up to the brain through fine capillaries. With this the brain is energized and made fit to receive enlightenment, whenever it takes place. Around this time the practitioner is possessed with extreme sexual desire and one's sexual organs are seen shaking and quivering with great intensity, whether one is male or female. In the case of males the penis becomes extraordinarily hard and large. Females are known to pass through similarly intense sexual desire, see for example the case of Irina Tweedy[27]. However, the wave passes quickly, taking from 30 seconds to one minute, if the practitioner holds on to him/herself firmly and watches the situation as a witness. No ejaculation or loss of seed takes place. What follows is felt as unconditional love, peace, tranquillity and bliss. The experience may repeat for months or more than a year. Another symptom is the collection of spit in the mouth till the amount is sizeable and then it is swallowed to reach a place where it is effective. A nervous system break down takes place between the eyebrow centre and crown centre. Sometimes one eye, another time two eyes appear to watch the practitioner on his inner screen. The tongue sticks to the palate most of the time, which is responsible for the secretion of rejuvenating vital fluids. Divine colors, divine tastes and divine smells, never found on earth, are often experienced.

(8) Now comes the point of *celibacy* that has always baffled researchers. After reaching the stage described in the above paragraph, a period of natural celibacy follows, which varies from person to person. For some it lasts for a period of two years, for some, five years and for others it becomes a permanent feature. It is rare that both participants have transformed at the same time. When the period of *celibacy* is over, the practitioner may

live the family life again, but there is a vast difference between the situation before and after. It is like a cyclist finding his bicycle still moving, although he has stopped peddling. Thus, one may be making love at times but it is not demanding or compelling, and one does not make any special effort for satisfaction. Opposite sex, special kinds of food, clothes, cars, houses or other modes of living are not as important for the person now because they have served their purpose and no longer hold an attraction. One accepts and experiences pleasure as a gift from God, without making any effort or craving. One is in the world but not of the world. He/she is free from the clutches of *maya* or illusion.

(9) A balanced development of the four sides of personality—physical, mental, emotional and spiritual—leads to a swift awakening of the Kundalini, with a minimum of problem and side-effects. From the beginning, this chapter has proposed a balanced development based on simultaneous applications of Hathayoga (asanas or postures for 45 minutes), Bhaktiyoga or devotional practices (prayer to God and chanting of mantras), Jnanayoga or practices for knowledge (reading scriptures and case histories of evolved persons, and constantly posing the question to oneself—who am I, where did I come from and where would I go?) and meditation or spiritual practices (connecting Soul to Supersoul through spiritual practices or *sadhana* leading to samadhi). Regulated family life works as the catalytic agent and it becomes the most important factor at this stage. Yogic postures provide sexual strength and retention of vital fluids so that lovemaking can go on for a long time. And after the successful awakening of Kundalini one temporarily becomes a natural celibate. When the masculine and feminine aspects or the intellectual and sentimental in a practitioner achieve a balance, an inner marriage takes place. This results in the

birth of a spiritual or psychic child (Lord Krishna in child form) that the practitioner sees clearly in visions, trances and dreams. The birth of such a child indicates the completion of the process of "individuation" in the practitioner, as observed by Carl Jung, perhaps the greatest philosopher of the west. Chinese call it the "holy child" as mentioned in their *Book of the Golden Flower*. After this stage one enjoys mental orgasm without sex play or ejaculation. These mental orgasms are the basis of unparalleled bliss, as seen on the faces of saints.

Appearance of God Almighty as the "spiritual child" is the confirmation of the fact that *jiva* or individual soul has become one with the Supersoul or Paramatma or Brahman and that he has broken the chain of repeated incarnations on earth. After physical death "spiritualized *jiva*" will transcend to *spiritual sky*, which is beyond the *material sky*. Three-fourth of the Cosmos is *spiritual sky* and one-fourth of it is *material sky* that contains innumerable solar systems and stars like ours, the highest of it being *Brahmaloka* or the planet of Brahma or Jehova, who is the third order potency after Lord Supreme (first order potency) and Supersoul (second order potency). There are innumerable spiritual planets called *vaikunthalokas* in the *spiritual sky*, one of which could be the abode of the spiritualized *jiva*, with no more births and permanent knowledge and bliss. All these points are elaborated in various sections of Chapter 3.

(10) On awakening the higher centres, from the fifth onwards, one sees blue, indigo and violet colors on the inner mental screen, the signs of spiritual maturity. The sixth or the eyebrow centre is most crucial; its opening is recognized with the appearance of golden to copper colors the size of a large pea on the inner screen. The sixth centre is where the practitioner's ego is shattered into a thousand pieces to qualify for achieving libera-

tion. The practitioner witnesses one's ego's death as a physical death in one's consciousness, vision or dreams. One may see one's dead body being carried, sometimes a person may be killed and sometimes one may see a dead body lying somewhere. Sometimes the face of the dead person may resemble that of the practitioner, but it is not necessary. Sometimes an inner voice says the practitioner is dead, stating his/her name clearly. Dr. Elizabeth Kobler Ross experienced death as a result of going through the pain of her suffering patients, one by one. She asked for help and a shoulder to cry on, but the answer came, "you will not get it." However, the experience of death passes soon and then there is a resurrection in the chosen land or heaven, with love, peace and tranquillity.

(11) Sensitivity of the practitioner is gradually increased with spiritual advancement. One begins to feel both good and bad things more intensely, although it is a different thing that nothing affects the person after a certain stage is reached. Physically I had to keep myself covered with nearly skintight undergarments to remain unaffected with the changes in cold or warm environment. Emotionally I was too sensitive to the hurt caused to others and would not rest until the hurt was compensated in some way. Mentally I would receive fine intuitive and other ideas from time to time. One learns to forgive others who hurt him/her and also to forgive him/herself, knowing that there is no single cause for an event to take place, it is the whole machinery which forces an event to take place. One learns to "let go" everything—every possession and every relation—becoming vulnerable and opening the way for God to come in. Appearance of the Guru or High Self in dreams and visions is a common feature for the guidance of the practitioner.

(12) My dreams have a special significance in my unfolding spirituality. The most important of my dreams are actual visits to spiritual planets that I have described as out-of-body experiences. I find such a planet self-illuminated, full of greeneries, fruit trees, flowers and lakes or canals. Beings of the planet possess light bodies. The moment one enters such a planet one's heart is full of inner happiness and bliss. In my opinion this should be the abode of liberated ones from the cycle of death and rebirth. However, one may have the choice to either inhabit a spiritual planet or to merge with the Great Void. There may be other choices too.

(13) Flying dreams are commonly accompanied with the process, and in most cases they are real Soul travel experiences to higher realms. This happens especially at the opening of the third or naval chakra. Nature provides first hand knowledge of these realms for which the practitioner has now qualified. Both Jesus and Mohammed and Yogis like Yogananda have talked about the mansions their father is having or the planes up there. There are colonies to be visited, people to be talked and landscapes to be seen. During and after such experiences one is invariably happy and peaceful. In more advanced stages the practitioners visit the spiritual planets and temples, churches or mosques where their karma is burnt and purification is carried out. Being with the people of light or in bodiless forms, are also experienced at times. Witnessing oneself as Atman or Soul, without a physical body, is the first hand proof of one's eternal existence. At times there are visits to the "spiritual planets" that are self-illuminated, having unusual beautiful surroundings, as one of the possible places of one's future life. At times one visits a planet where flying is a normal mode of living. Like that there are visits to planets with unusual conditions from the earth's point of view, but they are real.

(14) Dreams have another significance in the process of individuation. There are four stages of development, according to four forms of the cosmic energy: ignorance, sex, love and spiritual experience. In the first stage a man dreams of a savage woman; in the second stage one dreams of an enchanting woman, such as Cleopatra; in the third stage one dreams of a loving woman, such as Mother Mary and the child sucking milk; and in the fourth stage one dreams of a goddess like woman, such as Durga-the Indian Goddess or Sophia – the Greek Goddess of wisdom or Athena or Mona Lisa – the sinless beauty. These dreams tell a man's stage of spiritual development. I am saying this with my own experiences. A woman would similarly see a savage man, such as Tarzan; a romantic male, such as the poet Shelly; a loving man, such as a war hero or a social reformer; and an exalted man, such as Mahatma Gandhi or Jesus Christ, during the four stages of her development.

(15) Having completed most of the requirements the practitioner must give up all sources of dependence and become vulnerable, which opens the door within us for the entry of God. And then faith, surrender and sincere prayer for help bring the personal experiences with God in different forms. As a passing show one experiences the possession of paranormal powers in one's consciousness or dreams. These powers are natural means of existence on higher realms and the practitioner gets a glimpse of them as part of one's education. Taking interest in paranormal powers or *siddhis* is forbidden, since this can lead to falling down from spiritual goal, and then liberation would be never achieved. In fact, paranormal powers are manifested only if Kundalini gets stuck in one of the chakras, otherwise it is only a passing show. In final stages one experiences one's connection with the Infinite Void, which in fact

is the source of all creation. However, this experience is for very short periods of time. Buddha talked about the Void in a big way.

(16) Light and Sound are the twin pillars in the form of which the Ultimate Reality is found to express Itself. Nevertheless, at times one sees God in one's cherished form since the beginning, such as, Mother Goddess, Krishna, Jesus or Buddha. The objective light (*brahmajyoti*) is very shining but cool and peace giving, and it is supposed to be the manifestation of the unmanifestable, for the benefit of the practitioner. There are various forms in which Light can materialize. Similarly the Word or Logos or AUM appears internally and is heard by the practitioner through one's inner or spiritual ears. Sound too has many different forms. Appearance of light and sound indicate the high stage the practitioner has reached in one's spiritual journey. At times the Soul appears as a shining blue pearl or star, which is the sign of completion of the spiritual practices and achieving liberation.

(17) Spiritual development seems to be a "right brain" activity; I began to lose calculative and intellectual interests and began to develop intuitive interests. This further manifested in me as a stronger left side of my body.

(18) Looking at the classical methods, they are sure but slow, taking whole lifetime or even more than a lifetime, depending on the preparation of the practitioner. However, a hitherto hidden and fast method, passed only from mouth to mouth from Guru to disciple, is the method of Shaktipat, in which, Shakti passes from Guru to disciple, which awakens the dormant "spiritual energy Kundalini" of the disciple in a short time that results in Self-Realization in a much shorter period. I can say that with my own experience and experiences of those who have gone through it. The method is briefly described in the last chapter.

CHAPTER 2

WE ARE ALL GODS IN THE MAKING

Introduction

Yajur Veda says, "Aham Brahmasmi," meaning, "I am Brahma." Sama Veda says, "Tatvamasi," meaning, "That thou art." Atharva Veda says, "Ayam Atma Brahma," meaning "This Atma is Brahma." Rig-Veda says, "Pragyanama Brahma," meaning "Awakened Atma is Brahma." Sufi Muslim saint Mansoor after knowing the Truth said, "Anal Hak," meaning, "I am Allah." Jesus Christ under similar situation said, "I and my Father are one." Thus whether one is a Hindu, a Muslim or a Christian, realization of the Self means one and the same thing to all, that is, "he and God are identical." This statement needs a thorough understanding.

Chhandogya Upanishad states in the beginning there were two birds sitting on a tree. One bird was fully happy and satisfied with the tree on which she lived and enjoyed eating its fruits filling the appetite. The other bird looked around and on seeing the second tree flew to it and began to enjoy its fruits. After some time she noticed another tree around and was attracted by its beauty. She then flew to the third tree and ate fruits and lived there for a while. Then she jumped to the fourth tree, the fifth tree, and the sixth tree and in course of time it crossed over to thousands and uncountable number of trees. One day she stopped finding any interest in the new trees and its fruits and a sort of dissatisfaction began to grow in her. She began to think that the original tree was more satisfactory in every way. She began to long for the original tree and started to search for it. She tried all methods but failed and began to feel homesick. She looked forward to meeting some one who could show her the way back home. The first bird is God and each one of us, who are searching their original spiritual home, represents the second bird. Consciously or unconsciously we are all feeling homesick as the materialism and relations of the physical world do not provide real satisfaction. We have forgotten who we are and where we came from?

Shwetketu was the son of a well-known rishi. At the young age of 22 he finished studying most of the scriptures and returned home with a pride of it. His father was not happy to see this since humility is one of the basic virtues of the *jnanis* (knowledgeable persons). He asked Shwetketu if he has known that after which there is nothing left to be known. Now the young man was puzzled and looked at his father for the answer. Then the father told him that just as the goldsmith knows that every ornament is made of only one thing called gold, although the ornaments appear to be different; and just as the potmaker knows that every pot is made of the same mud, although the pots appear to be different; in the same way the jnani comes to know that all living beings are made of the same material called atmatattva (soul-matter). And God too is made of the same soul-matter. Knowing this the spiritual seeker becomes humble and peaceful and not arrogant.

Shankaracharya later wrote the famous book, *Vivekchudamani*, meaning the "crown jewel of wisdom" in which he has talked about the various aspects of Atman or Soul. Self-realization is the knowing of the Truth that this body changes in every incarnation but the Atman or Soul around which the body is made every time is permanent. This knowledge removes the fear of death once for all and the individual lives a full life for the first time. Cheerfulness, contentment and peace are the natural properties of Atman as well as God, and that is why the two are one. Permanence-knowledge-bliss is the natural property of Atman-God, and it is in this that the two are one, and it is with the acquirement of this knowledge that one exclaims *Aham-Brahmasmi, Anal-hak* or *I and my father are one.* Realization of the fact that the individual is not the body and mind that are perishable, but the Atman or Soul that is eternal, full of knowledge, is blissful and makes one exclaim that he or she is "one with god."

However, this is the beginning of "liberation" and not the end.

Thus we are all gods in the making. Godhood is a property which when attained by an individual makes him exclaim that he is one with God. Again we have to understand what we mean by the term God and what we understand by being one with Him. In *The Secret Doctrine* Madam H. P. Blavatsky says, "...the teachings belong neither to the Hindu, the Zoroastrian, the Chaldean, nor the Egyptian religion, neither to Buddhism, Islam, Judaism nor Christianity exclusively. *The Secret Doctrine* is the essence of all these."[1] *Book of Dzyan*, a collection of palm leaves made impermeable to water, fire, and air, by some specific unknown process, forms the basis of her work. According to her it is the first major work in several thousand years, which attempts to give the accumulated wisdom of the Ages. Her attempt has been to save archaic truths that are the basis of all religions; and to uncover, to some extent, the fundamental unity from which they all spring; and that the science of modern civilization has never approached the occult side of nature. The theory applies to the cosmology of our own planetary system and what is visible around it, after a Solar Pralaya (dissolution). Teachings pertaining to the Universal Cosmos cannot be given, since they could not be understood by the highest minds in this age, and there seem to be very few Initiates, even among the greatest, who are allowed to speculate upon this subject. Not even the highest Dhyani-Chohans have ever penetrated the mysteries beyond those boundaries that separate the milliards of Solar systems from the "Central Sun," as it is called. Therefore, that which is given relates only to our visible Cosmos after a "Night of Brahmaa."[2]

The Spiritual Hierarchy

The findings of various faiths and traditions from East to West and from time immemorial, can be summarized in the following:

1. There exists an Omnipresent, Eternal, Boundless, and Immutable PRINCIPLE, Parabrahman or Brahman, Rootless Root of All, Root meaning pure knowledge (*sattva*), eternal (*Nitya*) unconditioned reality or SAT (*Satya*); THAT—Absolute Being and a Non-being at the same time; some have called It—One Reality, Creator or the Absolute, on which all speculation is impossible, since it transcends the power of human conception. According to Mandukya Upanishad it is unthinkable and unspeakable. Buddhists, Socrates and some others however, have maintained that there is no Creator but infinitude of *creative powers*, which collectively form the external substance, the *essence* of which is inscrutable – hence not a subject for speculation for any true philosopher. It is sexless, unconditioned and eternal, and has two aspects: Parabrahman and Mulaprakriti.

2. Adi-Shakti—the direct emanation of Mulaprakriti, the eternal Root of THAT, is the female aspect of the creative Brahmaa, a Maya and the cause of human Maya. As Mulaprakriti it is undifferentiated and eternal, while as manifested (vyakta), it becomes differentiated and conditioned. Objectively, Parabrahman appears as Mulaprakriti, as if the latter is a veil thrown over the former. Pre-cosmic root-substance Mulaprakriti is that aspect of the Absolute that underlies all the objective planes of Nature.

3. The first manifestation of Brahman is Brahma (neuter), the impersonal unmanifested Logos, the precursor of the manifested, the "first cause", and the "Unconscious" of the European Pantheists. It is One, androgynous and phenomenally finite. He is Kalahamsa, the Eternal Swan, also referred as Hamsa-vaahana, meaning the one who uses swan as his vehicle. According to Hindus, Brahma is in every atom of the Universe.

4. Second (or manifested) Logo or Word is Brahmaa—the Creator, who expands himself later into gods and the entire visible Universe; Spirit-matter, Life, "Spirit of the Universe" separating himself into male and female, the Purusha and Prakriti, comparable to the esotericism of chapters ii, iii, and v of Genesis. The occultists call it male-female Jehovah, Yaah-Havaah. In its totality, Brahmaa includes Prakriti, both evolved and unevolved (Mulaprakriti), Spirit and time. Father-Mother are the male and female principles in root-nature, the opposite poles that manifest in all things on every plane of Cosmos, the resultant of which is the Universe, or the Son. Esoterically, Brahmaa is Father-Mother-Son, or Spirit-Soul and Body at once; each personage being symbolical of an attribute, and each attribute being a graduated efflux of Divine Breath in its cyclic differentiation, involutionary and evolutionary.

5. There is something, called "Fohat" by occultists, which translates "Divine Thought" into "Laws of Nature". Cosmic Ideation, Mahaa-Buddhi, Mahat or Intelligence brings forth "Manifested Universe," which is pervaded by duality as the very essence of its existence as manifestation. Opposite poles, such as, subject and object, spirit and matter, male and female, are therefore two aspects of One Unity in which they are synthesized, and they should not be regarded as independent realities. The One Reality thus exists in its "dual aspects" in the conditioned Universe.

6. The expansion and contraction of the Divine *essence* results in the formation and dissolution of the universe continually, which is also known as "breathing out" or exhalation and "breathing in" or inhalation of the Divine essence by Secret Books, or day and night of Brahmaa by Hindus. Fohat (the mysterious link between Mind and Matter) runs the Manus' (or Dhyani-Chochans) errands, and causes the ideal prototypes to expand from within—viz, to cross gradually, on a descending scale, all the planes from the noumenon to the lowest phenomenon, to bloom finally on the last into full objectivity—the acme of illusion, or the grossest matter[3]. The appearance and disappearance of the worlds, and an alteration like day and night, sleeping and waking, life and death, flux and reflux, ebb and flow, are according to the universal law of periodicity.

7. The Trinity: Before any Cosmic activity, Space is known as Mother. After Pralaya (dissolution), whether the great or minor Pralaya, the first that reawakens to active life is the plastic Akash, called Father-Mother, the Spirit and Soul of Ether. In Kabala it is known as Father-Mother-Son. In the Eastern philosophy it is called Atma-Buddhi-Manas, meaning Spirit, Soul, Intelligence. The three hypostates of the manifesting Spirit of the Supreme Spirit are called *Hiranyagarbha, Hari,* and *Sankara*; or Brahmaa, Vishnu, and Rudra or Mahesh; these are three purely metaphysical abstract qualities or divine avasthas (states) of formation, preservation, and destruction. It is here that Vishnu is greeted as first Avatar. It is here that the Christianity differs from Eastern thought. Whereas in East the Spirit (Brahmaa) of the Supreme Spirit (Brahman) separates into Trinity, orthodox Christian separates the personal creative Deity into the three personages of the Trinity, and he does not admit any higher Deity. In Eastern philosophy the creative god or the aggregate gods are said to be false or erroneous appearances of material form.

8. A perfect circle with the point (root) in the centre represents reawakening of the Cosmos, in the sacred symbolism. Christian mystics used the sign—cross inside the circle, meaning the Union of the Rose and Cross—to represent the great mystery of occult generation, which gave rise to the name: Rosi-crucians, that is, the rose and the cross! The real creed of the Brothers of the Rosie-Cross is the symbol with the "Pelican tearing open its breast to feed its seven little ones," which is a direct outcome from the Eastern Secret Doctrine. The seven stanzas in the *Book of Dzyan* refer to and describe the seven stages of the evolutionary process, talked about in the *Puranas* as the "Seven Creations" and in the Bible as the "Seven Days of Creation."

9. The only immortal and eternal principle in us is the Monad (Jiva), embedded with the opposites like spirit and matter in one, which is an indivisible and integral part of the Absolute, from which it emanates and into which it is absorbed at the end of the cycle. This Monad or Soul is on a seemingly eternal pilgrimage through the "cycle of incarnations," according to the Cyclic and Karmic law. There is the "fundamental identity" of all Souls with the Universal Over-Soul, which itself has an Unknown Origin. The Soul, being the spark of the Divine, has passed through all elemental forms of the phenomenal world of the period and acquired "individuality" through natural impulse and graduating from lowest mineral and plant to highest intelligence of the holiest archangel, under the influence of Karma.

10. Desire to exist in everything, from an atom to a sun, is a reflection of the Divine Thought propelled into objective existence, the real cause of which remains forever hidden; its first emanations are the abstractions that bring the existence of the material Universe which presents itself to the senses and intellect; and they underlie the secondary and subordinate powers of Nature,

which, anthropomorphized, have been worshipped as God by the common herd of every age.

11. Absolute and Life pulsated in Universe is sensed by "Opened Eye of Dangma", known as "The Eye of Siva" in India, or simply the "third eye." Dangma means a purified soul, one who has become the Jivanmukta (liberated while living), the highest adept or Mahatma. It is the inner spiritual eye, the faculty of spiritual intuition, through which the seer obtains direct and certain knowledge. The faculty manifested is not clairvoyance as ordinarily understood, that is, the power of seeing at a distance.

12. Although various schools of thoughts differ, and science has never been able to talk about it, Alaya is the "Soul of the World" or "Anima Mundi" or Emerson's "Over-Soul," according to esoteric teachings. It is known as Pradhan in *Vishnu Purana*. According to Yogacharas of Mahyana school Alaya is the personification of the Voidness and also the basis of every visible and invisible thing, and it reflects itself in every object of the Universe, like the moon in still water. Alaya is eternal and changeless on higher planes that are unreachable by either men or Cosmic Gods. However, it alters during the active life period with respect to lower planes, including our own. At such times both the Cosmic Gods and man with strong yoga or mystic meditation "are able to merge their soul with it," which is Nirvana according to some schools and "only next to Nirvana" according to other schools. Thus Alaya is both the Universal Soul and the Self of the progressed adept. One who is strong in the Yoga can introduce at will his Alaya through meditation into the true Nature of Existence.

13. Whereas Anaxagoras of Clazomenae, like Plato, had been researching on the principle that is absolutely separated and free from matter, the notion of *Jivatman* called

Motion, the One Life, already existed ages before the year 500 B.C. in India[4]. Furthermore, various speculations made by Hegel, German transcendentalists, Schelling and Fichte, Von Hartmann, and European speculations to Hindu Advaitin Doctorines, fall short of the reality. According to Vedantins, Spirit and Matter, or Purusha and Prakriti are but the two primeval aspects of the One and Secondless. The matter-moving Nous, the animating Soul, immanent in every atom, manifested in man, latent in the stone, has different degrees of power. This pantheistic idea of a general Spirit-Soul pervading all Nature is oldest of all, existing much before the speculations of Paracelsus or his pupil Van Helmont. Spirit, Soul and Matter: Soul is the vehicle for the manifestation of Spirit on a higher plane, and Matter is the vehicle for the manifestation of the Soul on this plane. A Mahatma in whom the unity of God and man has taken place, that is, the identity of the individual with the universal consciousness has taken place, attains the truth. Such a person exclaims, "Aham Brahmasmi" or "Anal-Haque" or "I and my Father are one." This feat has to be accomplished by every man himself.

14. Androgen is an important property that means being sexless in esoteric state and a balanced male-female in exoteric state.

SPACE, called VOID by the modern thinkers, is well defined by the ancients as "the *unknown container of all, the Unknown First Cause.*" Hindus call it Brahman, the ever unknowable, causeless cause of everything, being *first-rate* potency. It is limitless and its PRINCIPLES are "septenary," which manifest only grossest fabrics of *their subdivisions* in our phenomenal world. All the fundamental truths of nature were universal in antiquity. Taking the two most ancient religious philosophies on the globe, Hinduism and Hermetism, from the scriptures of India and Egypt, the identity of the two is easily recognizable[5]. Even the latest of them—the Jews—show in their Kabalistic teachings this idea, e.g., the seven-headed Serpent of Space, called "the great Sea."[6] A ray emanates from SPACE as "unmanifested Logos," called Brahma, which is the *second rate* potency. Sprung from darkness (Space) Brahmaa, the vehicle of Brahma, and the creator of universe and everything in it. He is, therefore, the *third rate* potency. Gnostics called the *first, second* and *third rate* potencies as Ain-Soph, Aion and Bythos. In the Bible it is first *Alhim,* then *Yahva-Alhim,* and finally Jehovah—after the separation of the sexes in chapter iv of Genesis. The very few learned Fathers of the Church, who were aware that Jehovah was a third rate potency and no "highest" God, knew this.[7]

In Egyptian mythology, the Eternal unrevealed Deity is called "Kneph", the first-order potency, which is shown as a snake-emblem of Eternity encircling a water-urn, with his head hovering over the waters, which is incubated with his breath. The Older and Younger Horus represent the second and third order potencies, respectively. Former is the *brother* of Osiris, and latter is the *son* of Osiris. The first Horus represents the "idea of the world" concealed and then born in darkness, while the second one represents the idea being carried by Logos and then clothed with matter, and assuming an actual existence.[8]

The limitless, unknowable and indivisible Absolute Point (Parabrahman) spreads itself over the endless space, and in this way forms a veil (Mulaprakriti), which conceals this Absolute Point. The trinity of Fire, Air and Water, and all the Forces of Nature collectively form the "Word," or Logos, which is the Voice of the Will of the Absolute Silent All. In the cosmogonies of all the nations, the creator "architects" fashion Cosmos out of Chaos, who are the collective *Theos,* male-female; Spirit and Matter. According to Genesis (ii, 4), "By a series (*yom*) of foundations (*yesodoth*) the Alhim caused earth and heaven to be." Also from Genesis (iv), first in Bible is *Alhim,* then it is *Yahva-Alhim,* and finally it is Jehovah, after the separation of the sexes. It is the symbol of the Unknown Deity, used in connection with the Creation of the Universe. These architects or movers or runners came to be known as messengers or *malaakhim* in Christianity. According to *Rig-Veda*, in Hinduism it is the Prajapatis or Rishis-The Lords of Being, who are the movers connected with terrestrial creation, and not Brahmaa. Brahmaa has thus three forms: as Prajapati, he is the creator; as Vishnu, he is the sustainer; and as Siva or Rudra, he is the destroyer. All these personified powers are not evolutions from one another, but so many aspects of the one and sole manifestation of the Absolute All.[9]

A word about Genesis would be quite appropriate here. It is suspected that its writings are not independent and original. "For who, after studying dispassionately the respective legends of Abram or Abraham, Sarai or Sarah, who was 'fair to look upon,' and those of Brahmaa and Saraswati, or Sri, Lakshmi-Venus, with the relations of all these to the moon and water; and specially one who understands the real Kabalistic meaning of the name Jehovah and its relation to, and connection with the moon—who can doubt that the story of Abram is based upon that of Brahmaa, or that genesis was written upon the old lines used by every ancient nation?"[10]

We endeavour yet to understand the three-tier system or the difference between the Deity, the Highest God, and the God or gods. The Deity, Parabrahman, is not God; it is Nothing, incomprehensible, nameless, and Darkness; the Ain-Soph of Gnostics, and Alhim of Bible. It is the "first-order potency" from which everything comes. A ray emanates from it as the unmanifested Logos, the Word, who is the Son of the Deity, the Brahma of Hindus, Aion of Gnostics, and Yahva-Alhim of Bible. It is the "Highest God," the Macroprosopus, the "second-order potency." In the Chaldean Kabala it is represented by Word or Hebrew "Dabaar," which becomes a plural number, or "Words"—"Debaarim," as it divides into Hosts of Angels or Sephiroths, but is still collectively ONE. It is without form or being, "with no likeness with anything else[11]." Alike in Hindu Puranas and Jews Kabala, the

Incomprehensible drops a seed, which becomes the golden egg, from which Brahmaa is produced, which is the second or manifested Logos, the Bythos of Gnostics and Jehovah of Bible. It is the "third-order potency," commonly called God, the Creator. In fact, it is next to God (the original unmanifested Logos)—the "Second God", the wisdom of the "Highest God." The triad in the Egyptian system is Kneph, older Horus—the brother of Osiris, and younger Horus—the Son of Osiris. The idea of the world brought forward by first Horus is given practical shape by second Horus.

With the notion of architect of the world, the word God came into being. Singular word God, embracing all the gods, represents the Creator of physical "Humanity," on the *terrestrial* plane; but surely it had nothing to do with the formation or "Creation" of Spirit, gods or Cosmos. Its source is phallic, as the sincere, open-spoken *linga* of India. The word God has come to the Latin races from Aryan *Dyaus* (the Day), to the Slovenian, from the Greek Bacchus (*Bagh-bog*); and to the Saxon races from Hebrew *Yodh* or *Jod*. The number 10 represents male and female, and Jod is the *phallic* hook. This explains the Saxon *Godh*, the Germanic *Gott*, and the English *God*.[12]

Thus God in every religion is the Logos or Creative Deity, the "Word made Flesh," who is the third-order potency called Brahmaa (or Prajapatis) in Hinduism, Jehovah in Judaism, and Bythos (the second Logos) in Gnosticism. Becoming a plural number, gods imply the directing active "Intelligences."

The Aryan, Hermetic, Orphic and Pythagorean cosmogonical doctrines, as well as those of Sanchoniathon and Berusus, are all based upon one irrefutable formula, viz., that the Aether (Akash) and Chaos (Space), or, in the Platonic language, mind and matter, were the two primeval and eternal principles of the universe, utterly independent of each other. The former was the all-vivifying intellectual principle; the chaos, a shapeless, liquid principle, without "form or sense," from the union of which two sprang into existence the universe, or rather the universal world, the first androgynous deity—the chaotic matter becoming its body, and aether the soul. According to the phraseology of a *Fragment* by Hermeias "chaos, from this union with spirit, obtaining *sense*, shone with pleasure, and thus was produced the *protogonos* (the first born) light." This is the universal trinity, based on the metaphysical conceptions of the ancients who, reasoning by analogy, made of man, who is a compound of intellect and matter, the microcosm of the macrocosm, or great universe.[13]

Plato and the Pythagoreans surmised that Chaos became the "Soul of the World." Hinduism teaches that the Deity in the form of *Aether* (Akash) pervades everything, and therefore it is called "the living fire" or "Spirit of Light." According to Plato it is the Highest Deity who built the universe. These ideas have given birth to the greatest picture allegory in which Vishnu is sleeping on Ananta-Sesha, the great Serpent of Eternity. Furthermore, a lotus is growing through the naval of Vishnu and Brahmaa is sitting in the lotus. A person does not rightly understand the picture, since there is no ancient to tell them the underlying idea behind it, so much so that the Western theology has made it the Devil. It represents the fact that Vishnu is the first-born Son of the unknowable Deity, and Brahmaa came into being later, as the architect of the universe. The idea is identical with Egyptian cosmogony, where "primeval element" covering the infinite abyss, animated by water and spirit of the Eternal, dwells alone in Chaos; and with Jewish Scriptures, where the history of creation opens with the spirit of God, wherefrom emanates another creative Deity.

Parabrahman being veiled by its extension Mulaprakriti; the former being ever unknowable, the latter manifesting for knowledge of seekers as Mother or a female figure. Gnostic system being mutilated and distorted by the Church Fathers, the second century chief of Marcosians—Marcus was the only Gnostic who gave out actual esoteric truth. In his own words, "Supreme Tetrad (name of Deity in four syllables made of 30 letters) came down unto me (him) from the region which cannot be seen nor named, in a female form, because the world would have been unable to bear her appearing under a male figure," and revealed to him "the generation of the universe, untold before to either gods or men[14]." The *Tetrad* shows to Marcus the Truth in the form of a naked woman, and letters every limb of that figure, calling her head A, her neck B, shoulders and hands C, D, etc. In this, Sephirah is easily recognized, the Crown (*Kether*) or head being numbered *one*, the brain or Hokhmah, *two*; the heart or intelligence (Binah), *three*; and the other seven Sephiroth representing the limbs of the body. The Sephirothal Tree is the Universe, and Adam-Kadamon represents it in the West as Brahmaa represents it in India.[15]

World not ready to receive and bear direct revelation, Marcus describes the revelation allegorically as follows: "When first the inconceivable, the Beingless and sexless (the Kabalistic Ain-Soph) began to be in labour (i.e., when the hour of manifesting itself had struck) and desired that Its Ineffable should be born (the first Logos, or Aeon, or Aion), and its invisible should be clothed with form, its mouth opened and uttered the world like unto itself. This word (logos) manifested itself in the form of the Invisible One. The uttering of the (ineffable) name (through the word) came to pass in this manner. He (the Supreme Logos) uttered the first word of his name, which is a *syllable of four letters*. Then the second syllable was added, also of *four letters*. Then the third, composed of *ten* letters; and after this the fourth, which contains *twelve* letters. The whole name consists thus of *thirty letters* and of *four syllables*. Each letter has its own accent and way of writing, but neither understands nor even beholds that form of the whole Name—no; not even the power of the letter that stands next to Itself (to the Beingless and Inconceivable) ... All these sounds when united are the collective Beingless, unbegotten Aeon, and these are the Angels that are ever beholding the face of the

Father (the Logos, the "second God, who stands next to God, "the Inconceivable," according to Philo.[16]

Isvara, or the Logos, cannot see Parabrahman, but only Mulaprakriti, says the lecturer in the *Four Lectures on the Bhagavad Gita*.[17]

Rig Veda says, "THAT, the one Lord of all beings....the one animating principle of gods and man," arose, in the beginning, in the Golden Womb, Hiranyagarbha—which is the Mundane Egg or "Effulgent Womb" or sphere of our Universe. According to *Manu*, Hiranyagarbha is Brahmaa, *the first male* (to be understood esoterically), formed by the indiscernible Causeless Cause in a "Golden Egg resplendent as the Sun." Brahmaa is surely androgynous, and allegorically separates into two halves—the male Viraaj (himself) and the female Vaach. Everything eventually emanated from the Divine Man: The Arupa (formless), the Rupa (with bodies), the Sparks, the sacred Animals, and the messengers of the sacred Fathers (the Pitris); within the Holy Four. The 4—represented in the Occult numerals by the Tetraktys, the sacred or perfect square is a sacred number with the mystics of every nation. It has one and the same significance in Brahmanism, Buddhism, the Kabala, and in the Egyptian, Chaldean and the other numerical systems.[18]

Numbers 3, 7 and 1065 are sacred and quite significant with regard to the phenomenal world, found common to different religions as common myth. Number 3 signifies the *triune*—primeval Vedic Trimurti—Agni (fire), Vayu (air) and Surya (sun). From this *triune* (Hiranyagarbha—Brahmaa) emanate "the seven Lords of Being—Prajapatis, lying concealed in Sarvatman (Supersoul) like thoughts in one brain." Sephiroths of Kabala are also seven in number. "The One from the Egg, the Six and the Five," give the number 1065, the value of the first born (later on the male and female Brahmaa-Prajapati), who answers to the numbers 7, 14, and 21 respectively. Total emanations from the Deity are 3+7=10, both in Veda and Kabala. In the *Mahabharata* the Prajapatis are 21 in number, or ten, six and five (1065), thrice seven. In

We Are All Gods in the Making

the Kabala the same numbers are a value of Jehovah, viz., 1065, since the numerals of the three letters which compose the name—Yod, Vau and twice He—are respectively 10, 6 and 5; or again thrice seven. Ten is the Mother of the Soul, for Life and Light are therein united," says Hermes. For number one is born of the Spirit and the number ten from matter (chaos, feminine); the unity has made the ten, the ten the unity (*Book of the Keys*). By means of the Temurah, the anagrammatical method of the Kabala, and the knowledge of 1065 (number: 21), a universal science may be obtained regarding Kosmos and its mysteries (Rabbi Yogel). The Rabbis regard the numbers 10, 6 and 5 as the most sacred of all.[19]

And now a very important number 31415—The Three, the One, the Four, the One, the Five—(in their totality—twice seven) representing numerically Dhyani Chohans of various orders, of the inner or circumscribed world. An American Kabalist has discovered the same number for Elohim. It came to the Jews from Chaldaea[20]. These Dhyani Chohans guard the boundary of the great circle of "Pass Not," called Dhyanipasa or the "rope of Angels,"[21] which separates the phenomenal from the noumenal Kosmos, so that it does not fall within the range of our present objective consciousness. 31415 is both the number of the circle and the mystic Swastika. Mathematically the ratio of the diameter to the circumference of a circle is 1 to 3.1415 or "pi."

Lipikas, the Recorders of the Karmic Ledger, make an impassable barrier between the personal Ego and impersonal Self, the Noumenon and Parent-Source of the former. Hence the allegory. They circumscribe the manifested world of matter within the Ring "Pass-Not."

Divine sons of immaculate mothers find a mention in most religions like common myth. "Being the husband of his mother" is one of the principal titles of the god. When the Son separates from the Mother he becomes the Father. Prajapati (Brahmaa) is known as first procreating male and "his Mother's husband." In Egypt too, Mut stands for Mother, and she was the mother and than the wife of Amen.

According to Roman Catholic Church, Anna conceived Mary without sin, and gave birth to her daughter in an immaculate way. Anna is derived from Chaldean Ana, meaning Astral light or Anima Mundi. Uma-Kanya (Virgin of light) is the name of goddess Durga, the wife of Siva, who is also known as Annapurna, the mother giving food to everyone. And again in *Mahabharata,* Karna—son of the Sun-God, was born to mother Kunti in an immaculate way.

Initiation and Nature of Gods

Confusion has been created about the attributes and genealogies of the "gods" in their theogonies, by the half-initiated Brahmanical and Biblical writers round the world. They are, nevertheless known to every *"twice-born"* (Dvija, or Initiated) Brahman, and the *Puranas* contain references to some of them in veiled terms, which no matter-of-fact Orientalist has yet endeavoured to make out, nor could he if he would![22]. It is very much in place now to talk about what we mean by initiation. Brahmans in ancient India were said to be initiated when they got their "dormant spiritual energy (Kundalini)" awakened and activated. An initiated person in Vedas is called "Dvija," meaning "born again" or "twice-born." The same terminology was used by Lord Jesus Christ when he said, "Only the 'twice-born' can enter the kingdom of God." Similar expressions can be found in other faiths and traditions. However, such an "initiated person" becomes one with his "creator god" or "Father." Remember Jesus saying, "I and my father are one." Only at this level a person can understand the Truth beyond. For others, however learned they may be, the spiritual facts may appear as unbelievable. It is for this reason that Mr. Sinnet said:

"For reasons which are not easy for the outsider to divine, the possessors of occult knowledge are specially reluctant to give out facts to Cosmogony, though it is hard for uninitiated to understand why they should be withheld."[23]

We Are All Gods in the Making

Why there is a vast difference between the understandings of initiated and uninitiated people can be understood through simple examples: 1. A man sitting in Baghdad or New Delhi under 45 degree temperature in summer and sweating heavily would find it unbelievable that the people in Scotland and Greenland are wearing warm suits; 2. A person sitting indoors cannot make out how pleasant it is to be in a cool breeze while it is raining outside, unless he himself stands outside. These are some crude examples. Let me give my own examples of beliefs and unbeliefs, before and after my initiation.

Since early childhood I was a religious person and until the age of 50 I had read *Bhagavad Gita*, *Mahabharata*, *Puranas*, *Kuran*, *Bible* and Egyptian's *Book of the Dead*. I used to believe theoretically in the words of Lord Krishna that each one of us is a dimensionless soul or Atman which cannot be cut by sword, cannot be wet in water, cannot be dried in air. I did not like to disbelieve Him yet I could not fully appreciate the idea of it. It was only after July 1987 when I got my Kundalini awakened that I witnessed myself as a "dimensionless being" in non-physical realms, passing very closely through a waterfall without getting wet and with the speed of thoughts. Only then I could really appreciate the words of Lord Krishna.

As an example of disbelief by non-initiates, I was in a party at a hill station where my son-in-law was an Air-Force officer. In an evening party the chief of station was telling the people that many spiritual practitioners will say that they are hearing a conch-like sound internally, and they will support it by many kinds of words, but it is ridiculous and unbelievable to us and we feel like laughing at that. Right at that time I was hearing the sound very loudly through my inner ears, which had awakened in me in 1987. He could laugh at me and I could laugh at him. It is this disbelief of things told by many saints for which they were killed, e.g., Jesus Christ by crucification, Buddha by being served poisonous mushrooms, Socrates by being made to drink poison, Dayanand Saraswati by being served milk with powdered glass mixed in it, Pythagoras assassinated by his disbelievers, and many more examples can be added to the list.

A large number of Brahmans in ancient India got initiated. They knew the Truth told to them directly by their "creator god" or Brahma or Prajapati. And it is through their writings that the Vedas, Puranas and other scriptures were created long time ago, which is unfathomable by either Orientalists or scientists. Talking about the mystery-language and its keys Blavatsky[24] says,

"It is maintained that INDIA (not in its present limits, but including its ancient boundaries) is the only country in the world which still has among her sons adepts, who have the knowledge of the seven *sub-systems* and the key to the entire system. Since the fall of Memphis, Egypt began to lose those keys one by one, and the Chaldea had preserved only three in the days of Berosus. As for the Hebrews, in all their writings they show no more than a thorough knowledge of the astronomical, geometrical and numerical systems of symbolizing all the human, and specially the physiological functions. They never had the higher keys."

All the fundamental truths of nature were universal in antiquity, and the basic ideas upon spirit, matter, and the universe, or upon God, substance, and man, were identical. Taking the two most ancient religious philosophies on the globe, Hinduism and Hermetism, from the scriptures on India and Egypt, the identity of the two is easily recognizable Gods have been the life and animating " soul-principle" of the various regions of the Universe. No one could range one's speculation *beyond* those *manifested* gods. The boundless and infinite UNITY has remained untrodden by man's thoughts, untouched by fruitless speculation, with every nation. However, there has been a brief conception of its diastolic and systolic property, of its periodical expansion or dilatation, and contraction; the appearance and disappearance of the worlds. The breath returning to the eternal bosom which exhales and inhales them—the anthropomorphized powers, or gods, their Souls, had to disappear from view with their bodies.

A breath of the infinite UNITY is the length of one creation, called Maha-Kalpa, which is the age of creator Brahmaa. The age of Brahmaa is 100 Years; each Year is made of 360 Days and an equal number of Nights. One Day of Brahmaa is equal to 4,320,000,000 mortal years. Thus the age of Brahmaa and hence that of one breath or a single creation is 311,040,000,000,000 mortal years. This is therefore the age or the life span of our *universe* or our *solar system* and hence of our *earth*[26].

In most of the faiths and traditions the spiritual hierarchy is divided in three orders of potencies. The first order potency is invariably the Unknowable Source of all, who creates around Him a cover of Female Energy, which is the second order potency; the first and second potencies then emanate a Ray from their union, which is the Creator of the Universe and its inhabitants; this Creator is the third order potency. Different religions have given different names to these three potencies as follows.

The Spiritual Hierarchy

S.No.	Religion	First Potency	Second Potency	Third Potency
1.	Vedic/Hindu	Parabrahman	Mulaprakriti Aditi / Vach Mothers of all	Brahma-Vishnu-Siva (Son of Purush and Prakriti) 7 Prajapatis Brahmaa (vehicle) Ishwara, Shabda
2.	Gnostics	Ain-soph	Aion	Bythos
3.	Egyptian	Kneph	Older Horus (an idea)	Younger Horus (practical shape)
4.	Chaldean	Ainsoph	Sephirah	Sephiroth Three Worlds of Emanations: Creation, Formation, Action-Earth or Our World
5.	Hebrew/Jews		Shekhinah	Adam-Kadmon Elohim, Jehovah (vehicle) Logos, Word
6.	Zohar	Hokhmah	Binah	Son

In every Cosmogony, behind and higher than the *creative* deity or god, is a superior deity, a planner, an Architect, of whom the Creator is but the executive agent. In the Vedas Brahmaa (androgynous) is the Creator, and he is the vehicle of Brahma (formless), who is the first-born, the first Ray emanating from Parabrahman and Mulaprakriti. Similarly, Jehovah the Creator is the vehicle and executor of Elohim, the planner. In fact, every entity has a dual existence, the grosser one being the carrier of the subtler one. And still higher, *over* and *around*, *within* and *without*, there is the UNKNOWABLE and the *unknown*, the Source and Cause of all these emanations…[27]

Thus Adam-Jehovah, Brahmaa and Mars are identical in the sense that they are the primitive or initial *generative powers* for the procreation of humans. Similarly, Syrian goddess Ashtart, Venus, Isis, Ishtar, Mylitta, Eve, Shekhinah and some others are identical with Aditi and Vach of the Hindus. All of them are the "Mothers of all living" and "of the gods." All the male gods are the "first born," first becoming the "Sun-gods" and then the "Suns of Righteousness," and the Logoi, all symbolized by the Sun. The gods themselves would not know the UNKNOWABLE; the maximum they could come to know was the Mulaprakriti, in one form or the other. This is the reason that, we always see Lord Siva sitting in meditation upon the ABSOLUTE, perhaps to know him, as closely as possible.

There is a notable difference between the *spirituality* of the two nations. Sephiroth (Elohim-Javeh, also) created Man, and they were the cause of the creation of the *earthly* Adam. Therefore in *Genesis* Elohim says, "Behold Man is become *as one of us*." This admits man's equality with the creator, and also the use of sex in the creation of man. However, in Hinduism, Brahmaa-Prajapati created Viraj and Rishis, spiritually, and hence they were called the "Mind-born Sons of Brahmaa." Therefore, *Phallicism,* at least in the earlier human nations, is out of question, in this mode

We Are All Gods in the Making

of mental production. Also, the creators were higher than the created men, the latter being called the sons of the former.

The gods created man on one hand, and maintained the "PASS NOT" ring on the other, so that the ordinary humans could not know and understand gods—their Fathers, unless they got the initiation and the ability to cross the "PASS NOT" ring. That is why Master Jesus, only on being initiated after long years of meditation, said, "I and my Father are one." However, there have been rishis and yogis who could go even beyond the gods. Buddha could be one such example who believed only in the "Light of the Void," which is higher than the creative gods or angels. The angels aspire to become men; a perfect man, a man god is above all the angels.[28]

Christ was one of the several world-reformers, a Saviour but for his direct followers, and only a great and glorious Initiate for the rest of all. Christian symbologists only tried to fit the birth time of Jesus of Nazareth with the great constellation—Sun entering the sign of the fish (*Pisces*)—to try to show that the elect Messiah had to be born. But if Jesus of Nazareth was that Messiah—was he really born at that "moment," or was he made to be so born by the adaption of theologians, who sought only to make their preconceived ideas fit in with sidereal *facts* and popular belief?[29] Everyone knows that the real time and year of the birth of Jesus are totally unknown. It should be noted that the forefathers of Jews have made the word *Dag* signify both "fish" and "messiah," who later denied this Christian claim. Long back, Brahmans connected their "messiah," the eternal Avatara Vishnu with a *fish* and the *great flood*. And lately the Babylonians equated their *Dag-on* with fish and messiah, the Man-Fish and Prophet!

The theologians have also meddled with the leading figures of the age of Brahmaa, that is, 4,320,000,000 mortal years, to suit their own preconceived ideas at various places.[30]

According to S. A. Mackey, the noted "philosopher, astronomer and shoemaker" of Norwich, "Christian theologians think it their duty to write against the long period of *Hindu Chronology*, and in them it may be pardonable; but when a man of learning crucifies the names and the numbers of the ancients; and wrings and twists them into a form which means something quite foreign to the intentions of the ancient authors; but, which, so mutilated, fits in with the *birth* of some *maggot* pre-existing in his own brain with so much exactness, that he *pretends* to be amazed at the discovery, I cannot think him so pardonable."[31]

CHAPTER 3

THE CREATION OF UNIVERSE AND MAN – COSMIC EVOLUTION

The Seven Races

Blavatsky postulated three new propositions regarding the evolution of mankind, which were in direct antagonism to modern science on one hand and to religious dogmas on the other; they were (i) the simultaneous evolution of seven human groups on seven different portions of our globe; (ii) the birth of the *astral,* before the *physical* body, the former being a model of the latter; and (iii) that man in this Round, preceded every mammalian—the anthropoids included in the animal kingdom.[1] She mentions that these proposals may antagonize and may not be acceptable to rigid believers of *Bible* and to the men of science, readily.

Hermes too in his *Divine Poimandres* points towards "Seven primeval men" evolving from Nature and "Heavenly Man"— Creative Spirits collectively. Babylonian legend of Creation inscribed on Chaldean tablets mentions seven human beings "with the faces of ravens" (black, swarthy complexion) created by the "Seven great gods." Kabala mentions the Seven Kings of Edom, who grew and increased in number, as members of the same family. Others who support this point are the Egyptian *Books of Thoth,* and *Book of the Dead,* and the Hindu *Puranas* with the seven

Manus. Also the tiles of Chandean-Assyrian accounts mention "seven primitive men," or Adams. Kabir (Adamas) born of the Holy Lemnos, the island sacred to *Vulcan,* was the archtype of the first males in the order of generation, and was one of the "seven autochthonous ancestors" or progenitors of mankind. Kabir's name is associated with the "Holy fires," which created on seven localities of the island of *Electris* or Samothrace.[2] Since *Genesis* was compiled by the Jews, who got their primitive knowledge of creation from Moses, who had it from the Egyptians, it would be sufficient to study the Babylonian and Assyrian cuneiform. First two chapters of *Genesis* are distinguished as Elohite and Jehovite creations, following the two Creations in the Babylonian fragments.

There have been four great Races preceding our Adamic race that were born, lived and died. They were named differently according to the varying language of the nation that mentioned them. For example, the land *Vendidad* or Airyana Vaejah, where original Zoroaster (Zarathushtra or Zartusht) was born, is known as *Sveta-Deep* or Mount Meru in Puranas, which is the abode of Vishnu; and, the Secret Doctrine has named it the "Land of the Gods" governed by the "Spirits of this Planet." Zarathushtra was the ruler of Varaa made by Yima in that land. There were thirteen Zarathushtras in succession, each being the reincarnation of the first one. The last of them founded the temple of Azareksh and wrote the primeval sacred Magina religion. In course of time Alexander destroyed all what Zoroaster had created.

In order to describe in brief the Races I to V, there have to be some names for them. We will use the names proposed by Blavatsky.[3]

I. The Imperishable Sacred Land – This "Sacred Land" is the only one whose destiny is to last from the beginning to the end of the Manvantara throughout each round. There are seven rounds in which the process of the universe is divided from its beginning to the end, spanned over several million years. The "first man" begins here and the last *divine* mortal, called *Sishta*, will dwell here, for the future seed of the humanity. Although very little can be said about it, a poetical description says that the "polestar has its watchful eye upon it, from the dawn to the close of the twilight of the 'Day of Brahmaa,' or 'a day of Great Breath'."

II. Hyperborean – The name for the Second Continent, stretching southward and westward from the North Pole for the second race to inhabit, known as Northern Asia now, was suggested by the oldest Greeks. It was a real continent where there was no winter in those days and no sorry remains for more than one night and day. According to Greeks the nocturnal shadows never fall upon it, as it is the *Land of Gods*, the abode of Apollo, where the Sun is never set for one half of the year. Its inhabitants were beloved priests and servants. It was a truth at that time although now it may be taken as a poetic fiction.

III. Lemuria – The gigantic third continent, so named by P.L. Sclater on zoological grounds between 1850 and 1860, extended from Madagascar to Ceylon and Sumatra, from Indian Ocean to Australia, including some portion of what is now Africa, has submerged in Pacific Ocean completely, leaving behind some islands which were then some of its highland tops; this included New Guinea, Solomon Islands and Fiji, according to A.R.Wallace, the naturalist. A difference of opinion exists between Sclater and Wallace; according to Sclater the third continent united Africa, Madagascar and India, but not Australia and India; while Wallace maintained that India and Australia did certainly exist, and at a time so very remote that it was certainly *pre-tertiary*, because Lemuria had vanished before the full development of Atlantis, and the latter sunk with its main portions disappearing before the Miocene period came to an end.

IV. Atlantis – The first three continents being prehistoric, this great fourth continent is the first historical land, whose "fragment" was the famous island of Plato, named Atlantis after its parent continent, which vanished some 850,000 years ago. Island of Plato, so named, was submerged in the waters of Atlantic Ocean between 10,000 and 12,000 years ago. The fleeing inhabitants settled in Central American countries, now known as Mexico, Guatemala and Honduras. I visited Guatemala in 2002 for this reason, so as to see the remnants of Atlanteans in person.

V. America – America together with Europe and Asia Minor, has been called the fifth continent by the Indo-Aryan Occultists. This is so, following the order of evolution of the Races. However, an alteration may be necessary if the geographical and geological order has to be followed. Face of the earth has changed many times since the destruction of the great Atlantis. For example, before the formation of the Straits of Gibralter, delta of Egypt and Northern Africa belonged to Europe. However, a further upheaval changed the face of the map of Europe entirely. According to *Zohar*, "These secrets (of land and sea) were divulged *to the men of the secret science,* but not to the geographers."

There are certain facts that may not be in agreement with Darwinian Anthropology and Biblical Theology. Ethereal prototypes of Atlanteans of the Primary age had nothing to fear from that which could hurt them. But the gigantic third-race titans of the Secondary age were fit to fight successfully the gigantic monsters of the air, sea and land. Occult sciences claim less and give more as compared to official science. For geological periods alone the learned men of the Royal Society have been differing with each other a lot. For example, according to Professor Winchell of Geology in America, 2,500,000 years must have elapsed before the Tertiary Age or Eocene period began. Whereas English Geologist Charles Gould talks about 15 million years since the beginning of Eocene period. Ages and periods in geology are not delineated but conventional, and no two geologists or naturalists are found to agree about the figures. As another example, authorities like Sir W. Thomson have changed about half-a-dozen times their opinion upon the age of the Sun and the date of the consolidation of Earth's crest. In Thomson and Tait's *Natural Philosophy,* only ten million years are allowed since the appearance of vegetable life. But Darwin estimated a minimum of 98 and a maximum of 200 million years since the consolidation of the crust. Some eminent men of Science therefore, corroborate figures given by Occult Science.

In any case, agreement or disagreement of the Naturalists about the geological periods is not so important as their agreement on the point that "during the Miocene age, the remnants of Second or Hyperborean Continent—Greenland and Spitzbergen—had almost a tropical climate." "During the Miocene age, Greenland (in N. Lat. 70 degrees) developed an abundance of trees, such as the Yew, the Redwood, the Sequoia, allied to the Californian species, Beeches, Planes, Willows, Oaks, Poplars and Walnuts, as well as Magnolia and a Zamia," says science, that is, Greenland had Southern plants unknown to Northern regions. (4) This "Land of the Eternal Sun", where the Greek's Apollo journeyed every year, was known to the Greeks in the days of Homer. How did the Greeks come to know about this blessed land, unaffected by winter and hurricane, where the sun never set and palm grew freely? Greenland at the time of Greeks was covered with perpetual snow. Certainly, the tradition must have descended to the Greeks from some people more ancient than Greeks themselves, who were familiar with those climatic details which were not known to the Greeks. This blessed land of eternal light and summer lied beyond Norway or Scandinavia, where the nights are short and days are long.

Archaic teachings, *Puranas* through their allegories, and the suspicion of modern science about a land beyond the polar seas, at the very circle of the Arctic Pole—all point towards the existence of a sea which never freezes and a continent which is ever green. It is therefore highly probable that, there was a time when Greenland was a tropical land, where people, now unknown to history, lived during the Miocene period of modern science.

Nature of Gods and the Seven Rounds

When a great Manvantara commences, Parabrahman manifests as Mulaprakriti and then as the Logos. The fourth in the chain is the Spirit-Guardian of our globe, is subordinate to the chief spirit (or God) of the Seven Planetary Genii or Spirits or Mystery-gods, whose chief was, *exoterically*, the visible Sun, or the eighth, and *esoterically*, the *second Logos*, the Demiurge. The seven, who became "seven eyes of the Lord" in the Christian religion, were the *regents* of the seven *chief* planets. Exoterically, the sun was the chief of the twelve great gods, or zodiacal constellations; and esoterically, the Messiah, the Christos, the subject *anointed* by the Great BREATH, or the ONE. The sun was thus surrounded by his twelve subordinate powers, also subordinate, in turn, to each of the seven "Mystery-gods" of the seven planets.

The invisible and visible worlds are the double links of one and the same chain. The *invisible Logos*, having seven hierarchies—represented or personified as the seven chief angels or rectors, forms one POWER, the inner and the invisible; so, the objective or *visible Logos* of the invisible and ever-subjective angels, having in the world of Forms, the Sun and the seven chief planets, constitutes the visible and active potency.

According to all the ancient Cosmogonies of Hermes, Chaldeans, Aryans, Egyptians, and Jews, the seven Higher ones were the fabricators of our solar system. The terrestrial spirits were the creators, the *regents* were the supervisors. The visible sun gives life to the planets; so, the Higher One—Spiritual Sun gives life to the whole kosmos.

Seven races in their evolution were born under the direct influence of the seven planets. The first race received its breath of life from the sun. Beings of the first and second races were androgynes, who became separate entities in the third race of humanity, a male and a female. The third race of humanity was under the direct influence of Venus—the *little sun* in which the solar orb stores its light.

The Creation of Universe and Man – Cosmic Evolution

Gods and men arose from one and the same Point—one universal, immutable, eternal, and absolute UNITY. It became: (i) Primordial substance or Force (centripetal and centrifugal, positive and negative, male and female, and so on) in the sphere of objectivity and Physics; and (ii) the SPIRIT OF THE UNIVERSE or Cosmic Ideation, called Logos, in the world of Metaphysics. This Logos is the apex of the Pythagorean triangle, representing symbolically in a dual way, the manifested Cosmos and unmanifested RAY.

Logos in Western Pantheism represents Unconscious Universal Mind—SUBJECT-side of manifested Being, and it is the source of individual consciousness. The potential latency in Parabrahman or One Reality transforms its "supramental thought of Logos" into energy, and thus objectivates Force. Mulaprakriti (root-nature) is the Primordial Cosmic Substance; it is the foundation of the OBJECT-side of things, and it is the basis of all objective evolution and Cosmogenesis. Force *succeeds* Mulaprakriti. Mulaprakriti without Force is non-existent for all practical intents.

The planner—Heavenly Man or Brahma or Elohim is the "*first Logos*," and the "first manifestation" of the deity's shadow is the "first-born"—executive/creator Brahmaa/Prajapati or Jehovah, called the "*second logos*," and the created Man was regarded in several systems as the "*third Logos*." (5)

There is a great difference between Logos and *Demiourgos*, former is the *Spirit* and latter is the *Soul*, one being the superior apprehending, the other the comprehending—one noetic and the other phrenic. The concealed thought is objectively expressed as Logos (*Verbum:* speech or word), just as a photograph objectively expresses hidden feelings or thoughts. DIVINE MIND reflects itself in Logos. Logos reflects itself in the Universe, and the Universe/world reflects itself in the Man. Egyptians regarded Sun as Logos, the guiding Force, and Demiurge the *creator* of our planet and everything pertaining to it—sevenfold Ray of light, for example, through which Logos becomes cognizant.

Going further into the nature of the Creator, it is neither good nor bad. Its differentiated aspects in nature make assume one or the other character. According to the '*Books of Hermes*,' none of the sun-gods have anything to do with the invisible and unknown universes disseminated throughout space.[6] This fact is symbolized by a Dragon and a Serpent, for Good and Evil, respectively; and, by the right-hand and left-hand magic, respectively on Earth.

In China the "men of Fohi" or "Heavenly Man" are called twelve *T'ien-hang* – twelve hierarchies of Dhyanis or Angels, with human faces and dragon bodies. In general, a dragon or a serpent represents divine wisdom or Spirit. In Scandinavia twelve AESIR of *Eddas* mean the same thing. Similar facts are found in the Druses of Syria. In each case the Sons of God create men. The dual (male and female) and triple (spiritual and psychic essence within) nature of man is at the origin of all these allegories.

Every Universe (world or planet) has its own Logos. Greek *Hermes-Sarameyas* is closely related to the Hindu *Sarama* Sarameya, the "divine watchman," watching over the golden flock of stars and solar rays. Corresponding to seven planets and seven spirits (Dhyanis/Creators) associated with them, there are seven regions on earth to be inhabited by seven races (or primordial human groups), created by the Dhyanis. Each of the seven regions on earth, and the race to be born on it, receives its vital force, life and powers—spiritually from its own special Dhyani, and physically from the planet of that Dhyani. Thus, the *first* race is born under the Sun; the *second* under *Brihaspati* (Jupiter); the *third* under *Lohitanga* (fiery-bodied), Sukra (Venus); the *fourth* under *Soma* (Moon, our Globe also, the Fourth Sphere born under and from the Moon) and *Sani* (Saturn)—the *krura-lochana* (evil-eyed) and *Asita* (dark); the *fifth* under *Budha* (Mercury).[7]

Like the duality of the Dhyani (spiritual) and his planet (physical), every man has an "inner man" or principle, and an "outer man" or physical form. Each man gets its specific quality from its primary—planetary spirit. Since all the seven principles are to be found in every man, in varying degrees of course, every man is *septenate*—a combination of principles, each having its origin in a quality of that special Dhyani. Every active power or force of the earth comes to her from one of the seven Lords. Thus, light comes through *Sukra* (Venus), who receives a triple supply, and gives one third of it to the earth. Scientifically, Venus receives from the sun twice as much light and heat as the earth. There is an occult as well as an astronomical meaning to the fact that the most radiant planet of all, the Venus, keeps two parts of the supply to herself and gives one third of it to the earth. Venus and earth are known as "twin-sisters," although the Spirit of Earth is subservient to the Lord of Venus.

Svastika represents male and female principles in Nature and much more. Astrologically and astronomically Venus is represented by a *Globe poised over a Cross* (Svastika bereft of its four arms), and the Earth, as a *Globe under a Cross*. Esoterically it means that, "Earth has fallen into production/generation of its species through sexual union." Westerners, however, had their own meaning of it saying that Earth and its species were redeemed *by the Cross* – while Venus (Lucifer-Satan) was trampling upon it.

According to exoteric Brahmanism, Venus is the most occult, powerful and mysterious of all planets, whose influence upon, and relation to, the Earth is most prominent. Sukra (Venus) is a male deity (Venus is bearded in mythology, to avoid confusion about being hermaphrodite) and he is the son of Bhrigu Rishi, one of the creative Prajapatis and a Vedic sage. Furthermore, Venus is Daitya-Guru, that is, Guru of the primeval giants. According to *Puranas,* the "double ones" (the Hermaphrodites) of the Third Root-Race descended from the first "sweat-born" through Sukra. The whole history of Sukra refers to the Third and Fourth Races.

The first *ideal* world (primitive Root-Race) was *self-generated* and *self impregnated* by the universally diffused Spirit of life. This was represented by an isolated diameter (female nature) in a circle, as a symbol. As the Races and all on Earth developed into their physical forms, they were androgynous, and the symbol became a circle with a diameter from which runs a vertical line, meaning that the male and female were not separated yet. The first and the earliest Egyptians represented this fact by the symbol of *Tau*. Later, when male-female were separated and fallen into generation, the symbol became a cross. Venus presided over the natural generation of man, which is symbolized by the sign of globe over the cross. Egyptians represented *Ankh* (life) by the ansated cross—a circle over the Tau—which is nothing but Venus (Isis); meaning, that all mankind and animal life has emanated from the "divine spiritual circle" and fallen into the generation of physical male and female. From the end of the Third Race onwards, the "ansated cross" and the "Tree of Life" in Eden had the same phallic significance. Moses—learned in the wisdom of priests of Egypt—introduced *Ankh* (life) from Egyptians to Hebrews. For Hebrews *Ankh* means my life, my being, which is Anochi (parallel to *Anukis*, the Egyptian goddess, a form of Isis). Ansated Cross (Venus) signified the existence of *"parturient energy* in the sexual sense", which was one of the attributes of Isis, the Mother of Eve, Havah or Mother-earth.

The presexual state of the Third Race is denoted by the ansated cross—Svastika, the "male and female sign," right in the central part of hermaphrodite goddess *Ardhanari* in the Madras Presidency, India. The same idea is carried by an ancient carving of the double-sexed Vishnu and Lakshmi standing on a lotus leaf floating on water, the water rising in a semicircle and pouring through the Svastika, signifying the generation/descent of man. Brahmaa sitting on a lotus, which is emerging from the naval of Vishnu, signifies the Creation of Brahmaa evolving from the *Nara*—the central point of the Universe.

The complete process from the beginning of the Universe to its completion is divided into seven Rounds, the present stage being the middle of the fourth Round at which we are

The Creation of Universe and Man – Cosmic Evolution

now. The development of the various Root Races created by the Dhyanis can be shown briefly as follows:[8]

Ist Round: An ethereal being, *non-intelligent,* but super-spiritual. In each of the subsequent races and subraces and minor races of evolution he grows more and more into an encased or incarnate being, but still preponderatingly ethereal. And like the animal and vegetable he developed monstrous bodies correspondential with his coarse surroundings.

IInd Round: He is still gigantic and ethereal, but growing firmer and more condensed in body—a more physical man yet still less intelligent than spiritual; for mind is a slower and more difficult evolution than the physical frame and the mind would not develop as rapidly as the body.

IIIrd Round: He has now a perfectly concrete or compacted body; at first the form of a giant ape, and more intelligent (or rather cunning) than spiritual. For in the downward arc he has now reached the point where his primordial spirituality is eclipsed or overshadowed by nascent mentality. In the last half of this 3rd Round his gigantic stature decreases, his body improves in texture (perhaps the microscope might help to demonstrate this) and he becomes a more rational being—though still more an ape than a Deva-man.

IVth Round: Intellect has an enormous development in this Round. The dumb races will acquire *our* human speech, on our Globe, on which from the 4th race language is perfected and knowledge in physical things increases. At this half-way point of the 4th Round Humanity passes the *axial point of the minor manwantaric circle.* (Moreover at the middle point of every major or *root race* evolution of each Round, man passes the equator of his course on that planet, the same rule applying to the whole evolution or the 7 rounds of the minor manwantara—7 rounds $\div$ by 2 = $3\frac{1}{2}$ Rds.) At this point then the world teems with the results of intellectual activity and *spiritual decrease."*

It should be noted that at the mid-point of third round primordial spirituality is eclipsed and man becomes more intellectual, rather cunning, than spiritual. Also, he had reached the apex of his physical form, acquiring a giant body, which begins to decrease from then onwards. At the mid point of the fourth round, which is the time now we are passing through, there is enormous intellect but spiritual decrease. This is the mid point also of the complete 7 rounds. So from now onwards the reversal of the activities should be expected. That is, intellectual decrease and spiritual increase. However, the process back to the original spirituality should take the same time as it has taken from the beginning of the universe, in the normal course. But for the past few millennia several yogis have achieved High Order Spirituality through yoga, meditation or other metaphysical activities, in different parts of the world. We will return to this topic in the next chapter.

The Brahmans in South India have maintained the following calendar concerning the evolution of the universe:[9]

I. From the beginning of cosmic evolution, upto the Hindu year Tarana (or 1887) – 1,955,884,686 years.
II. The (astral) mineral, vegetable and animal kingdoms up to Man, have taken to evolve – 300,000,000 years.
III. Time, from the first appearance of "Humanity" (on the planetary chain) – 1,664,500,987 years.

The changes of digits in the last three triplets of figures cannot be accounted for. Once the three hundred million years are subtracted, the figures ought to be 1,655,884,687. The figures quoted here are from the Tamil calendar. According to Swami Dayananda Saraswati, founder of the Arya Samaj, the date given is 1,960,852,987. However, the Occultists' account for the time from the first appearance of "Humanity" is 18 million years.

God, Monad (Jiva) and Atom (The Creation of Man)

The creation of man can be described in the following seven steps.

1. God (gods collectively), Monads (Jivas) and Atoms—the basis for the creation of everything else in the universe—emanated from one and the same source, the unknowable PARABRAHMAN.
2. Venus—guardian and life-giver of "Earth and men," guru of daityas or demons—cursed Vishnu (Logos incarnate) to be reborn on Earth seven times; and hence seven human races had to be created on earth.
3. In the beginning unacceptable beings were created many times by Nature, such as a being with a human head and the body of some animal; a being with several eyes, hands and legs; a being with animal head and human body, and so on.
4. The creators destroyed these forms and recreated men till the final shape of present humans came into being.
5. The first-borns of Brahma (or Elohim), the seven Prajapatis (collectively Brahmaa), were the deep spiritualists, who neglected the creation of men and were cursed to be reborn on Earth.
6. The second set of Prajapatis, or Jehovah (collectively); who were not really spiritual, without intelligence and with material ideas, created men in their own image. Therefore men as such were not spiritual but materialistic.
7. Brahmaa told the Creator Prajapatis that all created monads (Jivas), from lowest to the highest level, must gradually know the truth and God.

These points will now be elaborated in detail. The so-called Arch-Angels, Angels and Spirits of the West, copies of their prototypes, the Dhyani Chohans, the Devas and Pitris, of the East, are no real beings but fictions. Materialistic Science is inexorable at this point. "The exact extent, depth, breadth, and length of the mysteries of Nature are to be found only in Eastern esoteric sciences. So vast and so profound are these that hardly a few, a very few of the highest Initiates—those *whose very existence is known but to a small number of Adepts*—are capable of assimilating the knowledge[10]." "...the Esoteric Doctrine may well be called the 'thread-doctrine,' since, like *Sutratman*, in the Vedanta philosophy, it passes through and strings together all the ancient philosophical religious systems, and reconciles and explains them all.[11] *Sutratman* (thread-soul) in the philosophy of Vedanta means that the Atman (Spirit or Spiritual SELF) passes through the "five subtle bodies" like a thread. The "five subtle bodies," which cover the Atman one after another, finally producing the physical man are: *anandamaya kosh* (cover of bliss), *vigyanmaya kosh* (cover of scientific knowledge), *manomaya kosh* (mental cover), *pranamaya kosh* (cover of vital energies), and *annamaya kosh* (cover of the physical body), in that order.

For Roman Catholics, Satan is at the foundation of Cosmos, Christ in its center, and Anti-Christ at its apex. For both, the Hierarchy of Beings begins and ends within narrow frames of their respective theologies: one self-created *personal* God, and an Empyrean ringing with the Hallelujahs of *created* angels; the rest, *false* gods, Satan and fiends.[12]

God, Monad (Jiva) and Atom are the correspondences of Spirit, Mind and Body (*Atman, Manas and Sthula-Sarira*) in man. They are the "Heavenly Man" in their septenary aggregation, according to Kabala. "Terrestrial man" is therefore the provisional reflection of the "Heavenly Man." When a form is needed, Chohans (Dhyanis or *gods*) clothe themselves in the fabrics of Monads (Jivas) and Atoms, former being the souls of the latter. Thus Monads (Jivas) are *atomic souls* descending into concrete matter (taking on themselves the five covers described above, the physical body being the final cover), which marks the mid-point of their own individual pilgrimage. Losing their individuality in the mineral kingdom at this point, they begin to ascend through the seven states of terrestrial evolution to that point where a correspondence between the human and *Deva* (divine) is firmly established. Those who have developed highly clairvoyant faculties in themselves can see the life and behavior of these *atomic souls* in Space. Leibnitz, who was neither an Initiate nor a Mystic, came very close to the truth, and defined the evolution of the monads-though incorrectly, since he was only a philosopher, although having a high order of intuition.

The whole process can be briefed as follows: Spirit descending into Matter; equivalently-ascending into physical evolution; reascending from the depths of materiality towards its *status quo ante*, correspondingly dissipating its concrete form and substance up to the Laya State (state of final absorption—Samadhi), which is known as "the zero-point," and beyond, in science. Having known esoteric philosophy, the knowledge of these states is necessary for the practitioners. Scientists one after another, like Figuier and Dassier, are likely to follow in the "Intellectual fall." "They will be driven out of their position not by spiritual, theosophical, or any other physical or even mental phenomenon, but simply by the enormous *gaps* and *chasms* that open daily and will still be opening before them, as one discovery follows the other, until they are finally knocked off their feet by the ninth wave of simple common sense[13]."

Kepler, Leibnitz, Gassendi and Swedenborg came close to the truth, which was distorted; since it was alloyed with their own speculations in some predetermined direction. All the ancient, medieval, and modern poets have been anticipated in the exoteric Hindu books. Descartes *plenum* of matter differentiated into particles; Leibnitz' *Ethereal Fluid* and Kant's *Primitive Fluid* dissolved into its elements; Kepler's Solar Vortex and Systemic Vortices; in short, from the elemental vortices inaugurated by the universal mind—through Anaxagoras, down to Galileo, Torricelli, and Swedenborg, and after them to the latest speculations by European mystics—all this is found in the Hindu hymns and mantras to the "Gods, Monads and Atoms," in their fullness, for they are inseparable[14]. For example, the idea of Leibnitz's Monad being a living mirror and reflecting every other, was contained already in Sanskrit *Slokas* translated by Sir William Jones, which said that the creative source of the Divine Mind, "hidden in a veil of thick darkness, formed mirrors of the atoms of the world, and cast reflection from its own face on every atom...." The esoteric meaning of every Hindu cosmogony in the *Puranas* contains the theoretical knowledge. It is for the modern materialists to make science accept or not, the Eastern Occult views, which contain all the requisite material for filling those gaps; until then the mystery of "first creation" will remain unfathomable.

Finding an explanation, in the timeless Eastern scriptures, of the formation of whatever exists in the universe, there are two prominent names—Protyle and Svabhavat or (Fohat in Buddhism, Being in Chinese). Protyle is the undifferentiated cosmic matter in its infinitude, which is the "son" of the immaculate Celestial Virgin – Mulaprakriti, born again on Earth as son of Aditi or Eve, becoming humanity as a total—from androgynous Brahmaa or Jehovah to the Mankind below. Svabhavat is the "plastic material" filling the Universe, which is the root of all things. It is the abstraction of Mulaprakriti (Root-Nature). It is the body of the Soul, like ether would be to Akash (sky), the latter known as the informing principle of the former. Initiates and highly intuitive clairvoyants have seen the writhing like a snake of the Svabhavat or Fohat in space. Both these principles—Protyle and Svabhavat—emanated from the union of Parabrahman and Mulaprakriti. "Fohat runs the Manus' (or Dhyani-Chohans') errands, and causes the ideal prototypes to expand from within without—viz., to cross gradually, on a descending scale, all the planes from the noumenon to the lowest phenomenon, to bloom finally on the last into full objectivity—the acme of illusion, or the grossest matter."[15] This hidden "knowledge" or witnessing comes to the Initiates in the states of *samadhi* or *trance*. It is the knowledge part of Paramatman—known as "Existence-Knowledge-Bliss."

Acceptance and recognition of *protyle*, like invisible ether, which was a scientific necessity, would have turned the Chemistry developed from Avogadro to Crookes into a sort of new Metachemistry. *Vedas* and *Puranas* and the archaic Aryan work on occultism would have been vindicated by the discovery of such a radiant matter in space. The "allegories" in these Holy Scriptures contained hard scientific facts. For example, the three "first born" of the Mother (Aditi) and Father-Son-Husband (Daksha – a form of Brahmaa, the Creator)—were nothing but *Hydrogen*, *Oxygen* and *Nitrogen*. The characteristics of this triad of "first-born" were exoterically matching those of the three gases. So much so, that, in the context of the "atomic theory of evolution," the occult teachings are still found corroborated by exact science and its confessions, at least with regard to the "simple" elements, which now lie as degraded ones.

As another example in the Holy Scriptures, *Martanda* (the Sun) had evolved and aggregated, together with his smaller seven Brothers, from his Mother's (Aditi's) bosom—that bosom being *prima* mater, i.e. the primordial *protyle*. Esoteric doctorines teach the existence of "an antecedent form of energy having periodic cycles of ebb and swell, rest and activity"—and behold a great scholar of Science now asking the world to accept this as one of the postulates[16]. It has been shown that the "Mother," which is fiery and hot, becomes gradually cool and radiant, and it is the same thing that the scientists claim as their second postulate—a *scientific necessity*, it would seem—"an internal action akin to cooling, operating slowly in the protyle." According to Occult Science the "Mother" lies stretched in infinity (during *pralaya*, meaning the long period of rest) as the great Deep, the "*dry* Waters of Space," according to the quaint expression in the *Catechism*, and becomes *wet* only after the separation and the moving over its face of *Narayana*, the "Spirit which is invisible Flame, which never burns, but sets on fire all that it touches, and gives it life and generation."

In an attempt to get a glimpse of the secrets so darkly hidden, the first two very reasonable postulates need addition of the third postulate—that Leibnitz in his speculations, stood on a firm ground of fact and truth; the most notable of them being the postulate that there is nothing *inorganic* in Nature. Stones, minerals, rocks, and even chemical "atoms" are simply *organic* units in profound lethargy. There would be an end to their coma, and their inertia would become activity. Leibnitz had the metaphysical intuition, which was not possessed by Descartes, Kant or any other scientist. Vindicating the Occult teaching, Leibnitz endowed mental life to whole creation with infinite gradations, while Descartes denied soul to the animal.

Through a line from beyond between the ever-incognizable One Reality and invisible, yet comprehensible Presence of Mulaprakriti or Shekhinah vibrates the Sound of the *Verbum*, from which evolve the numberless hierarchies of intelligent *Egos*, of conscious and unconscious, *perceptive* and *appreciative* Beings, whose essence is spiritual Force, whose substance is the Elements and whose bodies are the *atoms*, whenever required. According to Henri Lachelier, that which exists outside of us in an absolute manner are Souls whose essence is force. The reality in the manifested world therefore is composed of a *unity of units,* which are immaterial and infinite, called "Monads" by Leibnitz, "*Jivas*" by Eastern philosophy and by a variety of names by Occultism, with the Kabalists and Christians.

There is a clear distinction between the Monads (Jivas) and Atoms. Atoms are not distinguished from one another, and are qualitatively alike; but one Monad differs from every other Monad, qualitatively; and everyone is a peculiar world to itself. Atoms on the other hand are absolutely alike quantitatively and qualitatively and possess no individuality of their own. Atoms are extended and divisible, while the Monads are *metaphysical points* and indivisible. Vindicating the mystic philosophy, Monads are representative beings, they reflect the universe like a mirror, and they are not mere passive reflecting agents, but *spontaneously self-active*. An adept can read everything, including the future in a Monad. This philosophy of Leibnitz had no distinction between the Elemental Monad and high Planetary Spirit, or even between the human Monad and Soul.

Occult philosophy separated Leibnitz's Monads into three distinct hosts: firstly, from the highest planes, are, "gods," or conscious spiritual *Egos*—the intelligent architects, who work after the plan in the *Divine Mind*. Secondly, the Elementals or *Monads (Jivas)*, who form collectively and unconsciously the grand Universal Mirrors of everything connected with their respective realms. Thirdly, the atoms, or material molecules, which are informed in their turn by their *appreciative* monads, just as every cell in human body is so informed. These three "rough divisions" correspond to *spirit, mind* (or soul) and *body*, in the human constitution.

The *Formless* (Arupa) Radiations, existing in the harmony of Universal Will, and being what we term the collective or the aggregate of Cosmic Will on the plane of subjective Universe, unite together an infinitude of monads (sparks)—each being the mirror of its own Universe—and thus individualize for the time being an independent mind, omniscient and universal; and by the same process of magnetic aggregation they create for themselves objective, visible bodies, out of the interstellar atoms[17]. Right from the moment of first differentiation (or separation from the Original Whole), atoms and Monads, in whatever form they are (associated or dissociated, simple or complex) are the *principles* (physical, psychic and spiritual) of the "Gods," who are themselves the Radiations of primordial nature. The higher Planetary Powers, therefore, appear to the eye of the Seer under two aspects: the *subjective*—as influences, and the objective—as mystic FORMS. Since Spirit and Matter are one, these FORMS become a *Presence* under the Karmic law. To be more specific, Spirit is matter on the highest *seventh plane* of existence; and matter is Spirit on the lowest point of its activity. Both, however, are illusion or Maya.

In Occultism atoms are called vibrations, and collectively they produce the sensation of "Sound" on the subjective side of the process. This sound cannot be perceived or seen by the scientist, who is involved in the discovery of the behavior of matter. But the psychic or a spiritual seer can see it, since his inner eye is opened and he can see through the veil of the matter. Atoms fill the immense Space; they propel their molecules into activity *from within* and their continuous vibrations produce MOTION and the correlation of Forces, because of which the wheels of Life go on perpetually. The ruling power, the consciously guiding noumenon, call it Angel or God, Spirit or Demon, is at the origin of every such force. The Seers see the motion of the interstellar shoals of atoms as dazzling specks of virgin snow in radiant sunlight. At times, the intensity of their motion produces flashes like the Northern lights. Thus there is a close relation between materialistic Science and Occultism, which is the missing link of the former. My own experiences with the Holy Sound and Light are elaborated in the first chapter.

One cannot arrive at the Truth, until one returns to the simplicity and fearlessness of the primitive ages. At that time men mixed freely with the gods, and the gods descended among men and guided them in truth and holiness. "Angels" in the *Bible* have several designations, e.g., "morning stars", "flaming fires", and "the mighty ones." St. Paul called them "Principalities and Powers," on seeing them in his cosmogonic visions. According to Bjerregaard, these can be known as impersonal existences as an influence, a spiritual substance or conscious force [18].

Venus

"Every sin committed on earth is felt by Usanas-Sukra. The Guru of the Daityas is the Guardian of the Earth and Men. Every change on Sukra is felt on, and reflected by the earth[19]." Sukra or Venus was the Guru of the Daityas (demons), the giants of the Fourth race, who defeated minor gods and obtained sovereignty of Earth, according to the Hindu allegory. Daityas of East are parallel to the *Titans* of Western allegory, connected with Venus-Lucifer, and Satan of Christianity. This common mythological allegory has great significance that will be elaborated later in the text.

There are more allegories which carry deep spiritual meanings behind them. Venus adopted Earth, the progeny of Moon, as a child. Gradually, Earth overgrew its parent Moon and created some trouble. Sukra was the son of the great Rishi and one of the seven Creator-Prajapatis Bhrigu. Because of its immense love for Earth, Sukra incarnated as Usanas and gave perfect laws that were gradually thrown away. At one point of time Sukra requested Siva to protect Daityas and Asuras, who were his disciples, against a fight with the gods. He also performed some Yogic rites for this purpose. This caused, according to the allegory, the axis of Venus getting inclined by about 50 degrees and getting enveloped by eternal clouds. Many occult philosophical meanings are carried by the allegory that Vishnu killed Sukra's mother, for which, Sukra cursed him to be "reborn seven times" on Earth. This caused the creation of "seven Races" on earth. One of the earliest popes in Rome was named as Lucifer, which suggests that the Christians too knew the fact that Sukra-Venus-Lucifer is both physically and mystically the light-bearer of Earth.

There are numberless planets or worlds in space with men and animals, all different and unique. Each one of them has a double nature—physical and spiritual. At the beginning of each Manvantara, light condensed into the forms of "Lords of Being," the first and highest in hierarchy, collectively called Jivatman or Pratyagatman issuing from Paramatman. The Greek philosophers called it Logos. Lower in hierarchy are the forms of condensing light that became gross matter on the objective plane—Creative Forces with and without forms, and lower Elementals without forms, which assume all possible forms according to the conditions that surrounded them. In the spiritual sense there is but one basis (Absolute Upadhi) for all creations on various planes, which evolve universally and cyclically during the entire period of the Manvantara.

"The Informing intelligences, which animate these various classes of Being, are referred to indiscriminately by men beyond the Great Range (India, as being the Trans-Himalayan region) as the Manus, the Rishis, the Pitris (Fathers and Progenitors), the Prajapatis and so on; and as Dhyani-Buddhas, and Chohans, Melhas (fire-gods), Bodhisattvas, and others on this side. The truly ignorant call them gods; the learned profane, the one God; and the wise, the Initiates, honor in them only the Manvantaric manifestations of THAT which neither our Creators (the Dhyani-Chohans) nor their creatures can ever discuss or know anything about. The ABSOLUTE is not to be defined, and no mortal or immortal has ever seen or comprehended it during the periods of Existence. The mutable cannot know the immutable, nor can that which lives perceive Absolute Life[20]."

Man, therefore, cannot know the beings higher than his own progenitors, nor shall he worship them, although he ought to know about his own creation on Earth. Yet, however, as stated elsewhere, there are facts "known to every *'twice-born'* (*Dvija*, or Initiated) Brahmana (the priestly division of India) and the *Puranas* contain references to them in veiled terms, which no matter-of-fact Orientalist has yet endeavoured to make out, nor could he if he would[21]. This implies that a normal mutable and living man cannot perceive Truth beyond the level of his own Creators, but a man who has become *"twice-born,"* in one way or the other, can perceive beyond his own Creators. Adiguru Shankaracharya has said in *Vivek-Chudamani* (The Crest Jewel of Wisdom): "One who is a *twice-born*, in whom the flow of vital-fluid (semen, in case of man) has reversed, is a walking God on Earth[22]." This is vindicated elsewhere as, "The angels aspire to become man; a perfect man. A man-god is above all the angels[23]."

Yet again, "the gods who had no personal merit of their own, dreading the sanctity of those self-striving incarnated beings who had become *ascetics* and Yogis, and thus threatened to upset the power of the former by their *self-acquired* powers—denounced them. All this has a deep philosophical meaning and refers to the evolution and acquirement of divine powers through *self-exertion*. Some Rishis-Yogis are shown in the *Puranas* to be far more powerful than the gods. Secondary gods or temporary powers in Nature (the Forces) are doomed to disappear; it is only the spiritual potentiality in man which can lead him to become one with the infinite and the absolute[24]."

Unless the light of the Eastern esoteric philosophy reads the Kabala, or whatever is left of it, Truth cannot be known. The Kabalists never cease to repeat that *primal intelligence* can never be understood. Hence the Ain-Soph—the "UN KNOWABLE" and the "UNNAMABLE"—which, as *it* could not be made manifest, was conceived to emanate manifesting powers. Therefore, human intellect can and has to deal with emanations alone. "Christian theology, having rejected the doctrine of emanations and replaced with direct, conscious creations of angels and the rest out of *nothing*, now finds itself hopelessly stranded between Supernaturalism, or miracle, and materialism. An *extra*-cosmic god is fatal to philosophy, an *intra*-cosmic deity, i.e. spirit and matter inseparable from each other—is a philosophical necessity [25]."

Nature in man became a compound of spirit and matter and led him to become what he is now; and now spirit that is latent in Matter should be awakened to life and consciousness gradually. The Monad (Jiva) has to pass through its mineral, vegetable and animal forms, before the Light of the Logos is awakened in the animal man. Therefore, before spiritual awakening he is referred to as Monad and only afterwards as man. Eastern philosophy recognizes evolution through "words." "Even the name of the first man in the Mosaic Bible had its origin in India, Professor Max Muller's negation not withstanding. The Jews got their Adam from the Chaldea[26]."

The astral through Kama (desire) is ever drawing Manas down into the sphere of material possession and desires. But if the *better* man or *Manas* tries to escape the fatal attraction and turns its aspirations to Atman—Spirit—then Buddhi (Ruah) conquers, and carries Manas with it to the realm of eternal Spirit.[27]

Each Manvantara has seven Kalpas (Rounds) to complete the rotation. Presently the Earth is in the middle of the fourth Round. At the commencement of each Kalpa or Round, the Earth (or the Jiva of the Earth) is reborn, just as a Monad (Jiva) is reborn in his mother's womb and gets a new human body, reemerging from space into objectivity. Then just as a snake casts off his old skin and gets a new one, it can be said that the Earth and human Monad also cast off their skin and get a new one. It is in this way that our Earth has cast off her old cover three times in three rounds, and the present cover (or skin) with new continents on its surface is the fourth one. There have to be seven new skins of Earth in this way; seven times the continents will get reshaped, till the rotation of Manvantara is complete in seven rounds. It is for this reason that the Earth is called *Sarpa Rajni* (Queen of the Serpents), and the Mother of all that is changing. Seven skins are the seven geological changes that accompany and correspond to the evolution of the seven root-races.

The organism of Man in every root-race is adapted according to its surroundings. Just as ours is material now, the first race was ethereal. The seven Creators produced seven primordial Adams. The first was Adam-Kadamon or Heavenly Man of the first chapter of Genesis, who was made in the image and likeness of God. He was the Sephirothal Host. Second Adam of second chapter was not made in the image or divine likeness of God; he was the Adam of Mindless first root-race, before he ate the fruit of wisdom. Third Adam belonged to the race that separated into male and female forms. These Adams are the correspondences of the Manus in Eastern philosophy, which are well elaborated therein.

The undifferentiated-changeless-immutable Nature (*avikara* and *sadaikarupa* Essence) awakened and changed, that is, it got differentiated into a state of causality (*avyakta*-unrepresented), and from "cause" (*karana*) it became its own discrete "effect" (*vyakta*-represented), from invisible it became visible. The smallest of small (*aniyamsam aniyamsam*—the most atomic of the atoms) became one and many (*ekanekarupa*); and produced the Universe as a garland of seven lotuses (Planets), our Earth being the fourth loka or planet. The "Unfallen" (*Achyuta*) then became "the Fallen" (*Chyuta*). This refers to the Creators-Dhyanis, who incarnated on earth in human forms of the *Third* Root Race; and, endowed men with intellect (*Manas*). Since the Dhyanis had to fall into generation in this way, they became "the Fallen" (*Chyuta*). The other Creators-Dhyanis-Prajapatis, who did not incarnate on Earth in human form, remained "Unfallen" (*Achyuta*).

Two very important personalities come to the notice in this round—Narada, the old Vedic Rishi and, Asuramaya, the great Atlantean. Narada was the son of Brahmaa (as in *Matsya Purana*), the progeny of Kasyapa Rishi and the daughter of Daksha (as in *Vishnu Purana*). He is the most mysterious character, known by Hindus as a great Rishi, who is forever wandering about the earth, giving good counsel; and, understood as one of the twelve *Messiahs*. Narada informed the vicious demonic King Kamsa about Vishnu incarnating in the form of Krishna, as the eighth child of Devaki, and for this reason both Brahmaa and Daksha cursed him. He on the other hand, sitting on the clouds in sky, lauded the birth of Krishna, when it took place. Narada is here, there, and everywhere, an active and ever-incarnating Logos. He as a "Messenger of Gods" or *Pesh-Hun* (Occultism) or *Angelos* (Greek), is the sole confidant and the executor of Karma, and he leads and guides human affairs from the beginning to the end of the Kalpa (Round). It is he who brings on wars and puts an end to them. He is sometimes known as strife-maker, while most of the times as Deva-Brahmaa. Jehovah is the only character in resemblance with Narada, with the difference that the former is known for saying, "I am the Lord God," while the latter had no desire to show such a complex, or any ambition or selfish motive; and, was always ready to serve and guide the progress and evolution of the universe.

Asuramaya was born in Atlantis, as per Hindu *Puranas*, perhaps at a place called Romaka-Pura in West. He was as great a magician as he was an astrologer and an astronomer. Most of the time calculations of periods such as Kalpa, Manvantara, and age of our universe, are due to him. "From the fragments of immensely old works attributed to the Atlantean astronomer, and found in Southern India, the calendar elsewhere mentioned was compiled by two very learned Brahmans in 1884 and 1885. The work is proclaimed by the best Pundits as faultless—from the Brahmanical standpoint—and thus far relates to the chronology of the orthodox teachings[28]."

There are two important points to be elaborated; they concern "failed creations" and "fallen angels," which are either not properly known or are misunderstood in most cosmogonies. According to Hindu *Puranas*, the Egyptian and Chaldean fragments, the *Genesis*, modern science and to a certain degree with the theory of evolution, there have been several "creations" before the last formation of the Globe, which changed its geological and atmospheric conditions, and changed also its flora, its fauna, and its men. Nature tried to produce forms; soft stones that hardened (*minerals*), hard plants that softened (*vegetation*), visible from invisible, insects and small lives. Earth shook all these off whenever they overran on her surface. At the first attempt to create men as a result of the "evolutionary impulse," after about 300 million years, according to *Rig Veda* and Occultism, the Nature produced monsters, half-human, half-animal and watermen, terrible and bad, which proved failures.

Brahmaa in *Puranas* is seen recommencing anew several creations after as many failures. Two great creations (not to be confused with seven Root-Races), padma (lotus) and varaha (boar) are mentioned. As Varaha Avatara (incarnation as boar) Brahmaa lifted the Earth out of the water, which is our present Globe. The creation is shown as a sport, an amusement (*Lila*) of the creative god. According to *Zohar* the primordial worlds perished as soon as they came into being[29]. Similar statements are found in Midrash and Rabbi Abbahu, saying that "the Holy One" had successively created and destroyed sundry worlds, before he succeeded in the present one[30]. *Genesis* I, 31, repeats the words, "This one pleases me" about the present world, in the usual distorted manner. Kuo P'o of China in *Sham-Hai-Ching* (*Wonders by Sea and Land*) writes about "men having two distinct face on their heads, before and behind, monsters with bodies of goats and human faces." At the time of the last emperor of Hsia dynasty, B.C.1818, Chung Ku carried his books in his fight to Yin, fearing that the emperor might destroy them treating of the ancient time.

In the Chaldean Cosmogony two distinct creations of animals and men are mentioned, the first having been destroyed as a failure. First, in the abyss of waters and darkness, called Thalatth (sea or water), resided most hideous beings—men with wings, four and two-faced men, humans with two heads, with the legs and horns of a goat, hippocentaurs, bulls with the heads of men, and dogs with tails of fishes. Various combinations of animals and men, of fishes, reptiles and other monsters with interchanging features are shown. Thalatth was the female element, which was conquered by the male element Belus: "Belus came and cut the woman asunder; and of one half of her he formed the earth, and of the other half the heavens; and at the same time destroyed the animals with her[31]." In view of Akkadians every object and power of Nature had its spirit. Triadic deities were formed by Akkadians normally of males or sexless; by Semites introducing sex; while for Aryans and the early Akkadians everything emanated through a Creator or Logos—not created by it.

Failed creations included locomotive qualities of the primary ethereal bodies of men, which could fly as well as walk, but who were destroyed because they were sexless and imperfect. Science will have nothing to say about these facts, or to metaphors and allegories pointing towards these possible facts of the remote past. However, modern human race has occasionally furnished us with monster specimens, such as, two headed children, animal bodies with human heads, and dog headed babies. This shows that if nature will still play such freaks now, which have been settled for ages, before she sorted out her species and began regular work upon them, it may appear like reversion in the language of science.

A clear conclusion can be seen now, that the nature left to itself can produce only the first two and lower animal kingdoms; it fails when the turn of man comes. Spiritual, independent and intelligent powers are needed for his creation, besides the physical body. Something higher than simply physical materials is needed to build the personalities of human Monads of former rounds.

The great French Naturalist A. de Quatrefages in his *Introduction a lelude des Races Humaines* proves that man has not altered one iota in his physical structure, while many races had already scattered during the Tertiary period and before. Every animal has been transformed except man which proves two things: his antiquity and that he is a *distinct Kingdom*. Man escaped transformation through changing geological conditions by his *psychic force*, and not his physical strength or body, which has been the case with animals. That human organism with all his characteristics, peculiarities and idiosyncrasies existed in that remote past when there was not one single specimen of the now-existing forms of mammalia, proves its fully developed existence prior to any other mammalia now known had even begun their appearance on this earth. Since all the human races are of one and the same species, this species is proved to be the most ancient, most stable and most preserving of all the now living mammalia. Darwinism is highly questionable in the light of these facts.

According to *Vishnu Purana*, which is certainly the earliest of all the scriptures of that name[32], Brahmaa appeared as male God for creation. He performed Yoga (*Yuyuje*) and "collected his mind into itself" (*Mano samadhatte*); and in this way his four bodies came into being: *Jyotsna* (dawn), *Ratri* (night), *Ahan* (day), and *Samdhya* (evening twilight), in that very order. With these four bodies, as explained by Rishi Parasher, he created four orders of beings: Gods (Dhyani Chohans), Demons (more material Devas), Progenitors (Pitris) and men. It is important to note that Demons were created before the angels or gods. The reason is that the first Cosmic aspect of Parabrahman, known as sat or universal soul, which is at the root of self-consciousness, is the principle mahat or Intellect or Universal Mind or manifested omniscience, and it is the first product of Pradhana (primordial matter). Demons, as they are called, are the *first positive poles of creation*, who are self-asserting and intellectually active principle. With the qualities of darkness pervading Brahmaa's assumed body, the first produced *asuras* (demons) issued from his thigh, after which the body was abandoned and was transformed into night.

Asu (breath), the "Breath of God" a similar meaning conveyed by Zoroastrian *Ahura* or Supreme Spirit, implied that Asuras were the *spiritual divine beings*, according to the *Rig Veda*. It is only later that they are shown issuing from the thigh of Brahmaa and *a-sura* was taken to mean "*not a god*," and that they became enemies of gods. Another reason for the demons being produced first is that every Cosmogony (including Aryan, Egyptian, Hesiod and Genesis) begins with the so-called "Secondary Creation," so that the mystery of the *manifested* Universe must remain "Darkness" to the finite intellect of Secondary Evolution. "The *Veda* contains the whole philosophy of that division, without having ever been correctly explained by our Orientalists, because it has *never been understood* by them[33]."

After Night, Brahmaa assumed the form of the Day and from his breath created gods having the quality of passive goodness. It is here that an allegory came into being, "by day the gods are most powerful, and by night the demons." Thus after positive activity, came negative passivity or goodness, from which issued Pitris, who were the progenitors of men. This "productive thinking" of Brahmaa during the process of creation, that he is the father of the world, is the mysterious *Yoga* power called *Kriya-Sakti*. Faith accompanied with Will makes things come to pass, as hinted by Mark (xi, 23). Later Brahmaa assumed the form of *Samdhya* (evening twilight), which is the interval between day and night. Next form assumed by the body of Brahmaa bore the *quality of foulness,* from which men were produced. That is why foulness and passion predominate the nature of men. This body when cast off became the dawn, the morning twilight or the twilight of Humanity, standing for the petra or father, collectively.

Brahmaa represents collectively the Lords of Being—Prajapatis. The four bodies assumed for creation by Brahmaa typify the four classes of creative powers or Dhyani Chohans, for the creation of everything in the universe, movable or immovable, including the world and men. First four chapters of *Genesis* represent the same idea, with their Lord and God being *Elohim* and *Eloah* (androgynous), respectively.

Kriya-Sakti is the "energy" of Mulaprakrati (Root-Nature), which is evoked and used by Brahmaa, through Faith and Will, for the creation of the Universe and everything in it. It is the yogic method by which one goes within oneself through concentration and gets the energy evoked. In the same way on Earth, Yogis experience the *Kriya-Sakti* at the successful completion of their yogic practices, and at that point their belief of "doership" is changed into "witnessing," which is the beginning of liberation or salvation. Greater details can be found in my former books on Kundalini[34],[35] and Shaktipat[36].

Coming back to the case of "Fallen Angels," it can be said that it has been wrongly interpreted and misunderstood both by Christian theologians and their followers on one hand, and those Hindu Brahmans who were greedy for power and ambition on the other. Christians settled with the belief that Satan and Fallen Angels were the earliest created; Satan being the first created, the wisest and the best of all of God's Archangels. Christians believed that only they knew the *truth* and *fact*; portraying all to be demoniacal; and, the *pagan* Scriptures, Orientalists and Mythologists-Christians or scientists were made to convey the same meaning, consciously or unconsciously. Initiates among early Christians remained silent, while others who did not know the truth, judged the hierarchy of Angels exoterically and disfigured the order of things. The *Asuras* were shown as "rebellious inferior gods," fighting the "popular higher ones," and the "eldest benevolent Logos" was shown as adversary or *Satan*. "But is this warranted by the correct interpretation of any old Scripture? The answer is, *most certainly not*[37]."

The Mazdean Scriptures of the *Zend-Avesta*, the *Vendidad* and others exposed cunning shuffling of the gods in Hindu Pantheon. The *Asuras* were restored to their legitimate place in theogony by ahura. Chaldean tablets discovered recently vindicated the good name of the "first divine emanations." The truth had passed from Babylonia to Pharisees, and from them to Christian Angelologists. Even the guardians of the Laws of Moses-Sadducees did not know of the rebelling Angels. They even rejected the idea that opposed the immortality of the human Soul. "In the Bible the only 'Angels' spoken of are the 'Sons of God' mentioned in *Genesis* vi (who are now regarded as the *Nephilim*, the Fallen Angels), and several angels in human form, the 'Messengers' of the Jewish God, whose own rank needs a closer analysis than heretofore given[38]."

Pharisees built their angelology on the accounts of Assyrian fragments of tiles on which Babylonian accounts of Creation are found. According to the "*Tablet with the story of the Seven Wicked Gods or Spirits,*" the "rebellious angels" were created in the *lower parts of heaven*, which ought to be a subjective plane in higher realms, not a cognizable one through our physical senses. In this way the Gnostics were closer to the truth; as compared to the non-initiated Christians who corrected themselves hundreds of years later; that our "visible world" – Earth was created by lower angels, the inferior Elohim, God of Israel being one of them. The king of the messengers of the God was Anu of Chaldean trinity. Both Anu (Chaldean) and Jehovah (Hebrew Kabala) were double-sexed, representing the dual aspect of male or spiritual and female or material, or the two antagonistic principles—Spirit and Matter. Thus the "Messengers of Anu" (who is Sin or Moon in Chaldean) are finally overpowered by the same Sin (*Argha*—the seed of all material life, or Moon in Kabala) with the help of Bel (the Sun) and Ishtar (Venus). Assyriologists regarded this *metaphysical fact* as a contradiction. However, there is more than one interpretation, since to the mystery of Fall has seven keys.

Theology shows two Falls: one, the rebellion of Archangels and their Fall, two, the Fall of Adam and Eve. Fall is an allegory, and both the lower as well as the higher hierarchies are charged with the crime, which according to the Occultism is not crime but "Karmic effects," belonging to the law of evolution—intellectual and spiritual (higher),

The Creation of Universe and Man – Cosmic Evolution 155

as well as, physical and psychic (lower). The higher—differentiating intellection or consciousness—seeking union with matter, at one end of the ladder of evolution; and the lower—the rebellion of matter against Spirit, or of action against spiritual inertia, on the other. Thus, simultaneously, "material angels" with animal passion, fought with Spirits of Darkness, while, the Spirits fought for supremacy of the conscious and divine spirituality on Earth. In the fight, Spirits lost to the power of matter; and the "lower material angels," who were devoid of intellect and spirituality, but were physical and materialistic, created the world and men. The allegorical "War in heaven" is identically reported in Hesiod as "War of the Titans against the Gods", and in the Hindu Puranas as "War of the Asuras or Tarakamaya against the gods," except the names being different. The fact is that the aspects of the stars show that "all the planets except Saturn were on the same side of the heavens as the Sun and Moon," and hence were his opponents (the nearest date for such a conjunction to have taken place was 945 B.C.). And yet it is Saturn, or the Jewish "Moon-god," who is shown as prevailing, both by Hesiod and Moses, neither of whom was understood. Thus it was that the real meaning became distorted[39].

All the rebellious sons of Brahmaa are represented as holy ascetics and Yogis in the Aryan allegory. They are reborn in every Kalpa (round) and they try to impede the work of human procreation. The great Rishi *Narada*, a son of Brahmaa, interferes and twice frustrates the aim of Daksha (creator-*Prajapati*), when the latter brings forth 10,000 sons to people the world. He persuades the Sons to remain holy ascetics and eschew marriage. Since *Narada* had refused to marry and obtain progeny, Brahmaa cursed him earlier, and now Daksha cursed him to be reborn as a man. It can be seen that *Narada* belongs to that class of Brahmaa's "first-born," who proved rebellious to the law of animal procreation, and hence they had to incarnate as *men*.

The supposed "rebels" therefore are the ones who were compelled by Karmic law to incarnate anew, and hence their inferior brethren on astral plane were given the responsibility of creation. Many of them refused to create since they were *arupa* (formless), presumably the Adepts and Yogis of long past Manvantaras, and not having the requisite materials (astral body). However, later on, as *Nirmankayas* (body-makers), they sacrificed themselves for the good and salvation of the Monads (*Jivas*) that were waiting for their turn, and which otherwise would have had to linger on as animal-like humans for countless ages.

Plentiful of "Fires," "Sparks," and "Flames" can be found in ancient scriptures and documents. They are clearly enunciated in the *Book of Concealed Mystery* and in the *Idra Zuta Qaddisha* (Lesser Holy Assembly). Among the sparks of the Prior Worlds, "Vibrating Flames and Sparks," from the divine flint, the *workmen* proceed to create man, "male and female" which "Flames and Sparks" (Angels and their Worlds, Stars and Planets) are said, figuratively to "become extinct and die," that is to say, remain *unmanifested* until a certain process of nature is accomplished[40]. The Kabala has also proved well that these Hebrew Elohim, Sparks, and Cherubs are identical with the Devas, Rishis and the Fires and Flames, the Rudras and the forty-nine Agnis of the ancient Aryans. The passage however, needs an elaborated explanation.

From *pre-existing material* and under the *law of evolution*, "worlds and men" have been repeatedly formed and destroyed, until our Earth (and in the same way other planets and their men) and its animal and human races became what they are now, in the present cycle. This resulted from the equilibrised compound of Spirit and Matter, of the positive and the negative, of the male and female. The creating Elohim kept on arranging his form on this sexual plane *astrally*, until man became his *prototype*— male and female physically. According to the law of *Balance* in Kabala, the atoms and organic forces, descending on the differentiated plane of Earth, had to be arranged in proper order intended by Nature. This process continued until the present stage of materialism, in which, the "male and female" reached its final perfection.

Male Sephiroth—Wisdom, known as *Hokhmah*—had to diffuse itself *in* and *through*, female *Binah*—Understanding or intelligent Nature. The First Root-Race of men that was sexless and mindless, was disapproved and hidden, until the time came when instead of dying, the first race disappeared in the second race, just as some lower lives and plants do in their progeny. Through complete transformation the First became the Second Root-Race, instead of the former being extinguished completely. It had to happen this way, since the *Holy City* had not been prepared yet[41]. And the "Holy City" meant the *Maqom*, the Secret Place or Shrine on Earth—the "human womb," which was the microcosmic copy and reflection of the *Heavenly* Matrix—Chaos or female space in which the male Spirit fecundates the germ of the Son—the visible Universe. Showing the importance of the Emanation of Male and Female Principles in the *Zohar* it is made clear that the Wisdom from the *Holy Ancient* "does not shine except in male and female, on this earth."

Hokhmah-Wisdom-Father and *Binah*-Understanding-Mother by connecting with one-another they bring forth, diffuse and emanate Truth. In other words, "Yod" connected with "Heh" resulted in impregnation and production of the Son. This is the completeness of the Whole[42]. According to the Rabbis also this was the "completeness" of the phallicism, the divine being dragged into the animal, the sublime into the grossness of the terrestrial. Such graphically gross presentations do not exist either in Eastern Occultism or in the primitive Kabala—the *Chaldean Book of Numbers*. "Catholic writers have unwisely written about the phallic symbols, because the profound metaphysical meaning is too much to grasp for the modern champions of that religion. They are in duty bound to destroy their oldest churches, and change the form of the cupolas of their own temples. The Mahadeva of Elephanta, the Round Tower of Bhagalpur, the minarets of Islam (rounded or pointed) are the originals of the *Campanile* column of San Marco at Venice, of Rochester Cathedral, and of the modern Duomo of Milan. All of these steeples, turrets, domes, and Christian temples, are the reproductions of the primitive idea of the *lithos,* the upright phallus[43]."

On Variety of Creators and the Process of Creation of Man

Whether it was a miraculous creation out of nothing, according to the dead letter of *Genesis*, or a first man born of a fantastic "missing" link so far—the common ancestor of man and "true ape." At this point Occult philosophy teaches that the first human stock was projected by "Higher and semi-divine Beings" out of their own essences. It was a double evolution in two contrary directions: spiritual, psychic, intellectual and animal evolution from the highest to the lowest; and, at the same time, physical development from simple and homogenous to more complex and heterogeneous, to fabricate the being now known as man. However, this required various ages of diverse nature and degrees of spirituality and intellectuality. There has been one ever-acting and never-erring law from one Manvantara (eternity) to the other—ever furnishing an ascending scale for the manifest (*Maha-Maya* or great Illusion), but plunging Spirit deeper and deeper into materiality on the one hand, and then *redeeming it through flesh* and liberating it. This law is seen to use Beings from other and higher planes, men, or *Minds* (Manus), according to their karmic exigencies. "At this juncture, the reader is again asked to turn to the Indian philosophy and religion[44]."

The producers of the *first stock of men*, called Fathers (*Pitaras* or *Pitris*) in India, presented themselves in bones and flesh as the first humans—the first *Manushyas* on Earth—

becoming themselves the first generation, with physical bodies and lower principles. They were the *"lunar* Beings." Then, the "Solar Angels" endowed, metaphorically or literally, "conscious, immortal EGO" to men. These "Solar Angels" are called Lords (*Nathas*), who are noted for their "persevering ceaseless devotion" or *Pranidhana*. These Lords belonged to the *fifth* principle (*Manas*), which originated the system of Yogis, who made *Pranidhana* their *fifth* observance (yam, niyam, asana, pranayama, pratyahar or *Pranidhan*, dharana, dhyana, and samadhi), according to *Yoga-Sutra*. Although there is a little difference in the meanings of pratyahar (withdrawal of senses from the world) and *Pranidhan* (persevering ceaseless devotion), the two imply the same *fifth* observance in the process of Yoga. These Lords are regarded identical with *Kumaras, Agnishvattas,* and *Barhishads* in India.

The great Initiate Philosopher Plato truly defined the "human soul" or EGO as "a compound of the *same* and the *other."* When the "Higher Self" merged with and in the Divine Monad (*Jiva*), it is called EGO or Man, and yet it is the *same* as the OTHER—the Angel, who incarnated in him, as the same with the universal MAHAT. It is that "something" in us that produces our "thoughts," e.g., a breath, a fire, ether, quintessence, slender likeness, intellection, a number, harmony – as observed by *Voltaire*, and the great classics and philosophers. In this and various other ways, Mind was endowed to the mankind.

Pitris have seven divisions or classes, three incorporeal or without forms (*Arupa*), and four corporeal or having forms (*Rupa*); and two kinds, the *Agnishvattas* and the *Barhishads*. Since the pitris are of two kinds, there could be a double and a triple set of each kind. According to *Manava-dharma-Sastra* (iii, 196), the Barhishads are the Pitris of the Demons or the corporeal beings. They gave birth to their astral doubles and then they were reborn as the Sons of *Atri*. The Agnishvattas are the pitris of the gods. They are reborn as the Sons of Marichi, who is a son of Brahmaa.

According to *Vayu Purana* the seven orders of pitris were originally the *first gods,* known as *Vairajas* and were beheld in the spiritual sky by Brahmaa through the eye of yoga. As mentioned in the *Vishnu Purana,* these *Vairajas* were the gods of the gods, and that the gods worshipped them. They were identified with the *elder Agnishvattas* and *Rajasas* (or *Abhutarajasas*), having no form at all. As said in *Vayu Purana,* the region inhabited by the Agnishvattas is called "Virajaloka." Virajaa is Brahma, and hence the *Arupa* (incorporeal or formless) Pitris, being the sons of Viraja, are called Vairajas. It is understood that Vishnu incarnated in and through them.

Another class of the sons of Viraja is called *Manasas,* with whom the Agnishvattas are ever associated, along with the Rajasas. Hari, best of gods, was born of *Sambhuti,* as the divine Manasa, originating with the deities called Rajasas in the Raivata Manvantara (*patriarchal* period). Sambhuti was a daughter of Daksha, and wife of Marichi, who was a son of Brahmaa and father of Agnishvattas. Thus *Manasas* and *Rajasas* are two classes that included the *Kumaras, Asuras,* and other rulers and *Pitris,* who incarnated in the third root race.

There is a great misunderstanding about thirty-three crores, or 330 millions of gods in India. In fact, they may be all "devas" but not "gods," in the high spiritual sense one attributes to them. It is an unfortunate blunder generally committed by Europeans. Deva is a kind of spiritual being, and since the same word is used in ordinary parlance to mean god, it does not mean that we have and worship 330 millions of gods.

Deities of a certain mystic class have different names in different manvantaras. Brahmaa created twelve great gods, called *Jayas,* to assist him in the work of creation in the very beginning of the Kalpa. These gods were lost in samadhi and neglected to create, and hence they were cursed to be repeatedly born in each manvantara till the seventh—they are known as *Ajitas, Tushitas, Satyas, Haris, Vaikunthas, Sadhyas*

The Creation of Universe and Man – Cosmic Evolution 161

and *Adityas*. According to *Vishnu Purana* (Vol. II, p. 226) these gods were known as *Tushitas* in the second Kalpa, and as *Adityas* in this *Vaivasvata* period. However, they are identical with the *Manasas* or *Rajasas*, and these with the incarnating Dhyani-Chohans. They belong to the class of *Jnana-devas* (knowledgeable gods). Besides Yakshas, Gandharvas, Kumaras and others of the kind inhabiting the astral plane, there are *Vairajas, Kumaras* and *Asuras* belonging to the class of *Jnana-devas*, called by Occultists as Manasvin, the wise and the foremost of all. These *Jnana-devas* would have made men *self-conscious* and spiritually intellectual beings, had they not been "cursed" to fall into generation, and to be reborn themselves as mortals for neglecting the duty of creating men.

Mind is the dividing point between the corporeal and incorporeal pitris, ancestors of men, who are so sacred that they are worshipped with offerings made to them by Brahmans whenever a son is born in the family. However, the pitris are not the ancestors of the present living men, but those of the great *human* races, which preceded our races of men, and were far superior to our present day pygmies, both physically and spiritually. Mind is a "thinker" as it comes from the Sanskrit word *man* (to think); which probably originated from the Latin *mens*, Egyptian *Menes*-Master Mind, and Pythagorean *Monas* or conscious "thinking unit." *Manas* or Mind is the *fifth* principle in man. Hence the shadows that are "mindless" are called *amanasa*. This dual group of the *seven classes* of progenitors or Pitris, divided by Mind, needs a philosophical explanation.

All *Puranas* are unanimous in saying that the three orders of pitris are *arupa* (formless), while four are *rupa* (with forms). The first group being intellectual and spiritual, the second devoid of intellect and material. Pitris of first group—born in the body of night—were called *Asuras*, while those of the second group were produced from the body of twilight. According to *Vayu Purana* the fathers of second group were gods, who were doomed to be born as fools on Earth. Although it is not clear whether these pitris were sons of gods, or of Brahmaa or instructors of their own fathers; since the legends are perhaps purposely mixed up; but certainly they were the creators of men on the seven divisions of earth. Pitris of the first group, although called "non-gods" (*asuras*) by Brahmans, were the highest *Breaths* (as called by the Occultists), who refused to build man, but endowed him with mind. The word *Asura* means "spiritual, divine" in *Rig Veda* and is used for the *three highest gods*—Varuna, Indra and Agni, before Brahmanical Theo-Mythology destroyed the true meaning of things in the Archaic Scriptures.

The Agnishvattas are the "Fire Dhyanis," who form the "Heart" of the Dhyani Chohanic Body, having incarnated in the Third Race of men, making them perfect. There is a mysterious relation between this angelic Heart and that of man, who is a reflection or copy of the model or prototype *above*, on the terrestrial plane *below*, in all the departments—physical, psychic and spiritual. It is therefore that the mystic number "seven" of the order of pitris is repeated in the anatomical structure of man. Human heart has *four lower* cavities and *three higher* divisions, i.e., a septenary division of human principles into two groups, the higher and lower, answering strangely to the same division of pitris (*three* incorporeal-higher and *four* corporeal-lower), and specially the Fire Dhyanis. The seven nervous plexuses of the body radiate seven rays. And, the human skin has seven distinct layers.

The progenitors projected their shadows and made man of one element (ether), then they reascend to Maharloka (Mental Plane), whence they descend periodically at the renewal of the world, to give birth to new men. The subtle bodies remained without understanding (Manas), until the Suras (Gods) now known as Asuras (not Gods) came into being.

Asura is the lord *Asura Visvavedas*, the all-knowing or omniscient lord in the Mazdean or Magian religion, as found in the *Zendavesta*. The Indo-Iranian "Asura" is sevenfold, and

The Creation of Universe and Man – Cosmic Evolution

combined with the name "Mazdha," it is the sevenfold Asura the Lord or Lords collectively—*Asura Mazdha*, later called *Ahura Mazdha*, who is the *bestower of intelligence*[45]. This connects the *Amshapendas* with Asuras and incarnating Dhyani Chohans, with Elohim, and the seven informing gods of Egypt, Chaldea, and all other countries.

Various cosmogonies have denounced the first and *mind-born* sons, the *Logoi*, for their refusal to create men, which was not because of their pride for not sharing the celestial power of their essence with the children of Earth, but for avoiding creating the "germ of sorrow." This was not understood by the later representatives of religion, who exaggerated the matter and used this excuse for obtaining hold over the people's mind. The intellectual group of Suras (gods) won over the non-intellectuals, who engaged themselves in "profitless ceremonial worship based on blind faith"—the fact, ignored by orthodox Brahmans—and immediately the former were declared *Asuras* (no-gods). Brahmaa cursed them to be repeatedly born as men. Christians degraded them as demons. Zoroastrians and Chaldeans denounced them as Spirits of Darkness. Ahriman destroyed the Bull created by Ormazd—the emblem of terrestrial *illusive* life and the germ of sorrow—and without understanding that the perishing finite seed must die for the plant of spiritual, eternal life to sprout and live, Ahriman was declared the enemy, the devil. Typhon cuts Osiris into fourteen pieces to prevent his peopling the world and thus creating misery, and Typhon was proclaimed as the Power of Darkness. In this way the worshippers of Form made demons of the Angels of Light, who showed men the way to regain their original status of divinity through *self-conscious* efforts.

The three *arupa* (formless) pitris, endowed with intelligence and not the elementary substance, were doomed by the law of karma and evolution to incarnate repeatedly on Earth. Some of these great ones came from the former Manvantaras, and their appearance on the globe was very useful for the multitudes, since these were *Nirmanakayas* (the builders). Accordingly, many of them appeared in the *third Manvantara* (third root race) as kings, rishis and heroes, as mentioned in all the *Puranas*. Aryan mystics concealed the truth (astronomical, physical and divine) under various allegories, after the destruction of Atlantean *giants* and *sorcerers*, since this tenet related to the *precosmic* theogony. This "fact" is not so easy to be grasped by the people in general, so the priesthood disfigured it and used it to keep a hold on the multitudes. Christians forgot their own highest Archangel, St. Michael having conquered the Dragon of Wisdom and of Divine self-sacrifice (mastering and assimilating the wisdom), who was the first to refuse to create, and was later miscalled and calumniated as Satan. Christian theologians could not understand the paradoxical language of the East and its symbolism, and there ensued endless confusion. *Willing* and *unwilling* angels or the *creators* and those who *refused to create*, were badly mixed up.

The four classes of pitris, or the pitar-devatas, those possessed of the physical creative fire, clothed human Monads (Jivas) with their own astral selves, and became the first race themselves, sharing its destiny and further evolution. These creating gods said, "Man must not be like one of us", as they would not since they could not, endow men with the spark of reason and self-consciousness. It is the other class of Devas, known as Prometheus in Greece, who were responsible for intelligence and spirituality in man, and had no concern with the physical body.

One class of Creators built external form of man, the other gave him its essence, which developed into human *Higher Self* due to his personal exertion. Sri Aurobindo called it the Psychic Being[46]. However, man could not be made perfect, because sinless, like its Creators, since he was destined to be created by material creators, who gave him what they had, and that is why the first-born had to refuse to do so. Following the eternal law, the first-born pure gods could project out of themselves only *shadowy* men, who were less ethereal and spiritual, and less *divine and perfect* than themselves, called shadows. Thus the first humans were a pale copy of its creators; even in their ethereality they were too material to belong to the hierarchy of gods, who were too spiritual and pure to be men, who had in them all the *negative* (Nirguna) perfections. There is neither light nor darkness in the realm of truth. Good and Evil are the twin produce of Space and Time under the effect of Maya, and hence they must coexist in order to come into being, each generated and created out of the other. Both must be known and appreciated before they can be perceived. Their division, therefore, was necessary for the mortal humans. And now, as *perfection* must grow out of imperfection, the *incorruptible* must be born out of corruptible, the latter has to be taken as the vehicle by men to arrive at the former.

If Adam and Eve are admitted to be ignorant of good and evil before the eating of the forbidden fruit of knowledge, how could they be expected to know that *disobedience was evil*? If omnipotent and perfect God created witless primeval human, then his creation was aimless and even cruel. "But Adam and Eve are shown, even in *Genesis*, to be created by a class of lower divine Beings, the *Elohim*, who are so jealous of their personal prerogatives as reasonable and intelligent creatures, that they will not allow man to become 'as one of us.' This is plane, even from the dead-letter meaning of the Bible. The Gnostics, then, were right in regarding the Jewish God as belonging to a class of lower, material and not very holy denizens of the invisible world[47]." Christian theology followed the Hebrew esoteric account of the creation of man, and could not explain a man devoid of mind being produced by God, the Creator, nor explain the punishment given to Adam and Eve for a supposed crime they did not commit.

The materialistic man was thus left to himself to achieve merit through struggle, and its creator were at the foot of the ladder of spiritual being. For the production of such wretched races, in a spiritual and moral sense, no high divinity could be made responsible, but only angels of a low hierarchy, to which class they regarded the Jewish God, Jehovah. Much before the laws of Moses, were the Gnostics, many of whom being Initiates, who held the "Mysteries of Life" in Nazara (ancient and modern Nazareth), and their doctrines are reflected in the teachings presented here.

Ancient Cosmogonies have mentioned mankind different from ours. Plato has spoken of a *winged race of men* in Phaedrus. I am pleasantly surprised to remember one of my lucid dreams in which I was at such a realm where winged people were living. People could walk or fly as they wished. Aristophanes talked about an androgynous race with round bodies. All the animal kingdoms mentioned in *Poimandres* are double-sexed[48]. In *Popol-Vuh* the first men are described as a race "whose sight was unlimited, and who knew all things at once," thus showing the *divine knowledge of Gods*, not mortals [49].

Various human races, called shadows, were born, each of his *own color and kind*, each also *inferior to his creator*, since the creator was a complete being of his kind. The Heavenly Man, according to *Poimandres*, created seven primitive men, all partaking the qualities of Seven *Governors* or Rulers, the former in this way being the reflection and synthesis of the latter. Same mystical lines and personifications are found in all well-known myths: *Vedas* and *Puranas*, Mazdean Scriptures and the Kabala. "Seven pillars of the world, its supports" of Scandinavian *Aesir*, seven Greek *Kosmokratores*, "Seven Workmen or Rectors" of *Poimandres*, the seven Rishis and Pitris of India, the seven Chaldean gods and seven evil spirits, the seven Kabalistic Sephiroth synthesized by the upper triad, and the seven Planetary Spirits of Christian mystics—all present identical mythical facts.

According to Scandinavian myth, *Aesir* slew the giant Ymir and from its remains he created the earth, the seas, the sky and the clouds, the whole visible world; and, the outer form of Man from the Askr or ash-tree. Lodur gave blood and bones to the Man; Odin endowed him with life and soul, and finally Honer furnished him with intellect (*manas*) and conscious senses. Issuing of the men of the generation of bronze, the Third Root-Race from the Hesiodic Ash-tree, and the creation of Quiche, *third* race of men from *Tzite* tree of the *Popul-Vuh*, are identical[50]. It is amazing to see the identity of Norse Yggdrasils, the Hindu Asvattha, the Gogard, the Mazdean tree of life, and the Tibetan Zampun, with the Kabalistic Sephirothal Tree, the Holy Tree made by Ahura Mazdha, and the Tree of Eden[51]. Moreover, the fruits of all these trees, call it *Pippala* or *Haoma* or the prosaic apple, are verily the "plants of life." It explains that the "prototypes of our races" were dormant in the microcosmic tree, which grew and developed within and under the great macrocosmic tree, and according to *Dirghatamas*, "Pippala, the sweet fruit of the tree upon which come *spirits who love the science*, and where the gods produce all marvels."

Among the luxuriant branches of all these mundane trees dwells the "Serpent", as observed in Gogard. The Serpents of the manifested Wisdom dwell in the microcosmic tree, which are the *reflections* of the Serpent of Eternity and of absolute Wisdom dwelling in the Macrocosmic tree. The dwelling serpents (conscious *Manas*) in the *tree* of Man are the connecting links between Spirit and Matter, or, Heaven and Earth. In recent years much research has been done on the "Serpents of Wisdom", see for example, *The Serpent Power*, by Sir John Woodroffe[52]. More prevalent name in the Eastern philosophy for "The Serpent Power" is "Kundalini," and a vast literature is available on this subject, see for example, the works by Gopi Krishna[53], Swami Satyananda Saraswati[54], Swami Sivananda Radha[55], and B.S.Goel[56]. My own books have appeared over the years[57, 58, 59, 60].

The gist of the matter coming through all the cosmogonies on earth is that the "lower group of Angels, the creators" produced Man but failed. The "higher group of Angels, the Logoi" attempted to endow Man with "conscious immortal spirit, reflected in Mind (*Manas*)" alone; they too failed and were punished to reincarnate on Earth repeatedly for the whole Manvantara. The orthodox priests in all religions took advantage of this and presented themselves as middle authorities to God, to keep a hold on people. The "fruit" of the Tree of Knowledge, the Serpent of Wisdom, or Kundalini remained *forbidden*, and the Voice of reason and consciousness remained associated with the Fallen Angels or Devil or Satan. The *Svastika*, the most sacred and mystic symbol in India, later called as "Jaina-Cross" by the Masons, not getting identified with the Christian Cross, was dishonored too. People forgot the great shining *Serpent* on the head of Vishnu (*eternal Deity*), the great seven-headed serpent called Shesha (*Ananta or* timeless*)* on which rested Vishnu, and the hood of *Serpents* on the head of great Egyptians.

The *Svastika* being the most philosophically scientific and comprehensible is found to head the symbols of most religions. In the *Chaldean Book of Numbers* it is the "Worker's Hammer" that strikes sparks from the flint (Space), which become the worlds. In Scandinavian myth it is "Thor's Hammer," used by the dwarfs against the Giants or the *precosmic* Titanic forces of Nature, and the former could not be subdued by the Gods. As "storm-hammer," Svastika or *Mjolner* helped in the purification of *Aiser* (holy gods), through passions and sufferings in their earthly incarnations, till the gods were fit to dwell in Ida in eternal space. And then the sons of Thor used *Mjolner,* not as a weapon of war, but as the hammer to consecrate the new heaven and the new earth[61].

The *Svastika* was born under the mystical conceptions of early Aryans, and was placed by them at the head of the Serpent Ananta (timeless), which is the very threshold of eternity. It shows from beginning to end the universal creative Force, evolving from pure Spirit and ending in gross Matter. It is the summary of the whole work of *creation*, from

The Creation of Universe and Man – Cosmic Evolution

Parabrahman to materialistic science. As "Hammer of Creation" in the Macrocosmic work, *Svastika* with its four arms bent at right angles, represents continual motion and revolution of invisible Kosmos, with all its Forces. On Earth it represents the rotation of world's axes and their equatorial belts in the cycles of Time. The two lines in the symbol represent Spirit and Matter, and the four hooks suggest the motion in the revolving cycles. The right hand being raised at the end of the horizontal arm points towards heaven, and the downward hand at the left points towards Earth. In this way, Man is shown to be a link between Heaven and Earth. The upward and downward arms are inscribed with the letters *Solve* and *Coagula* on the *Smaragdine Tablet* of Hermes. Thus *Svastika* is an Alchemical, Cosmogonical, Anthropological, and magical sign at the same time and contains the key to the seven great mysteries of Cosmos. However, the scholastic interpretations of medieval Anthropomorphists have brought the spiritual death of the most suggestive symbol of all. "It is also the key to the cycle of Science, divine and human; and he who comprehends its full meaning is forever liberated from the toils of *Mahamaya*, the great Illusion and Deceiver. The light that shines from under the divine hammer, now degraded into the mallet or gravel of the Grand Masters of Masonic Lodges, is sufficient to dissipate the darkness of any human schemes or fictions[62]."

Teachings of archaic wisdom are found in the prophetic songs of the three Norse Goddesses, as summarized by Dr. W. Wagner in his *Asgard and the Gods,* which tells about the seventh Race of our Round that is yet to come. Adam and Eve will climb up higher, to rise in knowledge and wisdom, in piety and deeds of love, step by step, from one heaven to another, until they become fit to be united with divinities in the house of Alfather. The same allegorical message can be found in the Esoteric *Buddhism* (or Wisdom), and in the myth of Prometheus, examined in the light of Hindu *Pramantha*. Divine *Agni* (fire) with the Sanskrit speaking race, becoming *Ignis* with the Latins, was born from the conjunction of

Pramantha and Arani (Svastika) during the sacrificial ceremony. According to Adalbert Kuhn, this process of kindling fire naturally led man to the idea of sexual reproduction. In the *Rig Veda*, Visvakarman is the highest and the oldest of the Gods and their Father, and he is the *architect* or *carpenter* of the universe. Light begins to dawn even upon the materialists. So ancient and sacred is the symbol of *Svastika* that it was found under the ruins of the ancient city of Troy, showing that ancient Trojans and their ancestors were pure Aryans.

The Hermetic narrative and the allegories of Greek Prometheus corroborate *Poimandres* in that the "Heavenly Man," the "Son of the Father," who partook of the nature and essence of the Seven Governors, or *creators* and *rulers* of the material world, "peeped through the *Harmony*, and breaking through the *"Seven Circles of Fire,"* made manifest the downward born Nature[63]. It also explains the "Wars in Heaven", the Christian dogma of the *fallen angels*, and casting of the "rebels" into the depths of Hell, i.e., matter[64].

George Smith comments on an engraving on an early Babylonian cylinder of the sacred Tree, the Serpent, man and woman. There are seven branches of the tree, of which *three* are towards man, and *four* are towards woman—representing the seven root-races. It is towards the end of the *third* root-race that the separation of the sexes took place, and the so-called fall into generation began. The first three races were sexless, then hermaphrodite; and the later four were "male and female," distinct from each other. In the Chaldean account of Creation, the Dragon leads man to sin. The Dragon is the creature of Tiamat, the living principle of the sea and of chaos, which opposed the deities on the creation of the world[65], which appears to be wrong, as observed by George Smith. In fact, Dragon is an *animalised* male principle or Phallus personified; and Tiamat is the female principle or womb, as an "embodiment of the spirit of chaos" or of the deep or Abyss. The Spirit of chaos and disorder implies mental perturbation. The sensual, attractive and magnetic principle fascinates and seduces the "ever living active element," which throws the whole world into disorder, chaos and sin. It can be said that the Serpent seduced the woman, or the latter seduced the former, and both are included in the Karmic curse. However, the act of seducement is only the cause producing the natural result.

Genesis being younger, does not have complete accounts of the happenings, which are to be found in the older Chaldean fragments. George Smith observed that the gods (Elohim) could not bear the man of clay becoming a Creator. They became jealous and invoked all the evils that afflict humanity, on the head of the human race. They doomed man through being injured by the wisdom and knowledge, leading to family quarrels, to be disappointed in desires, to anger the gods and submit to tyranny, to make useless prayers and to commit future sin.

The "Father" of primitive physical man (his body) is the vital electric principle residing in the Sun. The "Mother" is Moon, who mysteriously influences human gestation and generation, which is regulated like the growth of plants and animals. The "Wind" or Ether, called the "nurse," transmits those influences from the two luminaries and diffuses them upon Earth. Finally it is "Spiritual Fire" that makes man divine and a perfect entity. In alchemy "Hydrogen" is the Spiritual Fire, while in esoteric philosophy it is the Ray emanated from its *noumenon*, and it is gas only on our terrestrial plane. Hydrogen is allied to *protyle*, and is the only existing form of matter in the *laya* state between the manvantaras or rounds. It is the "material" emanation from the "subjective" and purely spiritual entitative Being in the region of *noumena*. Our *five physical senses* are the progenies of the Elements "Water, Fire and Air," which are not directly hydrogen, but they are all generated by it. Thus hydrogen is "three in one," and there is a direct (occult) connection between our senses and these three elements.

All ancient beings taught the secrets of these "Fires" in their Mysteries. Kabiri, the most arcane of all the ancient deities, gods and men, great deities and Titans, are identical with the Kumaras and Rudras headed by Kartikeya, who is a Kumara himself. Kabiri and these Hindu deities were the personified sacred fires of the most occult powers of Nature. Aryan Race, whether Hindu or Greek, in Asia or in Europe, tried to conceal the true nature of these deities. It is uncertain whether the Kabiris or Kumaras were four or seven. However, the four Kabiris—Axiokersos, Axieros, Axiokersa, and Casmilos are identical with the four Kumaras—Sanat, Sananda, Sanaka and Sanatana. Vulcan and Brahmaa were the Fathers of these two sets of deities. Flame of the Wrath of Brahmaa created Rudra or Nilalohita (Siva). However, these are all correlative Forces and Fires, and hence one. Students with personal intuition can understand these mysteries, which can never be described in full. Alchemists and Occultists have rightly connected fire with every element. The ancients always wanted religion, natural sciences and philosophy to grow inseparably with each other. Our five physical senses pertain even to a lower creation than Pratisarga (secondary creation) of Puranas.

Vach (the Voice) is the female *Logos* of Brahmaa, a permutation of Aditi, "primordial light," in *Purana*. Bath Kol is the daughter of the *Divine Voice* or "primordial light", Shekinah, in the Kabala. Vach was called the "Mother of the Vedas," who entered into the Rishis and inspired them through her revelations. In the same way, Bath Kol inspired the prophets of Israel and Jewish High Priests. In Jewish mysticism, Bath Kol is an articulate preternatural voice from heaven, which revealed the sacred traditions and laws only to the "chosen people." Both exist today in their respective symbologies. Ancients associated sound or speech with Ether of space, of which sound is the characteristic. Thus Fire, Water and Air are the primordial Cosmic Trinity. "I am thy Thought, thy God, more ancient than the moist principle, the *light that radiates within Darkness* (Chaos), and the shining Word of God (Sound) is the Son of the Deity."[66]

"The opponents of Hinduism may call the above Pantheism, Polytheism, or anything they may please. If science is not entirely blinded by prejudice, it will see in this account a profound knowledge of natural sciences and physics, as well as of metaphysics and psychology. But to find this out, one has to study the personifications, and then convert them into chemical atoms. It will then be found to satisfy both physical and purely materialistic *Science*, as well as those who see in evolution the work of the 'Great Unknown Cause' in its phenomenal and illusive aspects[67]."

Evolution of the elements and the senses; or the heavenly and mortal physical man, had the following order on parallel lines[68]:

TABLE 2

Evolution of Elements and Senses

1.	Ether	. .	Hearing	. .	Sound
2.	Air	. .	Touch	. .	Sound and Touch
3.	Fire, or Light		Sight	. .	Sound, Touch and Color
4.	Water		Taste	. .	Sound, Touch, Color and Taste
5.	Earth		Smell	. .	Sound, Touch, Color, Taste and Smell

It can be observed that each element adds its own characteristics to those of its predecessor, as each Root-Race adds the characterizing sense of the preceding race. Thus the first race did not have the element of *fire* as yet. The evolution of creative and sentient principles in the gods and even of the creative deity and everything else proceeded from *Prabhavapyaya*. Accordingly, Vishnu was first called as *Purvaja* (pregenetic) and then the other names connect him in their descending order more and more with matter.

Gods or Devas (Dhyani Chohans) proceeded from the First Cause, called *Jagat Yoni* (the womb of the world), and then mankind emanated from these active agents in Cosmos. The first and second races were not physical beings but *Bhutas*, which proceeded from the original place wherefrom the elements sprang. Everything proceeds from and resolves in *Prabhavapyaya*. Even Brahma (Logos), Isvara or Purusha is manifested deity, and hence created, or limited and conditioned. Only Parabrahman, the unknowable ALL CAUSE, is beyond any limitation or conditioning whatsoever.

The first to proceed from Parabrahman and Mulaprakriti is *incognizable,* eternal Brahma (neuter or abstract), the *Pundarikaksha* (having eyes like a lotus, heart-pervading, supreme and imperishable). He has first *Sadaika Rupa* (changeless or immutable) nature, later he is addressed *Ekaneka Rupa* (both single and manifold). The cause becomes merged with his own effects; and esoterically his names have the following descending order[69]:

1. Mahapurusha or Paramatman – Supreme Spirit
2. Atman or Purvaja (Protologos) – The Living Spirit of Nature
3. Indriyatman or Hrishikesha – Spiritual or Intellectual Soul (One with the senses)
4. Bhutatman – The Living or Life Soul
5. Kshetrajna – Embodied Soul, or the Universe of Spirit and Matter.
6. Bhrantidarshanah – False perception—Material Universe.

The last name—false perception, means the erroneous apprehension of material universe, which, in fact, is illusion or *Maya*.

The evolution of the "essences" of Dhyani Chohans (Devas), in both the spiritual and material worlds, takes place in strict analogy with the attributes of Brahma. The characteristics of these "essences" are reflected in their turn, in *Man*, collectively, and in each of his principles. Furthermore, every one of his principles contains a portion of various *"fires"* and *elements* of the "essences," in the same progressive order.

CHAPTER 4

THE LIBERATION OF MAN

I would like to present here four profound methods or steps of liberation as presented by (1) Blavatsky, based on the synthesis of most of the popular religions on the face of Earth, (2) Swami Sri Yukteswar, Guru of Swami Yogananda Paramahansa, (3) Srimad Bhagavata Mahapurana, (4) Swami Prabhupad, founder of the Hare Krishna movement or the International Society of Krishna Consciousness. It would be seen that though the processes appear to be on some different grounds, yet the steps provided for liberation from the clutches of maya or illusion, and the results obtained therein, amount to be the same. Autobiography in Chapter 1 presents my own story as a corroboration of the steps shown by the four major traditions here.

Blavatsky

As seen earlier, physical nature's unaided attempts failed to construct a perfect animal leave alone the creation of man. The Fathers (Lower Angels) are all Nature-Spirits and the higher elementals possessed intelligence of their own, which was not enough to create a "thinking man." A *Living Fire* that could give self-perception and self-consciousness (*Manas*) to the human mind was needed. This explains the difference between the "informing principle in man"—the Higher Self or human monad—and the animal monad; the former endowed with *divine* intelligence, the latter having only the *instinctual* faculty, although both are one and the same. Those few men, in whom the "divine *Rebels*" incarnated themselves, possessed the "Higher Self", while others had only the "spark" thrown into them, which quickened their fifth principle. This accounts for the great difference between the intellectual capacities of men and races. However, it is that "spark" of intelligence (*Manas*) thrown into the *Manushyas* (men), which made them skip the intermediate worlds, in their impulse towards intellectual freedom, and attain their ultimate goal through self-exertion. Otherwise, the animal man would never have reached upwards from this earth. He would have performed the cyclic pilgrimage through all the planes of existence half unconsciously, if that "spark" was not given. The animals, not having that "spark," have to entirely go through that pilgrimage.

Thus, the rebels are our saviours, as they gave us intelligence or *Manas*, because of which we rebelled against the morbid inactivity of pure spirit. This made us self-conscious, thinking men, with the capabilities and attributes of Gods in us, both for good and for evil. It is the attractive force of the contrasts that the two opposites—Spirit and Matter—coexist on Earth and are felt in the self-conscious experiences and sufferings all the time.

According to Hermes in his *Tabula Smaragdina*, the Father of Man is the Sun, the Mother is Moon, the Wind is the carrier, the Spirituous Earth is the nurse, and the Spiritual Fire is its instructor or Guru. This fire is the "Higher Self" or spiritual ego that incarnates eternally under the influence of its lower personal selves, changing with every rebirth, full of *tanha* or desire to live. It is unfortunate that on the terrestrial plane the higher (Spiritual) Nature is in bondage to the lower. The personal ego may continue to goad the spiritual ego to the bitter end, until and unless the Spiritual Ego takes refuge in Atman, the All-spirit, and merges entirely into the essence thereof. All this can be properly understood only when the three wings of the mystery of evolution—spiritual, psychic and physical—are made familiar.

There are two factors that force evolution and propel Man to grow and develop towards perfection: firstly, the Monad (Jiva) – one that acts in Man unconsciously through a force inherent in itself and, secondly, the lower astral body or the *personal* Self. The former is inherently endowed with the "force" that is identical with the All-force. That very "force" in the Monad, which may also be imprisoned in a vegetable or animal body, is all-potent on the *Arupa* or formless plane. On the terrestrial plane it becomes inactive, just as the rays of sun do not select this or that plant, but wherever they fall upon, they bring growth of vegetation. In the same way, unless the Higher Self or Ego gravitates towards its Sun—the Universal Atman—the lower *Ego* or *personal* Self will continue to have the upper hand in every case. According to Buddha in *Dhammapada* (p. 153 and 154), it is this Ego with its fierce selfishness and animal desire, which is the maker of tabernacle, and makes man live a senseless life (*Tanha*).

Spirits of earth or astral selves built human body in which dwells the monad with its conscious principle – Manas. Atman alone warms the inner man, enlightens it with the ray of divine life, and imparts immortality to the reincarnating ego. Thus in the first three and a half root races, up to the middle or turning point, the astral shadows of the lunar *pitris* built physical form towards perfection, at the cost of a proportionate loss of spirituality. From this turning point onwards the Higher Ego reigns over the animal ego, and rules it whenever the latter does not carry it down. In other words, spirituality is on the ascending arc now. However, "selfishness" has so strongly infected the *inner man* with its *lethal virus*, that the upward attraction has lost its power on the "thinking reasonable man," and it impedes the steadily progressing evolution. Perhaps mankind was never so wicked, selfish and vicious than it is now. The proof can be seen in the civilized nations, where ethical character has more importance than art.

It is only in the human form that the Souls can progress spiritually, whereas the angels are "intransitive" by nature; man therefore has the potency to transcend the faculties of angels. This is the reason that souls "descend from air to be *chained to bodies*"[1]. According to Judaeus, "The air is full of Souls, *they descend to be tied to mortal bodies, being desirous to live in them*"[2]. Initiates in India believe that Brahman, the twice-born, rules the gods or devas. St. Paul said that, "Know ye not that we (the Initiates) shall judge angels[3]." New Testament proved that Jesus believed in rebirth and repeated reincarnations (till spiritual perfection is achieved).

Man initially evolved as a *luminous incorporeal form*, over which the lower forms and types of animal terrestrial life built the physical frame of his body. According to Zohar, "the Soul and the Form when descending on earth put on an earthly garment." Men were created as shadows by the *Devas* out of their own astral bodies. It is believed in the East that *Devas* have no shadows of their own. According to evolutionary law the Devas or Fathers as Monads were made to pass through all the forms of life and being on Earth and they were in "human form with divine nature" by the end of the Third Round. Yoga (union with Brahmaa) being the supreme condition of the passive though infinite Devas, they were called the "Sons of Yoga," or as by Tibetans, "Sons of Dhyana" since this condition of Yoga or Dhyana is the essence of Brahmaa. It contained all the divine energies including the creation of everything through the power of Yoga. According to Puranic text Brahma (Neuter) created the most powerful energies of God-Brahmaa, Vishnu and Siva as creator, sustainer and destroyer. "All the creatures in the world have each a superior above. This superior, whose inner pleasure it is *to emanate into them*, cannot impart efflux until they have adored"—i.e., meditated as during Yoga[4]. According to *Bhagavad Gita*, Brahmaa made it very clear to Narada that all men whatsoever might know the true nature of Vasudeva and learn to have faith in that deity.

An impenetrable veil of secrecy was thrown over the occult and religious truth taught after the submersion of the last remnant of the Atlantean race, some 12000 years ago, lest they should be shared by the unworthy, and so desecrated[5]. This is the reason that most of the sciences have become exoteric, e.g., astronomy, which has now only mathematical and physical aspect. Their dogmas and tenets are forgotten and the meaning is perverted. Yet, however, there is unanimous agreement between the scriptures of different nations, e.g., hermaphrodites and same trinity are found in all traditions. The secrecy led the Fifth Race to reestablish the religious mysteries and teach the ancient truths to new generations through veil of allegories. Divine wisdom had to incarnate on earth and go through the pain and suffering of personal experiences.

"It is worth noting that a sudden upsurge of various religious leaders took place around the world in or around the sixth century B.C. Confucious of China was born in 551 B.C. Buddha of India was born in 563 B.C., Pythagoras of Greece was born in 590 B.C., and Taoism was born in China with the birth of Lao Tzu in 604 B.C. Although born in the seventh century B.C., Lao Tzu reportedly lived for 200 years, meaning thereby that his impact was seen in sixth century B.C. Zoroaster of Persia existed in the sixth century B.C. Mahavir, the founder of Jain religion in India, was born in the sixth century B.C., and the Druids, the priestly caste of Celts, a Germanic tribe which spread in Europe and Asia Minor, came up in the sixth and fifth century B.C. This was no ordinary happening. Perhaps the Universal Mind wanted humanity on Earth to start the search for God. Since then the spiritual avatars like Jesus, Pluto, Plutonius, Socrates, Plato, Mohammed, Nanak, and hundreds of lesser-known personalities like Richard Maurice Bucke and Gopi Krishna have emerged in the recent years. Thousands of people around the globe have been getting enlightenment and the numbers are increasing [6]."

No entity, whether angelic or human, can reach the state of Nirvana, or of absolute purity, except through aeons of suffering and the *knowledge* of Evil as well as good, as otherwise the latter remains incomprehensible[7].

Man—*a god in animal form*—cannot be the product of material nature by evolution alone. Intellectual potentialities of man and animal differ vastly, as the Sun does from the glow worm. Man is an animal *plus a living god*. There is *divine* man within the earthly man. Purely and transcendentally spiritual conceptions are adapted only to the perceptions of those who "see without eyes, hear without ears, and sense without organs." *Puranas* have hinted at the dual creation of man. A similar concept is seen in the Bible, *Genesis* and *Epistles* of Paul. In the *Genesis,* Elohim is referred to as "Lord God" or Gods (the Lords) in plural: one of them makes the earthly Adam of dust, the other breaths into him the breath of life, and the third makes of him a *living soul* (ii, 7). According to Paul, "The first man is of the earth, earthly: the second [the last or rather highest] is from heaven[8]. " Thus man is a god in the making, he only needs the right way to do it.

The astral through Kama (desire) is ever drawing Manas down into the sphere of material possession and desires. But if the *better* man or *Manas* tries to escape the fatal attraction and turns its aspirations to Atman—Spirit—then Buddhi (Ruah) conquers, and carries Manas with it to the realm of eternal Spirit[9].

Directly or indirectly most religions have embodied the doctrine regarding the ring "Pass-Not" guarded by the Lipikas (celestial recorders), which has to be crossed before the Truth can dawn. According to the Vedantin sect of the Vishishtadvaita in India the soul gets released and achieves Moksha (liberation, a state of bliss) only when one is released from the "bandhan" (bondage). The *Jiva* or Soul, at the time of physical death, arrives at a place called Paramapada, which is not material, but made of Suddhasatva or the essence with which the body of Isvara or Lord is formed. The Jivatmans or Monads who have achieved Moksha by becoming Mukta (free) are no more subject to the qualities of either matter or Karma. However, if for the sake of doing good to the people on Earth, they choose to incarnate on Earth, they can do so voluntarily. The Jiva in its *Sukshma sarira* or subtle body traverses the central-nerve Sushumna and breaks through the Brahmarandhra or Head Centre. It then arrives at Paramapada through the path called Devayana, guided by the Supreme Wisdom acquired through Yoga. Nevertheless, there are innumerable Adhivahikas (bearers in transit, certain pure souls), e.g. Archis and Prajapatis, who aid the *jivas* in their spiritual journey.

The barrier Pass-Not, which is created by the "celestial-recorders" between personal Ego and impersonal Self, or between descending monads for incarnation and ascending men for purification, or between the finite and truly Infinite is broken only when the individual becomes a "twice-born", i.e. an Initiate. The hierarchy of angels or devas welcomes such souls and calls it the day "Be-With-Us." Egyptians used to call it the "Day Come-To-Us." It could better be called "Rest-With-Us," because it refers to that long period of "Rest" which is called Paranirvana. "The 'Monad,' born of the nature and the very Essence of the 'seven' (its highest principle becoming immediately enshrined in the Seventh Cosmic Element), has to perform its septenary gyration throughout the Cycle of Being and forms, from the *highest to the lowest*; and then again *from man to God*. At the threshold of Paranirvana it resumes its primeval essence and becomes the Absolute once more[10]."

Swami Sri Yukteswar

Swami Sri Yukteswar[11] wrote *The Holy Science* independent of any scriptures, through his own experiences of realization of Truth. He first wrote his own teachings in Sanskrit poetry, given in bold letters, and then from the Bible in English verse, given in *italics*, confirming the facts between Hindu and Christian traditions. My own comments and clarifications follow this after every verse. A masterpiece of work by him is presented here in brief for the purpose of this book.

Parabrahman (Spirit or God) is everlasting, complete, without beginning or end. It is one, indivisible Being.

Now faith is the substance of things hoped for, the evidence of things not seen (Hebrews 11:1).

Then said Jesus unto them, When ye have lifted up the son of man, then shall ye know that I am he (John 8:28).

The author means to say that the real substance, *Sat*, is Eternal Father, God or Parabrahman, whose properties are "sound, touch, sight, taste, and smell." Man identifying himself with material body made of these properties comprehends only the properties and not *Sat*, which is possible only when man becomes divine by lifting himself above the creation of darkness, illusion or *maya*.

In It (Parabrahman) is the origin of all knowledge and love, the root of all power and joy. *So God created man in his own image, in the image of God created he him; male and female created he them* (Genesis 1:27).

Sakti (Eternal Joy or *Ananda*), the producer of the world, and *Chit* (Omniscient feeling) making this world conscious, demonstrate *Prakriti*, the Nature of God, the Father. As man is the likeness of God, directing his attention inward he can comprehend within him the said force and feeling, the sole properties of his Self—the Force Almighty as his will, *Vasana*, with enjoyment, *Bhoga*; and the Feeling Omniscient as his consciousness, *Chetana*, that enjoys, *Bhokta*. This is the way man can comprehend God.

Parabrahman causes creation, inert Nature (Prakriti), to merge. From Aum (Pranava, the Word, the manifestation of the Omnipotent Force), come kala (time), desa (space), and anu (atom), the vibratory structure of creation.

These things saith the Amen, the faithful and true witness, the beginning of the creation of God (Revelation 3:14).

In the beginning was the Word, and the Word was God...All things were made by him; and without him was not anything made that was made.....And the Word was made flesh and dwell among us *(John 1:1, 3, 14)*.

Aum, Amen or Word is the beginning of the Creation. Repulsion and Attraction (Omniscient Feeling or Love) is the Omnipotent Force that manifests as vibration appearing as a peculiar sound called Aum, Amen or Word. Idea of change (Time or *kala*) and idea of division (Space or *Desa*) are the other aspects of aum, although truth is ever-unchangeable and ever-indivisible. Thus the Word, Time, Space and Atom are one and the same and mere ideas. His own self or the eternal nature of the Almighty Father manifests as word, aum or amen; and it is inseparable from and nothing but God Himself. One can understand this from the fact that the burning power is inseparable from and nothing but the fire itself.

The cause of creation is *Anu* or Atoms. Enmasse they are called *Maya* or the Lord's illusory power; each individual *anu* is called *avidya*, ignorance.

And in the midst of the throne, and round about the throne were four beasts full of eyes before and behind. (Revelation 4:6)

The four ideas—Word, Time, Space and the Atom—are represented by the Atoms, which are the throne of Spirit, the Creator, which shining on them creates the universe. Collectively the Atoms are called *maya* or darkness or illusion since they keep the Spiritual Light out of comprehension. Furthermore, since the process of reflection on Atoms makes man ignorant even of his own Self, each Atom is called *avidya* or ignorance. It is for this reason that these four ideas giving rise to all kinds of confusions are called the "four beasts" in the *Bible*. As long as man identifies himself with the material body he is inferior to the four ideas and is unable to understand this fact. As soon as he raises himself to the level above, he comprehends the Atom-inside and outside as well as the whole creation – manifested and unmanifested (before and behind).

The Omniscient Love aspect of Parabrahman is *Kutastha Chaitanya*. The individual Self, being Its manifestation, is one with It.

"In him was life; and the life was the light of men."

"And the light shineth in darkness; and the darkness comprehended it not."

"He came unto his own, and his own received him not." (John 1:4, 5, 11)

Attraction, the Omniscient Love (Premabijam Chit) is Life, the Omniscient Holy Spirit called the **Holy Ghost**, Kutastha Chaitanya or Purushottama that shines on Maya, Illusion or Darkness and attracts every part of it towards Divinity. However, Repulsion, Avidya, Ignorance, Darkness, Maya or its individual parts (present in men) are unable to either receive or comprehend the Spiritual Light, but reflect it. The Omniscient Nature of Eternal Father, God manifests as the Holy Ghost and is nothing but God Himself in substance. Therefore the "reflections" of Spiritual Rays are called the **Sons of God** or Abhasa Chaitanya or Purusha.

The Atom, under the influence of Chit (universal knowledge) forms the Chitta or the calm state of mind, which when spiritualized is called Buddhi (Intelligence). Its opposite is manas (mind), in which lives the jiva (the self) with ahamkara (ego), the idea of separate existence.

Like the iron filings getting magnetized in a magnetic field, the atom, *avidya* or ignorance gets spiritualized under the influence of universal love, *chit*, the holy spirit. Spiritualized Atom together with the consciousness or the power of feeling becomes *Chitta*, the Heart called Mahat. The idea of separate existence now appears in it that is known as *Ahamkar* (Ego), which is the "son of man." Spiritualized Atom has two poles that demonstrate attraction and repulsion, respectively. The former attracts the atom towards the real substance, *Sat*, and it is called *Sattwa* or *Buddhi*, the Intelligence that determines what is Truth. The latter repels the atom from *Sat*, and produces the ideal world for *ananda* or enjoyment and is called *Anandatwa* or *Manas*, the Mind.

Chitta, the spiritualized Atom, in which *Ahamkara* (the idea of separate existence of Self) appears, has five manifestations (aura electricities).

They (the five aura electricities) constitute the causal body of *Purusha*.

The five electricities, *Pancha Tattwa*, from their three attributes, *Gunas—Sattwa* (positive), *Rajas* (neutralizing), and *Tamas* (negative)—produce *Jnanendriyas* (organs of sense), *Karmendriyas* (organs of action) and *Tanmatras* (objects of sense).

These fifteen attributes plus mind and intelligence constitute the seventeen "fine limbs" of the subtle body, the *Lingasarira*.

The Repulsion part of *Chitta* produces five sorts of aura electricities from its five different parts—middle, two extremities and spaces intervening between the middle and the two extremities. These electricities are attracted towards *Sat* under the influence of Universal Love or the Holy Ghost, and produce a magnetic field called *Sattwa Buddhi* or Intelligence. Being the Root Causes of all creations, these five electricities are called *Pancha Tattwa* and constitute the "causal body" of *Purusha*, the Son of God. The five electricities, because of being in the polarized state as *Chitta*, also possess the three Gunas or attributes—Sattwa (positive), Rajas (neutralizing) and Tamas (negative)—of the *Chitta*.

Now the satisfaction of the desires of the heart takes place through the five senses: smell, taste, sight, touch and hearing. For this, three kinds of mechanisms of the five electricities have to work in unification—the positive attributes or the five organs of senses, called *Jnanendriyas*, working under the influence of *Manas* or Mind; the neutralizing attributes or the five organs of action, called *Karmendriyas*-excretion, generation, motion (feet), manual skill (hands), and speech – working under the influence of the life force or *prana;* and the negative attributes or the five objects of senses, called *Tanmatras*. Thus the idea for satisfaction first generates in Mind through five *Jnanendriyas*, then the action takes place through five *Karmendriyas,* and lastly the satisfaction takes place through five *Tanmatras.* Five Jnanendriyas constitute the body of the *Manas* or Mind, and five Karmendriyas constitute the body of the Energy or *Prana.* These fifteen attributes together with two poles – Mind and Intelligence constitute the fine material body or subtle body of *Purusha* (the Son of God), called *Sukshmasarira* or *Lingasarira.*

The aforesaid five objects, which are the negative attributes of the five electricities, being combined produce the idea of gross matter in its five forms: *Kshiti,* solids; *Ap,* liquids; *Tejas,* fire; *Marut,* gaseous substances; and *Akasa,* ether.

These five forms of gross matter and the aforesaid fifteen attributes together with *manas* (mind, sense consciousness), *buddhi* (discriminative intelligence), *chitta* (the heart or the power of feeling) and *ahankara* (the ego), constitute the twenty-four basic principles of creation.

And round about the throne were four and twenty seats; and upon the seats I saw four and twenty elders. (Revelation 4:4)

The five negative attributes of the five electricities—solid, liquid, fire, gaseous substance and ether—constitute the gross material body of *Purusha* (the Son of God), which is the outer covering called *Sthulasarira.* The twenty-four principles that completed the creation of Darkness or *Maya* are simply the development of *Avidya* or Ignorance. As mentioned earlier, this Ignorance is made of the four ideas: the Word, Time, Space and Atom. Therefore the creation has no substantial existence in reality and it is merely the play of ideas on the eternal substance *Sat* or God, the Father.

This universe is differentiated into fourteen spheres, seven *swargas* and seven *patals.*

And being turned, I saw seven golden candlesticks, and in the midst of the seven candlesticks one like unto the son of man...

And he had in his right hand seven stars...

The seven stars are the angels of the seven churches; and the seven candlesticks which thou sawest are the seven churches. (Revelation 1:12, 13, 16, 20)

The Liberation of Man

The whole universe beginning with *Sat* or God, down to the gross material creation is divided into seven different spheres called *swargas* or *lokas* or realms, as follows.

7th Sphere—*Satyaloka*: The highest of all is the sphere of *Sat*, God, which is indescribable, has no designation and is Nameless, and hence called *Anama*.

6th Sphere—*Tapoloka*: The division of the Holy Spirit that remains undisturbed by any limited ideas, and hence called Eternal Patience. Since it is "inaccessible" even to the Sons of God, it is called *Agama*.

5th Sphere—*Janaloka*: The realm of spiritual reflection, the Sons of God, originating the idea of separate existence of Self. Since no one in the creation of *Maya* or Darkness can comprehend it, it is called Incomprehensible or *Alakshya*.

4th Sphere—*Maharloka*: It is the division where Atom is created, upon which the Spirit is reflected, which gives rise to the creation of *Maya* or Darkness. Since this is the only link between the spiritual and material worlds, it is called the 10th Door or *Dasmadwara*. The significance of the door being tenth is that when the first nine doors in man (two eyes, two ears, two nostrils, one mouth, one opening of the generative organ, and one opening of the execrative portion) are closed, only then the tenth door can open.

3rd Sphere—*Swarloka*: This is the realm of magnetic aura, in which all the creation (including organs and their objects, and the fine material things) are absent, is the Great Vacuum, called *Mahasunya*.

2nd Sphere—*Bhuvarloka*: This division of electric attributes where only the fine matters are present and no gross matters of creation are found is said to be Ordinary Vacuum, called *Sunya*.

1st Sphere—*Bhuloka*: The lowest division of gross material creation that everyone can see and experience.

I have described my own experiences with the *Sunya* or vacuum in Chapter 1.

Since God created man in his own image, so the body of the man is also reflecting the universe in the form of seven divisions called *Patalas* or Churches, according to the *Bible*. There are "seven vital places" called *Chakras* in the body of the man where he perceives Spiritual Light while advancing in the right way towards the realization of his Self. Seven *Swargas* and seven *Patalas* constitute fourteen distinguishable stages of the creation, called the fourteen *bhuwans*. *Purusha* is covered by five *koshas* or sheaths.

Anandamaya Kosha: The first sheath that covers the Spiritualized Atom, called *Purusha* or the Son of God is *Chitta* or Heart, the Atom composed of the four ideas—the Word, time, Space and Atom—that feels and enjoys, and is the seat of *Ananda* or bliss.

Jnanamaya Kosha: The second covering is *Buddhi* or Intelligence that manifests as magnetic-aura electricities and is responsible for the determination of the truth. It is the seat of *jnana* or knowledge.

Manomaya Kosha: The third is the body of *Manas* or Mind composed of the organs of senses, as described earlier.

Pranamaya Kosha: The fourth is the body of *Prana* or life force, composed of the organs of action, as described earlier.

Annamaya Kosha: The fifth is gross matter, the outer covering of Atom that becomes *Anna* or food that nourishes and supports the visible world.

The creation of man with five sheaths is the completion of the manifestation of the Omnipotent Energy as the act of Repulsion from *Sat*. With the act of Repulsion being thus completed, the act of Attraction towards *Sat* now begins with the manifestation of the Omnipotent Love at the centre of the Heart. The Atoms begin to get attracted towards one another and by getting closer and closer they begin to assume ethereal, gaseous, fiery, liquid and solid forms. Thus begins the world of gross matter on earth.

First formation is that of the planetary system with suns, moons and various planets called the *Inanimate Kingdom*.

With the development of the Divine Love in this manner, the evolution of *Avidya*, *Maya* or Ignorance, which too is the manifestation of the Omnipotent Energy, reduces gradually and is withdrawn. With the withdrawal of the outer coating of gross matter around the Atom, called *Annamaya Kosha,* the next sheath made of *Karmendriyas* or the organs of action, called *Pranamaya Kosha,* comes in operation. Atoms embrace each other in this organic state and get more close to their hearts. This gives rise to the *Vegetable Kingdom* on Earth.

Next stage is the appearance of the sheath made of the *Jnanendriyas* or the organs of sense called *Manomaya Kosha,* when the *Pranamaya Kosha* is withdrawn. As a result the Atoms perceive the external world. Atoms of different nature attract one another and form bodies that are required for sensual enjoyment. In this way the *Animal Kingdom* is born.

At the withdrawal of the *Manomaya Kosha* the body of Intelligence made of electricities called *Jnanamaya Kosha* is perceived. The Atom now acquires the faculty of determination of the right and wrong. A rational being called *man* is thus created.

As the development continues and whenever the man is able to cultivate the Divine Spirit or Omniscient Love in his heart, after the withdrawal of the *Jnanamaya Kosha,* the innermost sheath made of four ideas known as *Chitta* or Heart comes to appearance. It is at this level that the *man* is said to become *Devata* or Angel.

If and when the last sheath *Chitta* is also withdrawn, there is nothing to keep *man* in bondage with the creation of *Maya* or Darkness. The *man* is then said to be free and called a *Sanyasi* or the Son of God. It is at this level that he enters the creation of Light or the Kingdom of God.

Just as the objects seen in our dreams are found, when we are awake, to be insubstantial, so our waking perceptions are likewise unreal—a matter of inference only.

The five "objects of sense" on *connection* with the five "organs of sense" through the five "organs of action" cause the perceptions in wakeful state, which in reality are mere ideas. It is the *Manas* or Mind that brings the said *connection* and it is the *Buddhi* or Intelligence that grasps the *connection*. All perceptions or connections of the wakeful state are therefore a "matter of inference" only, called *Parokshajnana*.

What is needed is a Guru, a Saviour, who will awaken us to *Bhakti* or devotion and to perceptions of Truth.

These things saith the Amen, the faithful and true witness, the beginning of the creation of God.... Behold, I stand on the door, and knock; if any man hear my voice and open the door, I will come in to him and will sup with him, and he with me.

There was a man sent from God, whose name was John.... He was not that Light, but was sent to bear witness of that Light.... He said, I am the voice of one crying in the wilderness, Make straight the way of the Lord (Revelation 3:14, 20 and John 1:6, 8, 23.).

Parokshajnana is true comprehension of the nothingness of the external world. One can then appreciate the witnessing of Light by John the Baptist, who bore testimony of Christ, after the development of love in the heart of the former. This is what happened to me in 1987 when I saw the column of Light, and later a Spiritual Guide or *Sat Guru* directed me in Brahma Loka in front of the temple of Brahma towards the centre of Bliss (Chapter 1). With the help and direction of a Spiritual Preceptor or Saviour, one's senses are directed inwardly towards the centre between the eyebrows called *Trikuti* or *Sushumnadwara*, which is the door to the inner worlds, where one hears the knocking sound of the Cosmic Vibration—the Word or *Aum* or *Amen*. Then one sees the luminous body of *Radha,* sent by God, and referred in the *Bible* as the forerunner or John the Baptist.

That was the true Light, which lighteth every man that cometh into the world.

Verily, verily, I say unto thee, Except a man be born again, he cannot see the kingdom of God (John 1:9 and 3:3).

The **Cosmic Sound** or the **Word** or **Aum** or **Amen** is like a stream originating from a higher unknown source and losing itself in the gross material world. Different sects have named it differently, e.g., Hindus call it **Ganga**, Vaishnavas call it **Jamuna**, Christians call it **Jordan**, Muslims call it **Kalma-I-Ilahi**, Sikhs call it **Shabad**, Pythagoras called it the **Music of Spheres**, and Paul Twitchell of Eckankar called it the **Audible Sound Current**. A man reaching the qualifying stage of spiritual development gets absorbed in this "holy stream of sound" through his luminous body, and becomes *baptized*. Thus *baptization* means hearing of the Cosmic Sound (through inner ears, and not the physical ones) and getting absorbed in it. Hindus call it *Bhakti Yoga*, which "unifies the individual soul" with "Universal Soul" or God through Love, the Attraction that is constantly drawing man toward the Kingdom of God. This is called the **second birth** of man, which is the only way to comprehend the "internal world" or the Kingdom of God. In July 1987 this Cosmic Sound got awakened in me, which I am hearing till today through the inner ears, and after that I had the inner journeys (Chapter 1).

On getting the real comprehension through direct experience called *Aparokshjnana*, the son of man begins to repent and turns his back from the gross material world, and gradually moves towards Divinity, God or the Eternal Substance *Sat*. With ignorance going away man begins to understand that *Maya* or illusion is only a game of ideas played by the Supreme Nature on His own Self, *Sat*.

Emancipation (*Kaivalya*) is obtained when one realizes the oneness of his Self with the Universal Self, the Supreme Reality.

Upon whom thou shalt see the Spirit descending, and remaining on him, the same is he which baptizeth with the Holy Ghost (John 1:33).

With the end of ignorance, the purified heart does not reflect but manifests Spiritual Light and becomes free, a *Sanyasi* or Christ the Saviour. Becoming one with Christ Consciousness (or Krishna Consciousness, for that matter) means getting absorbed in the Cosmic Vibration or Word or *Aum*, which is the reflected consciousness of Eternal

Father God in the creation. Krishna is said to be the "Logos Incarnate" for that reason, as stated by H. P. B. Blavatsky.

But as many as received him, to them gave he power to become the Sons of God, even to them that believe on his name.

Verily, verily, I say unto thee, except a man be born of water and of the Spirit, he cannot enter into the kingdom of God (John 1:12 and 3:5).

Thus the second baptization takes place when the son of man gets absorbed in the Spiritual Light, enters in the spiritual world and gets unified with *Abhasa Chaitanya* or *Purusha*, the Son of God. Man is now saved once for all from the bondage of *Maya* or illusion or Darkness. This is what happened to Lord Jesus of Nazareth when he exclaimed, "I and my Father are one." I had similar experiences when I as soul moved from the palace of Brahma, crossed a beautiful wide river as if moving on a hair like bridge, and entered the region of Bliss. There I felt as part of the blissful region, feeling one with it, absorbed in bliss. After a while I came out of it and felt that my individuality was not lost (Chapter 1).

To him that overcometh will I grant to sit with me in my throne, even as I also overcame, and am sat down with my Father in his throne (Revelation 3:21).

The "son of man," after entering the spiritual world in this way, becomes the "Son of God." He comprehends now the Universal Light or the Holy Ghost as a perfect whole and realizes the fact that he as Self is only an idea resting on a fragment of the *Aum* Light. His vain idea of separate existence is abandoned and he becomes one integral whole. Being one with the universal Holy Spirit of God the Father, he is unified with the Real Substance, *Sat* or God. This unification with the Real Substance, *Sat* or God is called *Kaivalya*. In other words this is "isolation" or "absolute independence" or "emancipation through oneness with God." My own experiences are described in Chapter 1.

The Goal
Hence there is desire for emancipation

Man can understand either by way of inference or through direct experience the true relation between himself and creation. With further understanding that he is completely blinded by the influence of *Maya* or Darkness, which makes him completely forget his real Self and is the cause of all kinds of sufferings, he wishes to be relieved from all these limitations, which is but natural. Getting **liberation** from the limitations or bondage of *Maya* therefore becomes the prime aim of his life.

Liberation is stabilization of *Purusha* (*jiva* or soul) in its real Self.

Rising above the idea of creation of *Maya* or Darkness, and going beyond its influence, man gets **liberated** from the limitations of *Maya* and is placed in the real Self or the Eternal Spirit.

Then there is cessation of all pain and the attainment of the ultimate aim (true fulfillment, God-realization).

The ultimate aim of the life of a man is accomplished through this liberation, which saves him from all the trouble and fulfils all the desires of his heart.

Otherwise, birth after birth, man experiences the misery of unfulfilled desires.

As long as the man identifies himself with the material body and is unable to get connected to his true Self, the desires of his heart are never satisfied. With the formula of "ant mati so gati", the placement of the person in a realm after death is according to one's last thoughts. After a specified time he is born again on earth to suffer and learn lessons through personal experiences. This process continues intermittently until one finds repose in the true Self.

Troubles are born from *Avidya*, ignorance. Ignorance is the perception of the non-existent, and the non-perception of the Existent.

Erroneous conception of the existence of that which does not exist is *Avidya*. Man believes that material world is the only real one, not knowing that it is the mere idea on the Eternal Spirit, which is the only Real Substance that cannot be comprehended by anyone in the created world through limited senses. This *Avidya* or ignorance creates several other troubles for man beside itself.

Avidya, ignorance, having the two-fold power of polarity, manifests as egoism, attachment, aversion and (blind) tenacity.

The darkening power of *Maya* produces egoism and (blind) tenacity; the polarity power of *Maya* produces attachment (attraction) and aversion (repulsion).

Egoism results from a lack of discrimination between the physical body and the real Self.

Attachment means thirst for the objects of happiness.

Aversion means desire for the removal of the objects of unhappiness.

The darkening power of *Maya* prevents man from knowing anything other than the material creation, and connects the Self with material body, producing *Asmita* or Egoism. Thus one begins to believe in the validity of material creation with a blind tenacity called *Abhinivesa* and a separate existence of oneself. This belief is responsible for the development of the Atom or the particles of the universal force. The polarized state of *Maya* produces attraction for some objects and repulsion for some others. The objects of attraction give pleasure and develop *Raga* or Attachment for them. Similarly, the objects of repulsion give hatred and pain, and develop *Dwesha* or Aversion for them. This is how *Raga* and *Dwesha* are formed.

The root of pain is egoistic actions, which (being based on delusions) lead to misery.

The five troubles—ignorance, egoism, attachment, aversion, and tenacity to the material creation—induce man to get involved in egoistic works, which brings sufferings.

Man's purpose is complete freedom from unhappiness.

The Liberation of Man

Once he has banished all pain beyond possibility of return, he has attained the highest goal.

Heart's immediate aim is *Artha* or the cessation of all sufferings. When sufferings are completely eradicated with no chance of recurring, it is called *Paramartha*, which is the ultimate goal of life.

Existence, consciousness, and bliss are the three belongings (of the human heart).

Ananda, bliss, is the contentment of heart attained by the ways and means suggested by the Saviour, the *Sat-Guru*.

Chit, true consciousness, brings about the complete destruction of all troubles and the rise of all virtues.

Sat, existence, is attained by realization of the permanency of the soul.

These three qualities constitute the real nature of man.

All desires being fulfilled, and the miseries removed, the achievement of *Paramartha* (the highest goal) is made.

Remember therefore from where thou art fallen, and repent. (Revelation 2:5)

Sat (existence); *Chit* (consciousness); and *Ananda* (bliss) are essential properties of human nature that are related only to his Self, and nothing else. Following the directions of a *Sat Guru* or Saviour, when man is able to direct his attention inward and is able to satisfy all desires of his heart, he achieves contentment, which is *Ananda* or bliss. Next, he is able to concentrate on any idea of his choice and know all its aspects. In this way he comprehends all the modifications of Nature up to its first and primal manifestation, the Word or *Aum* or Amen. Gradually *Chit* or consciousness of his own real Self appears. Being absorbed in the stream of the Word or *Aum* man is baptized and begins to repent and return to his own Divinity, the Eternal Father, whence he had fallen. Knowing one's own position and the nature of creation of *Maya*, creation loses control over man and he becomes free, and Ignorance begins to diminish in all its aspects. He now understands his own Self as a permanent real substance that can never be destroyed. In this way the existence of Self or *Sat* is made known. Thus all the three necessities of heart having been attained; Ignorance, the root of all evils been emaciated; troubles of material world and sufferings caused thereby cease once for all. The ultimate aim of the heart is fulfilled.

All fulfillment of his nature attained, man is not merely a reflector of divine light but becomes actively united with Spirit. This state is *Kaivalya*, oneness.

Believe me that I am in the Father, and the Father in me (John 14:11).

Ultimate aim being attained, the heart is now perfectly purified and hence actively manifests Spiritual Light, instead of merely reflecting it. Being anointed by the Holy Spirit, man becomes Christ, the Saviour. He now enters the Kingdom of God or Spiritual Light and becomes the Son of God. His vain idea of separate existence is now abandoned. He comprehends his Self as a part of the Universal Holy Spirit and unifies himself with the Eternal Spirit, or, becomes one and the same with God the father. This is the state of *Kaivalya*, which is the Ultimate Aim of all the beings in the created world.

My own experiences over the years confirm the above two paragraphs, as per details in Chapter 1. It is true that *Sat* or existence, *Chit* or consciousness and *Ananda* or bliss appear in that order. With the attention turning inward inner happiness (*Ananda* or bliss) and inner journeys begin to manifest. You come to know the higher realms and non-physical worlds and their inhabitants. This becomes a regular feature in dreams and trances. You see yourself as a dimensionless existence like a point (Self) without any kind of body, visits to various places and entering many spaces, even solid looking ones. You gradually understand your "Self" and the working of the Nature. This is the development of *Chit* or Consciousness. And finally, after crossing all kinds of barriers, and when you are least expecting it, you see yourself entering an ocean of blissful existence, such as, a very small piece of cotton entering and getting merged into a huge bulk of cotton, and after a while coming out of it. This involves a "highly blissful state" of being, and the understanding that "you are a part of the whole," having a permanent existence. You feel that you have always been so and will always be so. This is *Sat* or existence. This is the best possible explanation I can give, on the basis of my personal experiences.

The Procedure

Yajna, sacrifice, means penance (*Tapas*), deep study (*Swadhyaya*), and the practice of meditation on *Aum* (*Brahmanidhana*).

Penance is patience or evenmindedness in all conditions (equanimity amidst the essential dualities of *Maya*; cold and heat, pain and pleasure, etc.).

Swadhyaya consists of reading or hearing spiritual truth, pondering it, and forming a definite concept of it.

(Meditation on) *Pranava*, the divine sound of *Aum*, is the only way to Brahman (Spirit), salvation.

I know thy works, and charity, and service, and faith, and thy patience, and thy works; and the last to be more than the first (Revelation 2:19).

Patience or equanimity under both favorable and adverse circumstances, called *Tapas*; study with deep attention that is *sravana* and *manana*, called *Swadhyaya*, leading to the formation of faith in Self (whom am I, whence I came, where I shall go, what is the purpose of my coming etc.); and baptism or merging of Self in the stream of the Holy Sound (*Pranava*, the *Word* or *Aum*) called *Brahmanidhana*, which is the only way to attain salvation and to return to Divinity or our Eternal Father, whence we have fallen; constitute the three wings of *Yajna* or sacrifice.

Aum is heard through cultivation of *Sraddha* (heart's natural love), *Virya* (moral courage), *Smriti* (memory of one's divinity), and *Samadhi* (true concentration). *Shraddha* is intensification of the heart's natural love.

I know thy works, and thy labor, and thy patience, and how thy canst not bear them which are evil: and thou hast tried them which say they are apostles, and are not, and hast found them liars.

And hast borne and hast patience, and for my name's sake hast labored, and hast not fainted.

Nevertheless I have somewhat against thee, because thou hast left thy first love (Revelation 2:2-4).

There are four factors—*Sraddha, Virya, Smriti* and *Samadhi*—in that order, which are responsible for the spontaneous manifestation of the Holy Sound or *Pranava Sabda*. First requisite is the appearance of Nature's heavenly gift-heart's natural love, (*shraddha*) which normalizes the individual and invigorates the vital powers in him against the germs of diseases. Without this love man is unable to understand the foreign matters that have entered his system erroneously, causing suffering to his mind and body. This gives "a sound mind in a sound body" to the individual, enabling him to understand the Nature and its guidance. With this "love" he begins to understand his own Self and that of others around him, which brings him in the Godlike company of divine personages, which gradually leads him to salvation.

Moral courage (*Virya*) arises from *Sraddha*, directing one's love toward the guru, and affectionately following his instructions. Those who remove our troubles, dispel our doubts, and bestow peace are our true teachers. They perform a Godlike work. Their opposites (those who increase our doubts and difficulties) are harmful to us and should be avoided like poison.

Jesus answered them, Is it not written in your law, I said, Ye are gods.

I have said, Ye are gods; and all of you are children of the most High. (John 10:34 and Psalm 82:6)

Behold the Lamb of God, which taketh away the sin of the world. (John 1:29)

The Liberation of Man

The Real Substance, God, the Eternal Father Himself is the "Guru", and this creation is a mere idea – play on Himself, perceived in plurality by the manifold aspects of the play of Nature. Any object of this creation, whether animate or inanimate, significant or insignificant, that removes our doubts and miseries and bestows peace to us is *Sat* Saviour, its company is God-like and it deserves utmost respect from us. On the other hand any object that destroys our peace, throws us into doubts and miseries is *Asat*, which should be avoided at all costs.

People choose the objects of their Savior according to the stage of evolution they have reached. Ignorant people may have blind faith in and hence search their Savior in natural elements such as water, stone or a piece of wood. The learned may consider their deities to exist in heaven. The Yogis or adepts however, having transcended the objects of the material or external world, would realize their Divinity or Savior within their own Self.

The Godlike object should be taken as **Guru** and one should keep his company as many times and as long as possible. When his physical presence is not available, then he should be kept in the heart; we should try to be one with him in principle and should attune ourselves with him in this way. One should remember that a crowd is never a company. One should develop *Shraddha* towards the Godlike object by keeping his appearance and attributes fully in mind and by reflecting on them, and by following his instructions affectionately, like a lamb. From among the company of his divine brothers who help him in his spiritual progress, he can choose any one of them as his Saviour or Spiritual Preceptor or *Sat Guru*. By devoting his natural love to his Preceptor and developing *shraddha* in this way, one can attain moral courage or *Virya*.

Moral courage is strengthened by observance of *Yama* (morality or self-control) and *Niyama* (religious rules).

Yama comprises non-injury to others, truthfulness, non-stealing, continence, and non-covetousness.

Niyama means purity of body and mind, contentment in all circumstances, and obedience (following the instructions of the guru).

Absence from cruelty, dishonesty, covetousness, unnatural living and unnecessary possessions cultures *Yama*. Cleaning the body externally and internally from all foreign matters that on fermentation create diseases; clearing the mind from all prejudices and dogmas that produce the narrowness of mind and thus attain contentment in all circumstances; and obeying the holy precepts of the divine personages, cultures, religious observances or *Niyama*. *Yama* and *Niyama* are the foundations of moral courage.

Natural living depends upon the right selection of food, dwelling and company, which in turn depends on the natural instincts through the five senses of seeing, hearing, touch, smell and taste. Unnatural living from early childhood perverts organs of five senses in men and right selection may need observance, experimentation, and reasoning. Natural food is the one that aids in digestion and nutrition of the body, formation of good teeth and digestive canal and correct development of similar other systems.

Selection of natural food can be helped much by observing the kind of teeth given to men by Nature. "Carnivorous animals" have little developed incisors, smooth and pointed canines with striking length to seize the prey, pointed molars fitting closely side by side to separate the muscular fibres. "Herbivorous animals" have strikingly developed incisors, stunted canines and broad-topped molars with enamel only on the sides. "Frugivorous animals" have all teeth nearly of the same height and canines are little projected, conical and blunt so as to exert strength but not to seize any prey. Molars are broad topped and furnished with enamel folds to prevent waste caused by their side motions. Molars are not pointed meaning that they are not meant for chewing flesh. "Omnivorous animals" like bears have herbivorous-like incisors, carnivorous-like canines and molars are both pointed and broad-topped to serve a twofold purpose. Teeth in men do not resemble either carnivorous, or herbivorous or the omnivorous but of course they resemble frugivorous animals. This concludes that man is a fruit-eating animal. The fruitarian diet includes vegetables, nuts and grains as suggested by Swami Sri Yukteswarji.

Measurement of the length of bowels in men, observation of the organs of sense, nourishment of the young, cause of disease and children's development—all of them suggest that man is a frugivorous animal[12].

Passions and sexual desire need a special mention here. Excessive fasting, scourging or monastic confinement seldom suppress the sexual passions. However, this archenemy of morality can be overcome easily by natural living on non-irritant diet suggested above, which produces calmness of mind. Such a state of mind is favorable to mental activities, to a clear understanding and to a judicial way of thinking. Sexual desire, like all other desires, has a normal and an abnormal or diseased state. Unnatural living that accumulates foreign matter is responsible for the abnormal state. The thermometer of sexual desire accurately indicates condition of health of a man. In its normal state it makes man free from all disturbing lusts and it awakens a wish for appeasement only infrequently. Those who lead a natural life have sexual desire too in a normal way.

The sexual organ, which is a junction of important sympathetic and spinal nerve extremities, is the root of the tree of life. One who knows the proper use of sex can keep his body and mind in sound health and can live a pleasant life throughout. It is unfortunate that the subject of sexual health is regarded as unclean and indecent and hence it cannot be taught in open. Nature is thus veiled as impure, which is the opposite of truth and impurity lies only in the ideas of man. Thus the true knowledge about sex is not passed on to man, and he not knowing the dangers of the misuse of sexual power is compelled to indulge in wrong practices by nervous irritation caused by unnatural living. This causes troublesome diseases and premature death is the unfortunate result.

If you enter a crowded room after breathing fresh air on a mountaintop, a feeling of displeasure creeps in. A proper dwelling place would therefore be a mountaintop or a field or a garden or a dry place under trees, where the atmosphere is freshly ventilated. In the same way the company we should keep should be of those persons who magnetize us harmoniously and relieve our miseries by cooling our system, invigorating our vitality, answering our spirituality related queries, develop natural love in us and provide inner peace. Such a person is called *Sat* or saviour whose company promotes a sound mind in a sound body and the life span is prolonged. A person who produces opposite effects is *Asat* and his company should be avoided at all costs. A natural living helps in the practice of *Yama* and the purity of mind and body helps in the practice of *Niyama*, which are two basic essentialities of spiritual progress. Hence bondage disappears.

The eight bondages or snares are hatred, shame, fear, grief, condemnation, racial prejudice, pride of family, and smugness. Removal of the eight bondages leads to magnanimity of heart.

Thus one becomes fit to practice *Asana, Pranayama,* and *Pratyahara;* and to enjoy the householder's life (by fulfilling all one's desires and so getting rid of them).

Asana means a steady and pleasant posture of the body.

Pranayama means control over *prana,* life force.

Pratyahara means withdrawal of the senses from external objects.

There are eight obstacles (meannesses of human heart) on way to salvation—hatred, shame, fear, grief, condemnation, race prejudice, pride of pedigree, and a narrow sense of respectability. These obstacles are removed with the "firmness of moral courage" being attained. This leads to "magnanimity of the heart" (*Viratwam* or *Mahattwam*) that makes man fit for the practice of *asana*

The Liberation of Man

(steadiness and pleasantness in physical posture), *Pranayama* (control over *prana* or life energy), and *Pratyahara* (withdrawal of senses from the external world). With these practices man is able to enjoy the objects of senses intended for domestic life or *Grahasthashrama*. Otherwise life after life man remains unsatisfied and dies with unfulfilled desires every time, which brings him back to next incarnation. Once the desires are fulfilled completely, man transcends them and finds real interest in spiritual practices. Sri Aurobindo has clearly said that God's Realization is possible only when desires are eradicated, which can be done in two ways: either crush them to the roots or satisfy them to the full extent. The former method has chances of failure as shown by many living examples. Hence the latter method is the right one as advocated in this Para.

We have voluntary and involuntary nerves in our body system. Voluntary nerves are used at will and rested when fatigued through sleep and then they are fresh to work again the next day. Involuntary nerves are always in action irrespective of man's will for the whole life. When they are fatigued they too need rest, through great sleep (*Mahanidra*) or death. With this the circulation, respiration and other vital functions stop and the body begins to decay. When this great sleep is complete man awakes with unfulfilled desires and the same story repeats in the next incarnation. Thus salvation is never achieved. However, involuntary nerves can be rested and refreshed through *Pranayama*, the decay of the body can be delayed considerably and a longer life span with greater vigor can be used to work out the karma in the same lifetime. Life and death come under the control of the yogi; he experiences death while living in his physical body. Desires fulfilled, purification achieved, there may be no further rebirth and second death. This is what St. Paul meant when he said,

"*I protest by our rejoicing which I have in Christ (consciousness), I die daily.*"

"Be thou faithful unto death, and I will give thee a crown of life...He that overcometh shall not be hurt by the second death." (I Corinthians 15:31, and Revelation 2:10, 11).

At the time of enjoyment the organs of sense are directed towards the object of sense, and in doing so man is never satisfied as the desire increases twofold. However, if he redirects his sense organs inward towards the Self at the time of enjoyment, then his heart is satisfied immediately and the desire vanishes once for all. This is *Pratyahar* which works our earthly longings conclusively and saves man from repeated incarnations. Finally, the importance of *Asana* lies in the fact that a "steady and pleasant posture" is necessary to comprehend and feel a thing by the heart clearly.

Smriti, true conception, leads to knowledge of all creation.

Samadhi, true concentration, enables one to abandon individuality for universality.

Hence arises *Samyama* ("restraint" or overcoming the egoistic self), by which one experiences the *Aum* vibration that reveals God.

Thus the soul (is baptized) in *Bhakti Yoga* (devotion). This is the state of Divinity.

There was a man sent from God, whose name was John.

The same came for a witness, to bear witness of the Light, that all men through him might believe.

I am the voice of one crying in wilderness (John 1:6, 7, 23).

When man through the above practices begins to conceive or feel all things of this creation by his heart, it is true conception or *Smriti*. When man by fixing attention firmly on any object thus conceived becomes identified with it so much that he feels he was never separate, he attains the state of true concentration or *Samadhi*. When man directs all his sense organs towards the common center—sensorium or *Sushumnadwara*—which is the door of internal world, he perceives his God-sent luminous body of *Radha* or John the Baptist, and hears the knocking sound, the Word of God or *Pranava Sabda* or *Aum*.

This happened to me in that very order. In July 1984 when I was deeply engrossed in meditation my eyes got suddenly opened with a loud sound, and a column of cool bright light (*Radha*) stood before me. Then in July 1987 when I got up to attend the call of nature around 2 a.m, I heard a peculiar continuous sound (*Pranava Shabda or Aum*) that stays with me till today. For details please see the first chapter on my autobiography.

Man now believes in the true Spiritual Light, and having withdrawn from the external world, he concentrates himself on the Self, which is *Samyama*. This leads to absorption in the holy stream of the Divine Sound, which is "baptism" or *Bhakti Yoga*. Man now repents, turns back from the gross material world of Darkness or *Maya* and rises towards his Eternal father or Divinity whence he had fallen. He now passes through the door of sensorium or *Dasmadwara* and enters the next sphere that is the internal realm called *Bhuvarloka*. This entrance into the inner world is known as the "second birth" of man, who is now called a divine being or *Devata* or an Initiate.

Man is classified by the **five different states of the heart**: dark, propelled, steady, devoted, and clean. His evolutionary status is determined by the state of his heart.

In the dark state of the heart, man harbors misconceptions (about everything). This state is a result of *avidya*, Ignorance, and produces a *sudra* (a man of the lowest caste). He can grasp only ideas of the physical world. This state of mind is prevalent in Kali Yuga, the Dark Age of a cycle.

In the dark state of heart man misconceives the material world and considers it to be the only reality. This is contrary to the truth and is an effect of *avidya*. In this state man is regarded as *sudra*, belonging to the lowest caste meant to serve the higher class people so that he can elevate himself to the higher stage. This state of man is known as dark or *Kali*, and if the people in a solar system are all like this at a particular point of time, it is said to be the dark cycle or *Kali Yuga*.

Passing beyond the first stage in Brahma's plan, man strives for enlightenment and enters the natural *Kshatriya* (warrior) caste.

He is propelled (be evolutionary forces) to struggle (for truth). He seeks a guru and appreciates his divine counsel. Thus a *Kshatriya* becomes fit to dwell in the worlds of higher understanding.

Getting some enlightenment man compares his wakeful experiences with those of sleep state and finds them to be mere ideas. This propels him to find the truth about the universe itself. In the Kshatriya or military class man has a fighting nature that he applies to get an insight into the nature of creation and get the real knowledge about it. This state being the middle state between higher and lower called *Sandhisthala*, man becomes anxious for real knowledge and appreciates the need for mutual cooperation and love, which is the main requirement for gaining salvation. Energy of this love motivates man to keep company of those who clear his doubts, remove his troubles and provide peace. He avoids company of those having contrary nature and begins to study the Holy Scriptures and literature concerning divine personages. He now appreciates the value of faith and may be fortunate to find his Spiritual Preceptor or Savior or *Sat-Guru*. Under the guidance of holy precepts he learns to concentrate his mind and direct his sense organs towards the sensorium or *Sushumnadwara*, which is the door to the inner worlds. This enables him to perceive the luminous body of *Radha* or John the Baptist, and hear the holy sound of the Word or *Aum* or Amen. Getting absorbed in the Sound or baptized in it he passes through inner spheres or *lokas* in his backward journey towards the Eternal Father or his Divinity.

The worlds or *Lokas* of creation are seven: *Bhu, Bhuvar, Swar, Mahar, Jana, Tapo,* and *Satya* (These earths, and the "earthly" stage of man's consciousness, are called *Bhuloka*).

The seven spheres or stages of creation called *Swargas* or *Lokas* by the Oriental sages are: *Bhuloka,* the sphere of gross matter; *Bhuvarloka*, the sphere of fine matter or electrical impulses; *Swarloka*, the sphere of magnetic impulses and auras; *Maharloka*, the sphere of magnets, the atoms; *Janaloka*, the sphere of Spiritual Reflections, the Sons of God; *Tapoloka*, the sphere of the Holy Ghost, the Universal Spirit; and *Satyaloka*, the sphere of the Eternal Substance *Sat* or God. The first three of them (*Bhuloka, Bhuvarloka,* and *Swarloka*) constitute the material creation, the kingdom of Darkness or *Maya; Maharloka,* the middle one, the sphere of Atom, is the door between the material and spiritual creation; and the last three (*Janaloka, Tapoloka,* and *Satyaloka*) constitute the spiritual creation, the Kingdom of Light. *Maharloka,* the door of communication between the lower and higher worlds is the way to Divinity, called the tenth door or *Dasmadwara* or *Brahmarandhra.*

Entering *Bhuvarloka* ("air" or "the world of becoming") man becomes a *Dwija* or "twice born." He comprehends the second portion of material creation—that of finer, subtler forces. This state of mind is prevalent in Dwapara Yuga.

When man on baptization repents, withdraws himself from the gross material world (*Bhuloka*) and begins his backward journey to the Eternal Father through the inner world of fine matter (*Bhuvarloka*), he joins the class of twice-born or *Dwija*. He now comprehends his internal electricities, the second portion of creation, composed of fine matter. It is now clear to him that the external world comes into appearance due to the "union" of five organs of senses with the five organs of action, which is caused by his "mind." This "union" falls down with the stopping of the "mind." And the death of "mind" is the birth of "wisdom."

This is the *Dwapara* state of man; and when the people in general in a solar system belong to this category, the system is said to be in Dwapara Yuga. In this state the heart becomes steady. With continuous immersion in the holy stream of sound, man achieves the pleasant state in which his heart abandons completely the external world and rests in the internal world alone.

In *Swargloka* ("heaven") man is fit to understand the mysteries of *Chitta*, the magnetic third portion of material creation. He becomes a *Vipra* (nearly perfect being). This state of mind is prevalent in Treta Yuga.

Through devotion man withdraws from the world of electric attributes, *Bhuvarloka*, and comes to the world of magnetic attributes, *Swargloka*, and is able to comprehend *Chitta* or Heart, which is the magnetic third portion of creation. *Chitta* is the spiritualized Atom, Ignorance or *Avidya*, which is a part of Darkness or *Maya*. Comprehension of *Chitta* makes man understand the whole Darkness or *Maya*, and the entire creation, since *Chitta* is a part of *Maya* itself. Man is supposed to have achieved perfection at this stage, and is called the *Vipra*. This human state is called *Treta*, and if the people in general belong to this state in a solar system, it is called Treta Yuga.

Through true repentance man reaches *Maharloka* (the "great world"). No longer subject to the influence of ignorance and *Maya*, he attains a clean heart. He enters the natural caste of the *Brahmanas* ("knowers of Brahma"). This state of mind is prevalent in Satya Yuga.

Onward journey to God brings him to *Maharloka*, the sphere of magnet, the Atom, where Ignorance and external world having been transcended, man acquires a clean heart. He now comprehends the Real Substance, the Spiritual Light or Brahma, which is the last and permanent spiritual portion of the creation. Man now belongs to the highest spiritual class called *Brahmana*. It is the *Satya* state of humans, and the period is called Satya Yuga if people in general belong to this category in a solar system.

Not merely reflecting but manifesting Spiritual Light, man rises to *Janaloka*, the Kingdom of God.

Then he passes into *Tapoloka*, the sphere of *Kutastha Chaitanya*.

Abandoning the vain idea of his separate existence, he enters *Satyaloka*, wherein he attains the state of final release or *Kaivalya*, oneness with Spirit.

Heart being purified, man no more reflects but manifests now the Spiritual Light, the Son of God. Being consecrated or anointed by the Spirit in this way, he becomes Christ, the Saviour. With this second baptization or absorption in Spirit, man rises above the creation of Darkness or *Maya* and enters into the creation of Light, the Kingdom of God or *Janaloka*. This is the state of *Jivanmukta Sanyasi* that was attained by Lord Jesus of Nazareth as he said:

Verily, verily, I say unto thee, Except a man be born of water and Spirit, he cannot enter into the Kingdom of God.

Jesus saith unto him, I am the way, the truth, and the life: no man cometh unto the Father, but by me (John 3:5 and 14:6).

Man now realizes the fact that he is merely an idea resting on a fragment of the universal Holy Spirit of God, the Eternal Father. He sacrifices his self at the altar of the Holy Spirit or God, as he understands that this is the real worship of God. As the vain idea of separate existence is abandoned, he is in a way dead or dissolved in the universal Holy Spirit and arrives in the region of the Holy Ghost or *Tapoloka*. Becoming one and the same with the universal Holy Spirit of God, man is unified with God Himself and reaches *Satyaloka*. Here it is now very clear that the whole creation is merely an idea-play of his own nature and the only thing that exists in the universe is his own Self. This unified state is known as the Sole Self or *Kaivalya*. Lord Jesus observed:

Blessed are the dead which die in the Lord from henceforth.

I came forth from the Father; and am come into the world: again I leave the world, and again go to the Father (Revelation 14:13 and John 16:28).

The Revelation

Adeptship is achieved by purification of man's three bodies. It is also attainable through the grace of the guru.

Purification comes through Nature, penance, and *mantras*.

Through Nature there is purification of dense matter (the physical body); through penance, purification of the fine matter (the subtle body); through mantras, purification of the mind.

Man becomes an adept when material body is purified by things generated along with it by Nature; subtle or electric body by patience under both favorable and adverse situations; and magnetic body, the spiritualized Atom, Heart or *Chitta* by *mantra*, which regulates the breathing and purifies the mind. One can learn the process of purification humbly from the divine personages who witness Light and bear testimony of the Krishna or Christ consciousness.

Through the holy effect of the *mantra*, the *Pranava* or *Aum* sound becomes audible.

The sacred sound is heard in various ways, according to the devotee's stage of advancement (in purifying his heart).

The Spiritual Preceptor or *Sat Guru* guides the devotee and brings the regulation of breath because of which the holy word or *Pranava* or *Sabda* or *Aum* becomes audible spontaneously. With the appearance of the natural *mantra*—the Word or *Aum*—the breathing is automatically regulated, decay of the material body is checked and the ageing process slows down.

With the level of the purification of heart or *Chitta* the form of *Pranava* keeps changing. According to Sri Herald Klemp of *Eckankar* it varies from lowest to highest level in the form of thunder, roar of the sea, tinkling bells, running water, buzzing bees, single note of a flute, wind, humming sound, thousand violins, music of woodwinds and Hu.

During the course of meditation over the years I heard all these sounds internally myself and nearly in this order. For details please see my book, *The Journey Back to Our True Home through Spiritual Energy – Kundalini*[13]. For various kinds of lights, sounds, and other symbols that appear during continued meditation please see my book, *Secrets of Shaktipat*[14].

One who cultivates the heart's natural love obtains the guidance of a guru, and starts his *sadhana* (path of spiritual discipline). He becomes a *pravakta*, an initiate.

With the growth of pure love in his heart, man attracts the help from beyond and naturally finds the company of *Sat* and keeps away from *Asat*. In course of time he finds his Spiritual Preceptor or *Sat Guru*. God-like company of his preceptor grows an inclination or *Pravriti* in the heart of the disciple to save himself from the clutches of Darkness or *Maya*. He gradually becomes an initiate or *Pravakta*, and the practices of *Yama* and *Niyama* take place naturally for him, which are necessary to attain salvation.

I found a series of earthly gurus, without many efforts, who helped me in my spiritual progress, one after another. Furthermore, I got the *Darshan* (seeing in form) of my inner *Sat Guru* in a trance while meditating in San Francisco, who latter helped me also in *Brahmaloka* (plane of Brahma) to guide me beyond, where all of us existed without any forms. Complete details are given in the first chapter on my autobiography.

By the practice of *Yama* and *Niyama*, the eight meannesses of the human heart disappear and virtue arises. Man thus becomes a *Sadhaka*, a true disciple, fit to attain salvation.

Practice of *Yama* and *Niyama* removes the eight meannesses from the heart and brings magnanimity, which enables him to assume ascetic posture and meet other requirements laid by his *Sat Guru* to attain salvation. Following the directions of *Sat Guru* and with continued practices he becomes a *sadhaka* or true disciple.

He progresses in godliness, hears the holy *Aum* sound, and becomes a *Siddha*, a divine personage.

As described earlier, the disciple advances through various stages of meditation, conceiving different objects of creation in his heart, and by finally turning inward to the Self, he perceives the cosmic sound, the Word or *Pranava*, which makes his heart divine. The Ego, son of man or

Ahamkara gets merged or baptized in the holy stream; the disciple then becomes a divine personage, an adept or *Siddha*.

Then he perceives the manifestations of Spirit, and passes through the seven *Patala Lokas* (or centres in the spine), beholding the seven *rishis*.

And being turned, I saw seven golden candlesticks; and in the midst of the seven candlesticks one like unto the son of man... .And he had in his right hand seven stars.

The mystery of the seven stars which thou sawest in my right hand, and the seven golden candlesticks. The seven stars are the angels of the seven churches; and the seven candlesticks which thou sawest are the seven churches.

These things saith he that holdeth the seven stars in his right hand, who walketh in the midst of the seven golden candlesticks (Revelation 1:12, 13, 16, 20, and 2:1).

Through baptization or *Bhakti Yoga,* that is, absorption of Ego in the holy Sound, man withdraws from the plane of gross matter (*Bhuloka*) and enters into internal plane of fine matter (*Bhuvarloka).* There he perceives the manifestations of the True Light or Spirit as seven stars in seven centres, the astrally shining places or golden candlesticks. These stars are called angels or *rishis,* which appear one after another in his right way to Divinity. These seven centres are seven vortices of energy, called *Chakras*: *mooladhara* or root centre (coccygeal), *swadhishthana* (sacral), *manipura* or naval centre (lumbar), *anahata* or heart centre (dorsal), *visuddha* or throat centre (cervical), *ajna* or eyebrow centre (medulla oblongata), and *sahasrara* or crown centre (brain), in the ascending order. The first five of them are on the spine. It is at these seven centres or churches where the Spirit becomes manifested and Ego or son of man passes towards the Divinity.

And there was a rainbow round about the throne.

And I saw in the right hand of him that sat on the throne a book written within and on the back side, sealed with seven seals. (Revelation 4:3 and 5:1)

On baptization or *Bhakti Yoga* or *Surat Sabda Yoga* the son of man or Ego or *Surat* passes through the seven *Chakras* and acquires the knowledge, which makes him understand the true nature of the universe. On withdrawal of the self from the region of fine material (*Bhuvarloka*), man enters into the source of all matters – fine or gross (*Swarloka*). There he finds luminous astral form around his heart, Atom, the throne of Spirit, the Creator, having five electricities and two poles (Mind and Intelligence) of seven different colors like the ones in a rainbow. The source of all objects of senses and of organs of senses for enjoying them is this region of five electricities, mind and intelligence, which is described as a sealed casket of knowledge, a book with seven seals. Here man achieves satisfaction of his desires because he is in possession of all objects of desires, and hence he acquires complete knowledge thereof.

Then, because of yoga knowledge and power, man obtains supremacy over the seven *swargas* (heavens). He achieves salvation by dissolving the four original ideas (the "four *manus*" or primal thoughts by which creation sprang into being).

From *Swargloka* the son of man arrives at *Maharloka*, which is the place of magnet or Atom, having four components (ideas of manifestation): the word, time, space and particle or atom. The son of man or Ego is created for the first time in *Maharloka*, which therefore produces the idea of separate existence, and hence it is the plane of ignorance or *Avidya*. The four ideas of manifestation—the word, time, space and atom—are known as the four manus, which are the origins or sources of man. Since the son of man or Ego creates the idea of separate existence, which is ignorance, man is said to be the offspring of ignorance. On arrival at *Maharloka* on his journey backward to God, man comes to know the act of the creation of Ego that produced the idea of separate existence, which he now transcends and achieves salvation.

Being thus victorious over the powers of darkness and ignorance, man becomes one with God.

Verily, verily, I say unto you, he that believeth on me, the works that I do shall he do also; and greater works than these shall he do; because I go unto my Father (John 14:12).

Maharloka (region of magnet or atom) being the mid-region, it is the door between material and spiritual creations, called *Dasmadwara* or *Brahmarandhra*. On arrival at this door, the son of man or Ego comprehends the Spiritual Light and gets baptized in it. On passing through this door he comes above the ideational creation of Darkness or *Maya,* and on entering into the spiritual world he receives the true Light and becomes the Son of God. He now becomes possessed of all the ascetic majesties or *aishwaryas* of eight kinds:

Anima, the power of reducing one's body or anything else to a size as small as one likes, even as small as an atom or *Anu*.

Mahima, the power of magnifying one's body or anything else as large (*mahat*) as one likes.

Laghima, the power of making one's body or anything else as light (*laghu*) in weight as one likes.

Garima, the power of making one's body or anything else as heavy (*guru*) as one likes.

Prapti, the power of obtaining anything (*apti*) he likes.

Vasitwa, the power of bringing anything under control (*vasa*).

Prakyama, the power of satisfying all desires (*kama*) through one's will power.

Isitwa, the power of becoming Lord (*Isa*) over anything.

Knowledge of evolution, life, and dissolution thus leads to complete emancipation from the bonds of *Maya,* delusion. Beholding the self in the Supreme Self, man gains eternal freedom.

To him that overcometh will I grant to sit with me in my throne, even as I also overcame, and am set down with my Father in his throne (Revelation 3:21).

The Liberation of Man

On possessing the aforesaid ascetic majesties or *aishwaryas*, man fully comprehends the Real Substance, the Eternal Spirit, the Father as Unit or Perfect Whole, and his Self as a mere idea resting on a fragment of the Spiritual Light thereof. Transcending the vain idea of separate existence of his Self, he unites with the Eternal Spirit or God, the Father. This unification with God is known as *Kaivalya*, which is the ultimate goal of humanity.

Self-realization Fellowship concludes the book, *The Holy Science* of Swami Sri Yukteswar with stanza 2 from third canto of *The Lay of the Last Minstrel*, by Sir Walter Scott:
"Love rules the court, the camp, the grove,
The men below and saints above;
For love is heaven and heaven is love."
The whole text shows the fact that "Love is God" is the central message of Swami Sri Yukteswar. In the Trinity—Father, Son and The Holy Ghost—The Holy Ghost is nothing but "love," which as the "latent force" makes everything happen in the universe. It is not a noble sentiment of the poet but an aphorism, which explains that at every step it is love that brings forth the transcendence to the next step. Various methods are shown only to cultivate "love" and to culture it properly to achieve its development. It is by developing "love" for divine personages that man finds his Saviour or *Sat Guru*, who finally unites man with the Eternal Father.

In an Urdu poem it is rightly said that everything that happens in the world is due to the force of "love," so much so that it is "love" that converts man into God or Angel or *Devata*.

Patanjali's Yoga Sutras

In the sixth century B.C. the great sage Patanjali presented the eight-fold path (*ashtangayoga*) to bring man to Divinity or to become one with the Father. These steps are exactly the same as taught by Swami Sri Yukteswar, with a little variation in the end.

Table 1

Steps	Patanjali	Swami Yukteswar
1.	Yama	Yama
2.	Niyama	Niyama
3.	Asana	Asana
4.	Pranayama	Pranayama
5.	Pratyahara	Pratyahara
6.	Dharana	Smriti
7.	Dhyana	Samadhi
8.	Samadhi	

The sixth step of Swami Yukteswar is *Smriti*, meaning memory (of divinity). When man acquires his memory of what he was in the beginning, he goes into *Samadhi* or final absorption, which is oneness with God, the Father. Patanjali achieves the same goal in two steps: *Dharna* meaning determination, and *Dhyana* meaning concentration, which brings forth the final absorption or *Samadhi*.

I find that these are really the stages a disciple or a seeker or a devotee goes through in his spiritual journey, knowingly or unknowingly, whatever faith or tradition he may belong to. In my autobiography presented in the first chapter it would be seen that I too followed the same steps subconsciously, although I never knew about them while involved in my spiritual practices.

Srimad Bhagavata Mahapurana

The three modes of nature called *gunas* are *Sattva*, *Rajas* and *Tamas*. Humans keep rotating between theses modes according to the variations made by nature. Under Sattva one has the righteous or religious bent of mind and all good activities including spiritual ones take place in this mode. Under Rajas one becomes full of worldly activities and is

The Liberation of Man

goal oriented. Under Tamas one does not like to do anything and remains inert and unproductive. Therefore spiritual, worldly and no activities are performed by the person according to the Sattvic, Rajasic or Tamasic mode of nature working on him at the time. In the real sense therefore a person should neither be appreciated nor condemned for his so called good or bad work, as it is not he but the mode of nature that is responsible for the activity. Through Yoga and Meditation or otherwise a person increases Sattva mode and suppresses other two modes and hence he is able to perform only righteous or spiritual activities all the time. Thus a Jiva or "individual soul" is said to be bound or emancipated accordingly as its being subjected or not to the influence of the three *gunas* or "modes of nature" controlled by the Lord, and has nothing to do with his essential nature.

Man is naturally inclined towards the enjoyment of sexual pleasure, flesh and wine. No rules enjoin him to indulge in them. A certain check is provided over these tendencies by scriptures permitting sexual commerce with one's wedded wife, meat-eating at the end of an animal sacrifice, drinking of wine during a sacrificial ceremony in the case of those who are addicted to these. The real intention of scriptures is to turn man away from them. The only fruit or proper use of wealth is Dharma or righteous action or piety which gives knowledge and direct realization and forthwith leads to supreme peace or liberation. Those who use wealth for their own comfort or of family members forget death, the formidable enemy of their body. Animal sacrifice is allowed for the adoration of the deities and is not permissible to kill them for meat. In the same way, sexual relation is allowed with one's wife for getting an issue and not for the sake of enjoyment. These are some of the rules of Dharma or righteousness. Those who hate others, in whom also dwells the same Self or Lord, hate the Lord Himself and, being deeply attached to their mortal body and other relations, fall into hell or repeated births and rebirths. One of the Testaments in Christianity requires to "love your neighbor," which is denied by most people you ask from. Those who do not pursue the path of liberation kill their own self, are devoid of peace of mind, regard ignorance as knowledge, confusing action for knowledge, do not experience fulfillment and, being frustrated in their aims and thwarted by the Time-Spirit, become miserable. Those who are averse to the Lord are obliged against their will to forsake their home, wealth, children and friends, gained with great difficulty, and enter the dark hell.

According to *Srimad Bhagavata Mahapurana* a *kalpa* has one hundred rotations of the four *yugas* or ages—Satya, Treta, Dwapara and Kali. In each *Yuga* the Lord assumes different colors, names and forms and is worshipped in different modes. In the Satya age He had white complexion, four arms, wore matted locks and was clad in barks and deerskin. Men in that age had a calm mind, no feeling of animosity towards anybody, were friendly towards all creatures and looked upon all with an equal eye. They propitiated the Lord through Tapas in the form of contemplation and by their control of mind and the senses. In the age of Treta the Lord was of Crimson hue, had four arms, wore a triple cord about His loins and had golden locks. He was propitiated by sacrifices through the Vedic lore as an embodiment of all deities. In the Dwapara Age the Lord was of dark brown complexion, remained clad in yellow silk, wielded in his arms His own weapons and emblems—conch, discus, mace and lotus; wore the kaustubha gem and was distinguished by the marks of Srivasta (a color of white hair on the right side of his bosom). To know the ultimate Reality the Lord in that age was worshipped as characterized by the regalia proper to a monarch, such as the umbrella or fly-whisk, as indicated in the Vedas and Tantras. For example men may say, "hail to you, Vasudeva; hail to Sankarasana and hail to You, the almighty Lord, as Pradyumna and Anirudha." Hail to the Sage Narayana, the almighty, all-pervading, all-embodying Ruler of the universe, dwelling in the heart of all. Thus the people will adore and praise the Lord of the universe in the Dwapara Age. Lastly, in the present Kali Yuga the Lord is to be worshipped through sacrifices mostly consisting of chanting of names of the Lord and singing His praises. The Lord is of dark color, though bright in lustre, perfect in limbs, adorned with ornaments, furnished with His weapons and waited upon by His attendants.

Thus the Lord is worshipped differently in different ages for knowing the Truth and getting liberation. Elderly and discriminating people appreciate the merits of Kali age and extol this age, in which merely by chanting the names of the Lord one can attain all the desired objects, which could otherwise be had through many virtues only. Chanting of His names bestows perfect peace and as a sequel to which the cycle of birth and death comes to an end. For this reason those living in Satya, Treta and Dwapara yugas seek birth in the Kali age. Renouncing the notion of separateness from the Lord, one who wholeheartedly and completely resorts for protection to the protecting Lord is no more a servant of or debtor to the deities, rishis or others, relations or deceased ancestors. If such a person incurs any sin for any reason, although he is incapable of sin as a rule, the Supreme Lord enshrined in his heart, washes off all that sin. Even those who keep thinking of the Lord with a feeling of enmity while sleeping, sitting or eating, had His gait, graceful movements and glance, etc. imprinted on their mind and accordingly attained similarity to His form. What to say of those whose mind is attached to Him.

Jiva or Individual Soul, a reflection of the Lord, is in bondage from time immemorial through ignorance; the Lord brings about the release through knowledge in the form of Self-realization vouchsafed by Him. Let us see the distinction between Jiva and the other one who is liberated (viz., God), characterized by contrary properties (viz., sorrow and joy respectively), though coexisting in one and the same individual. Jiva and God (inner controller of the Jiva) are distinct from the body like the two birds dwelling on a tree yet apart from it, kindred (spiritual in substance) and settled as constant companions in the same nest (of the heart) on the tree (of the body) by force of Maya or divine will. Jiva partakes of the fruit (joy and sorrow) in the peepul tree of the body (as a result of good and bad karma); while the other (viz., God), though going without food (joy and sorrow) is always superior to the former in strength of wisdom. The enlightened one (viz., God), who does not partake of the fruit of the tree, knows Himself as well as the other (the Jiva); but not so the one who partakes of the fruit. The one in ignorance (the Jiva) has been in bondage from eternity; while the other with knowledge (viz., God) is ever free. An enlightened soul (a Jivanmukta or the one liberated while still living) is not tied to the body even though he remains in the body due to Samskaras, like the one who has awoke from the dream. One with perverted intellect remains identified with the body, as the dreamer remains identified with the dream body, though not actually present in it. The enlightened one feels that it is the Gunas (modes of nature) themselves in the form of the senses that apprehend their objects, which are made up of the same substance, while he does not feel that he is apprehending them. The ignorant Jiva remains tied to the body due to his Prarabdha (destiny), erroneously thinking that he is the doer, while in fact, it is the Indriyas (which are modifications of Gunas) that are the performers of the actions.

Thus remaining free from passion while (lying) in bed, sitting, moving about, bathing, seeing, touching, smelling, eating and hearing, etc. and allowing the (three) Gunas (in the form of the senses) to enjoy the various objects of the senses, the enlightened soul does not get bound (by such actions) like the ignorant man[15] (p. 562). King Parikshit questioned the great sage Sri Suka as to why a great devotee like Priyavrata, son of Vyvasvatha Manu, who was free from attachment, should take to householder's life, in spite of his serene and happy mind under the shelter of the glorious Lord's feet. Sri Suka replied, "Just as the strings run through the nostrils govern the oxen, human beings are controlled by the knots of Guna and karma, as ordained by him. One should enjoy the fruits of his Prarabdha Karma, though he has realization, which only helps him not to acquire or add to Karma or Vasana, leading to more bodies or births. To one, who has subdued his senses and is devoted to the Lord, householder's life could do no harm. He who has conquered the six enemies, is safe as in a stronghold. Priyavrata was one such and could rule the world, renouncing all attachment, and then return to his essential nature[16] (p. 140). "Sri Ramana Maharishi replied to a question as follows, "I am the body' idea will become extinct only on Self-realization. With its extinction the *vasanas* (desires of sensual enjoyment) become extinct and all virtues will remain ever. *Samskaras* are said to persist even in a Janna, but they are *bhoga hetu* (leading to enjoyment only) and not *bandha hetu* (leading to bondage)[17] (p. 492)." On being doubted that the fakes may pretend to be *sadhus* but lead vicious lives, saying it is their *Prarabdha*, Maharishi said that the one who has given up the idea of being the doer cannot repeat, "This is my Prarabdha." And again, "He who is liberated from the body and is himself perfect abides in enjoyment like a worldly man full of desire created by the past karma (does). But he lives quietly as a spectator, free from desires and changes, like the centre of a wheel[18]. According to Gopi Krishna, "Sufficient sleep, proper food, moderate sexual indulgence, temperance, an active altruistic life, conformity to sublime ideals and healthy principles, noble and benevolent traits of character–these are the essentials of a life spent in concordance with the demands of evolution[19].

Though continuing in his psych-physical organism (which is modification of Prakriti or Nature), the enlightened one remains unattached to it like the sky, the sun (which remains unattached to the water in which it is reflected) or the wind (which remains unattached though blowing everywhere). He turns away from the sense of diversity as all his doubts have been removed by his penetrating intellect whetted by all-round detachment. He remains unfettered by the three Gunas operating through the body, though dwelling in it. One who has transcended the sense of good and evil and sees equality everywhere neither praises nor condemns anyone. Revelling in his self, a man given to contemplation may roam around like a stupid fellow. Being well-versed in the Veda but without knowledge or realization of Brahma, one has ended in labour alone. One should retire from all activities and focus one's mind on the Lord, doing all allotted duties disinterestedly for the sake of the Lord. With unflinching devotion to the Lord one becomes His worshipper and finally attains to His state.

Having attained the state of purity one becomes compassionate to all, harms none, is forbearing, truthful, faultless of mind, equipoised in all circumstances-good or bad, beneficent to all, unaffected in judgement by the pleasures of senses, self-disciplined, soft by nature, perfect in moral, resourceless and effortless, solely dependent on the Lord, lives on a scanty meal, given to contemplation and vigilance, remains unexcited and firm even when there is room for excitement; has conquered the opposites such as, cold and heat, greed and infatuation, hunger and thirst; does not seek honor though bestowing it on others. Having known the truth about the Lord, he worships Him alone by beholding, touching and adoring His representations like images, etc. visits holy places and initiates others into Vedic and Tantric ways of knowing the Truth. He remembers that being made known through one's own lips spends a virtue.

The Liberation of Man

According to Srimad Bhagavata Mahapurana the Lord advises that one should worship Him as the conscious Self through undifferentiated vision. One should concentrate on Lord Vishnu's four-armed personality equipped with a conch, discus, mace and lotus. Ordinarily there is no royal road to His realization other than the discipline of devotion preceded by association with the righteous. Neither the Yoga according to eight limbed Yoga-Sutras of Patanjali nor Sankhya philosophy nor righteousness; study of the Vedas or japa (chanting) of the Divine Name, austerity and renunciation nor pouring oblations on the sacred fire and works of public utility (digging wells, laying gardens, etc.) nor gifts. Observing fasts, worship of gods, muttering secret spells, resorting to holy places, undertaking sacred observances and self-abnegation gain Him over as does Satsanga (assembly of holy men) capture Him, which puts an end to all kinds of attachments. There are innumerable examples of men who ascended His abode in this manner. Full of passion for Him as their lover, nay, paramour attained to Him, the Supreme Brahma, through the fellowship of the righteous. He reveals Himself in the six chakras (vortices of energy along the spine) in degrees and finally the practitioner attains Self-realization.

Sattva, Rajas and Tamas are the three modes of Nature and not the Self. By developing the quality of Sattva one should control the other two and then Sattva itself. When Sattva becomes predominant one develops real Devotion to the Lord. Ten factors that are responsible for the development of a particular Guna are—scripture, water, people, place, time, occupation and birth, the object of contemplation, mantra and purificatory rites. Men of mature judgement approve the factors responsible for Sattva, look with indifference the factors for rajasic and condemn the ones for Tamasic. Making use of sattvic things promotes righteousness leading to devotion to the Lord, and finally the wisdom culminates in self-realization.

Yoga taught by the Lord to Brahma—the secret formula, is revealed here for the benefit of the mankind. Although men know that the pleasures of senses lead to calamities, yet they doggedly pursue and enjoy them. The reason is that Rajas, although born of Sattva itself, brings up again and again the perverted notion of "I" with regard to body and related matters in the heart of the deluded soul, which pervades the mind and is the root of sorrow. Perverted mind first brings the notion about an object being worth enjoying and then finds out how to enjoy it. Dwelling on the excellent aspect of that object a passion arises in him, which is indeed difficult to arrest. Deluded by the impetuosity of Rajas one loses control over senses and is overpowered by desire, and hence embarks upon actions followed by sorrow in the end. The mind of a *man of discrimination* is also distracted and infatuated by Rajas and Tamas at times, but he collects his mind again with effort, remembers the evil inherent in the pleasures of senses and does not get attached to them. Controlling the breath and securing steadiness of posture, one should slowly compose the mind and concentrate on the Lord thrice daily at fixed times. He should not feel bored even if success deludes for sometime and continue with the process. Just as the *swan* is credited with the virtue of separating water from milk when mixed together, one should alienate the sense-objects from the mind. Yoga taught by the Lord to Brahma and other sages comprises of "withdrawing the mind from everything else and duly and directly establishing in Him."

As a result of the enquiry into the truth one should bear in mind that anything grasped by the mind, expressed through speech and perceived through vision and other senses is nothing other than the Lord Himself. Sense-objects and the mind both constitute the body (an adjunct and not the essence) of the Jiva or Individual Soul, which is essentially the same as the Lord. As such there is no real affinity between the Jiva and, the sense objects and mind, which can therefore be easily transcended by the Jiva by contemplation on its divine essence, its identity with Brahma. Sense-objects get imprinted on the mind in the form of latencies because of repeatedly enjoying them. By becoming one with the Lord and realizing one's own true nature, the Jiva should give up both the mind and the sense objects. Jiva should know that he is conclusively distinct from and witness of the three states of wakefulness, dream and deep slumber; which are the states of the mind and not the Jiva, resulting from the preponderance of the three Gunas—Sattva, Rajas and Tamas respectively. Jiva should shake off this identification with Buddhi or Intellect, which is the source of transmigration of the soul and its attachment with the three states of wakefulness, dream and deep slumber. Eventually a divorce follows between the sense-objects and the mind. Getting established in the fourth transcendent state of *witnessing,* one does not continue sleeping as a fool even though he is awake, just like a man who is waking in a dream. Know that everything else is unreal except the Self and the three states of mind are superimposed on the Lord appearing as the Jiva by His deluding potency. Cutting at the root of egotism the basis of all doubts (e.g., whether the body and the soul are one or different) with the sword of wisdom whetted by reasoning, the precepts of saints and Sruti texts, one should betake oneself to the Lord seated in his very heart.

Looking at the objective world as an illusion created by the mind one should understand the threefold division of the body, the Indriyas and the objects wrought by the projection of the three Gunas having an illusory appearance. One's thirst for enjoyment having ceased once and for all, he should keep quiet and effortless and remain absorbed in the realization of one's own blissful nature. Even though the body is perceived as a distinct reality at the time of taking food or doing other bodily functions, its once being dismissed as unreal other than the Self does not delude us any longer, although its impression on the mind may continue till the end of life. Although the realization of the

Self comes through the use of the body itself, yet its importance has been lost forever. However, body will survive till the exhaust of Karma. Having climbed the highest ladder of Yoga through concentration of mind, known as Samadhi (absorption of mind into the Universal Spirit), and having realized the truth, one does not recapture the lost attachment for the world and connected things in it, such as wife, children, property, power, position and other material things. This is the secret of Sankhya (path of knowledge distinguishing Matter from Spirit) and Yoga (philosophy of Patanjali) expounded by the Lord. Lord advises everyone to recognize Him as Yajna (Lord Vishnu Himself) arrived on earth to unfold the secrets of Dharma, the righteous course leading to Liberation. Under all circumstances He is the supreme goal of Yoga and Sankhya. All virtues like evenmindedness and non-attachment (being eternal since they are not the products of the three Gunas) find shelter in the Lord, who is transcendent and free from desire, the beloved friend, rather the very Self of all.

Happiness enjoyed with the Lord as their own Self cannot fall to those who have their mind set on sense-pleasure. All the four quarters are full of joy to him who has nothing to call his own, has fully subdued his mind and senses, whose mind is equipoised (free from likes and dislikes) and fully gratified with the Lord. Such a person does not aspire even for the position of Brahma, much less for the realm of paradise ruled by Indra, still less for the sovereignty over the entire globe or mystic powers acquired through Yoga, nor does he care for cessation of rebirth divorced from the Lord. Neither Brahma (His own son) nor Lord Siva (His own Self) nor Goddess Sri (His better half) is so dear to the Lord as a devotee. Lord's all-blissful character is realized by only exalted souls who have nothing to call their own, whose mind is fixed on Him, who have subdued their passions and are fond of all living beings and whose understanding is unclouded by desires or the ones who are free of wants.

Though attracted by objects of senses, such objects because of the powerful devotion to the Lord do not generally overpower Lord's devotee, who has not yet been able to conquer his senses. Just as fire reduces a pile of wood to ashes, so does devotion to Lord burns one's sins. Nothing captivates the Lord, as does intense devotion with reverence, which absolves even those who cook and eat the flesh of dogs. Devotion is known through hair standing on end or through one's heart melting or through tears of joy, which alone purifies the mind. Such a person speaks in a voice choked with emotion, who weeps incessantly at the thought of separation from Lord, who sometimes laughs when reminded of Lord's pastimes, who sings unabashed at the top of his voice and dances out of joy—purifying the whole world. Just as gold is purified in fire so does Karma burn off through devotion and the devotee attains oneness with the Lord. The greater the purification by listening to and recounting Lord's auspicious stories, the greater the discernment of the realities of Self by the Jiva, just as the eye perceives a minute object better on meditation.

Mind dwelling on sense objects gets attached to them; even so, mind contemplating on Lord gets absorbed in Him alone. One should abandon the company of women and of men delighted in company of women, secure a lonely place and unweariedly think of the Lord. No affliction and bondage results from attachment to others as does from the company of women and men delighted in the company of women.

Process of Meditation

Seated on a seat of moderate height (neither too high nor too low) with the body erect in a comfortable posture placing both the hands (with palm upwards) on the lap and steadying the gaze on the tip of the nose, having fully controlled the senses, one should cleanse the passages of life-breath by three processes of breath-control—*puraka* (slow inhalation), *kumbhaka* (retention of breath) and *rechaka* (slow exhalation) and then reverse the order. Manifesting in mind through the instrumentality of the life-breath the sound of Pranava (the sacred syllable OM), as extending uninterruptedly, fine as a fibre of the lotus stalk, from the *muladhara chakra* or root-centre near anus to the *sahasrara* or crown centre of the head, should be followed with a sharp nasal sound continuous as the ringing of a bell. If the whole exercise of breath-control is being joined with Pranava and repeated ten times thrice a day, then one attains control over breath in a month's time. One should then visualize the heart in the shape of the lotus bud turned upside down with its stalk upward, like the flower of a plantain in an inverted position, with eight open petals and pericarp turned upwards. One should picture in the mind in succession the sun, the moon and fire as existing in the form of circles on the pericarp; then mentally behold Lord's form in the centre of fire and contemplate upon it happily. Lord should be conceived as symmetrical, gracious, having a charming countenance, having four long beautiful arms, a very shapely and graceful neck, lovely cheeks and a bright smile; with brilliant alligator shaped earrings adorning well-matched ears, clad in golden raiment, dark brown as a cloud, bearing marks of Srivasta (a white curl of hair) and Sri (a golden streak) on both sides of the chest; decked with a conch, discus, mace and lotus and wreath of sylvan flowers, feet shining with anklets, distinguished with the effulgence of Kaustubha gem, graced all over with glorious diadem, wristlets, girdle and armlets; charming of every limb, pleasing to the heart, with a countenance and eyes enlivened with grace and very soft to the touch. One should concentrate the mind on each limb individually and then on the whole figure.

A wise man should mentally withdraw the senses from their objects and then withdraw the mind too from all objects using intellect, which is the driver of the chariot of the body, and then focus attention on the Lord. After going through all the limbs one should fix the thoughts exclusively on Lord's face wearing a winsome smile. After the mind has gained a firm hold on the countenance, it should be diverted and fixed on Lord's all-pervading Self, like the sky that is encompassing but unattached to all; and then even that should be transcended, becoming one with Lord the Absolute, and then cease to think of anything else, not even the distinction between the subject and the object. With his intellect thus established in the Lord he sees the Lord in himself and himself actually merged in the Lord, the Universal Soul, like the light in the fire. On concentrating the mind through most intense meditation as aforesaid, the misconception regarding matter (body being self), knowledge (ascribing knowership to Self) and action (attributing activity to Self) will soon disappear from the mind of the practitioner.

Sri Ishopanishad and Swami Prabhupada of ISKCON

Knowledge about the First Cause or Supersoul and its relation with Soul are elaborated in Sri Ishopanishad—Upanishad about Ishwar or God. It explains the meaning of self-realization in very clear terms. A.C. Bhaktivedanta Swami Prabhupada, founder of the International Society for Krishna Consciousness has interpreted and commented upon the 18 mantras or stanzas that cover the whole book[20]. The matter is presented here in brief.

Veda means the original knowledge. In conditioned state our knowledge is subject to many deficiencies, which is the difference between a conditioned soul and a liberated soul. First deficiency is to commit mistakes, e.g., Mahatma Gandhi and John F. Kennedy were warned not to go out that day when they were assassinated, but they erred and paid the price. Second deficiency is to be illusioned by *Maya*, i.e., identifying oneself with the body, which is illusion. Third deficiency is the cheating propensity. Without knowing the truth one thinks that he is intelligent and writes books on philosophy. Fourth defect is that our senses are imperfect, which cannot acquire true knowledge. Hence *Vedas* should be accepted as they are.

Vedas are not the compilations of human knowledge. They came from the spiritual world, from Lord Krishna. Brahma was the first living creature who was the first to be instructed in the Vedic knowledge by Lord Himself. Brahma imparted it to his son Narada and other sons and disciples, which was further distributed to their disciples. Thus Vedic knowledge is passed on from one generation to another through the disciples from disciplic succession. Even if one experiments one would finally come to the same knowledge. Science is endeavouring and it may arrive at the same conclusions may be after a million years or more. There are three kinds of evidences: *pratyaksha* (direct evidence, which is not good because of imperfect senses), *anumana* (inductive knowledge, i.e. Darwin's speculations) and *sabda* (knowledge from authoritative sources, i.e. program guide from radio station, which is perfect). Vedic knowledge is *sabda-pramana* or *sruti*, that is, by aural reception. It is transcendental, from beyond this universe, as compared to material knowledge that comes from this universe.

There is spiritual sky where the planets and inhabitants are eternal, beyond manifestation and non-manifestation. This is Vedic knowledge that cannot come through experimentation. Krishna is the highest authority on it, accepted by all classes of men. There are two classes of transcendentalists, who deal with the Vedic knowledge. One class is called impersonalists, Mayavadi or Vedantists, led by Adi Guru Sankaracharya. The other class called Vaisnavas includes Ramanujacharya, Madhavacharya and Vishnuswami. Both have accepted Krishna as the Supreme Personality of Godhead. The impersonalists preach impersonalism and impersonal Brahman. However, they have also accepted that Narayana is Krishna, beyond cosmic manifestation, who came as the son of Devaki and Vasudeva

The Liberation of Man

for the benefit of the mankind, as is the belief of the other class known as Vaisnavas. Both classes accept what Krishna has said and this is Krishna Consciousness. Another scripture called *Brahma Samhita* states that one could even travel in an airplane running with the speed of mind for millions of years and yet find that spiritual sky is unlimited and unapproachable. The only way to spiritual worlds is through a bona fide spiritual master, a *guru*, who has rightly heard the Vedic message from the right source and is firmly established in Brahman.

Aim of Vedic research is to know and find Krishna. *Brahma Samhita* states that Krishna has innumerable forms, but they are all one. They are not fallible like our forms are with a beginning and an end. He is every where, all-pervading, original, the oldest, and yet looking like a young boy of fifteen or twenty years. He was not less than a hundred years of age, having great grandchildren, yet appearing like a boy as the charioteer of Arjun from *Bhagavad Gita*.

Originally there was only one *Veda*, and people were so intelligent and sharp in memories that they could understand and remember it after hearing it for once from the mouth of the spiritual teacher. But five thousand years ago Vyasadeva thought that people in the coming Kali Yuga would be short-lived, less intelligent and poor in memory, and hence he wrote down the Vedic knowledge after dividing it into four parts—*Rig Veda, Atharva Veda, Sama Veda* and *Yajur Veda*. He gave charge of these *Vedas* to his disciples. He was especially concerned with the upliftment of women folk and *dvija-bandhus*, the persons born in knowledgeable *brahamana* race but not qualified as a *brahamana*. Vyasadeva compiled *Mahabharata*, eighteen *Puranas* and *Upanishads* as part of the *Vedas* for these persons. Then he summarized all Vedic knowledge for scholars and philosophers in what is called the *Vedanta-sutra*, which is the last word of the *Vedas*.

Sage Vyasadeva personally wrote the *Vedanta-sutra*, under the guidance of Narada, his spiritual master or Guru Maharaja, yet he was not satisfied. He also wrote the perfect *Vedanta* commentary, *Srimad Bhagavatam*. Then Narada explained to Vyasadeva that *Vedanta* means "ultimate knowledge," which is Krishna. Krishna Himself said, "I am the compiler of the *Vedanta-sutra*, and I am the knower of the *Vedas*." *Vedanta-sutra* hints at what is Brahman, the Absolute Truth: "The Absolute Truth is that from whom everything emanates." This is the summary, while the full details are given in *Srimad Bhagavatam* or *Srimad Bhagavata Mahapurana*. The Absolute Truth must be consciousness. He is self-effulgent (*sva-rat*). Those after Vedic knowledge should try to understand it from *Srimad Bhagavatam* and *Bhagavad Gita*.

Invocation

The Personality of Godhead is perfect and complete, and because He is perfectly complete, all emanations from Him, such as this phenomenal world, are complete wholes (equipped with everything). Whatever is produced of the Complete Whole is also complete in itself. Even though so many complete units emanate from Him, the complete balance is still remaining in Him.

The Complete Whole, or the Supreme Absolute Truth is the complete Personality of Godhead. He is *sat-chit-ananda-vigraha*. Vigraha means form, hence He has a form. Realization of impersonal Brahman is realization of only *sat* feature, and realization of Paramatma is realization of *sat* and *chit* features, hence incomplete. He should be realized in all His features: *sat* (eternal existence), *chit* (knowledge) and *ananda* (bliss). He has immense potencies, all of which are as complete as He is e.g., this phenomenal world. The world is made of 24 elements, which are complete to take care of it, till its temporary manifestation is annihilated. Human form is also a complete manifestation of the consciousness of a living being, and capable of realization of the Complete Whole, with all facilities available. If the chance is missed one may have to repeat the cycle of 8,400,000 species through which it has evolved. Illusory representation of completeness is sense enjoyment, which can never provide lasting satisfaction. All kinds of services such as, social, political, communal would remain incomplete until they are dovetailed with the Complete Whole, and then each of the attached part will be complete in itself.

Mantras

Mantra 1

The Lord controls all that is animate or inanimate in this universe. One should accept only that much of the things that are set aside as his quota, and one should not endeavour to gain the wealth of anyone else.

Ishopanishad is part of the *Yajur Veda,* and hence it contains information about the proprietorship of all things that exist in the universe. Lord's proprietorship over everything is confirmed in the seventh chapter of *Bhagavad Gita* (7.4-5), where *para* and *apara prakriti* are discussed. The elements of nature—earth, water, fire, air, ether, mind, intelligence and ego—all belong to the inferior, material energy (*apara prakriti*), whereas the living being, the organic energy is His superior energy (*para prakriti*). Both of these energies have emanated from the Lord and He is the controller of everything that exists. He is the controller, sustainer and dictator of everything. He is the possessor of all potencies, the knower of everything and the benefactor of everyone. He is full of inconceivable opulence, power, fame, beauty, knowledge and renunciation.

One should therefore know clearly that no one except Lord Himself is the proprietor of all things. Things have been nicely arranged and quota set aside by the Lord, e.g.

cow is made to give milk to humans but she does not drink it herself. Our houses are made of things like earth, wood, stone, iron and cement which are produced by Lord's energy and not by us, we can only transform and shape them differently. A laborer cannot be proprietor. Quarrel between laborers and capitalists in modern society have taken an international shape. This should be discouraged in the light of the knowledge of *Ishopanishad*. Communists, capitalists or any other party claiming proprietorship over the resources of nature can have no peace since they are entirely the property of the Lord. Unless this fact is recognized, nuclear bombs are likely to ruin all parties involved. Similarly, man killing animals for the satisfaction of his uncontrolled taste buds is responsible for breaking the laws of nature and eventually gets punished. Animals do not transgress the laws of nature, e.g., tiger does not eat rice or wheat or drink cow's milk since he is given animal flesh as food. Lower life forms such as animals, birds and reptiles adhere to the laws of nature, in eating, mating and so on. As such there is no question of sin or Vedic teachings for them but for humans, who are responsible. A vegetarian should not be proud of being so, as vegetables too have life. Yet, however, Lord states in *Bhagavad Gita* (9.26) that He accepts vegetarian food from the hands of a devotee. Therefore humans should offer food to the Lord in devotion and then eat the remnants as blessed food.

The root of sin is deliberate disobedience of the laws of nature. One who knows the laws of nature, and who is not influenced by unnecessary attachment or aversion is sure to be recognized by the Lord and thus become eligible to go back to Godhead, back to the eternal home.

Mantra 2

Continuously working in this way one may aspire to live for hundred years, for that set of work will not bind him to the law of karma. There is no alternative to this way for man.

The Liberation of Man

Both individually as well as collectively in the form of community or nation one wants to prolong living as much as possible. In fact, man is eternal by nature but due to his bondage in material existence he has to change his body over and over. This is transmigration of souls due to *karma bandhana* or bondage of karma. Other life forms may continue but once one attains a human life he has the chance to free himself from the chains of karma. *Bhagavad Gita* states that acting according to one's prescribed duties in scriptures is *karma*, actions that free one from the cycle of birth and death is *akarma* and actions with misuse of one's freedom that glides one into lower life forms is *vikarma*. Ordinary men act to achieve higher status in the world or in heaven, but intelligent men know that both good and bad work equally binds them to material miseries. Hence they seek such liberating activities that will free them from the reactions of both good and bad work. *Bhagavad Gita* or *Gitopanishad* says that one has to execute prescribed duties according to Vedic literature before attaining the state of *naiskarmya* or *akarma*. This literature regulates the working in such a way that one finally realizes the authority of the personality of Godhead or Krishna. Then one is said to have attained the stage of positive knowledge and then the three modes of nature—goodness, passion and ignorance do not affect and one is no more bound to the cycle of birth and death.

Acts of sense enjoyment extended to society as altruism, socialism, communism, nationalism or humanitarianism are attractive forms of karmic bondage. Only by the devotional service to the Lord, with God-centered or *isavasya* activities one can become karmaless. According to Krishna (*Bhagavad Gita*, 2.40) just a few of God-centered activities can save one from falling into the cycle of repeated births among 8,400,000 species. Such activities become a form of *Karma yoga* (*Bhagavad Gita*, 18.5-9). Even if such activities remain half-finished one is guaranteed a human form in next birth.

This gives another chance to improve one's position on the path of liberation. One is recommended to read *The Nectar of Devotion* by Srila Rupa Goswami to know details of God-centered activities.

Mantra 3

Whoever is the killer of the soul enters into the planets known as the worlds of the faithless, full of darkness and ignorance.

Those who act with responsibilities are called *suras* or godly persons, while others who neglect responsibilities are called *asuras* or demons. Only these two types of humans exist in the universe. *Rig Veda* states that *suras* aim at the lotus feet of the Supreme Lord Vishnu and act accordingly. Human form is achieved after millions of years of evolution in the cycle of transmigration. The material world is likened to an ocean, human body to a solid boat, saintly teachers of Vedic scriptures to expert boatmen, and facilities of the human body to favorable breezes that help the boat ply smoothly to its desired destination. One who does not utilize the facilities for Self-realization is called *atma-ha* or a killer of the soul, who enters the darkest regions of ignorance to suffer perpetually.

Human form of life is given not to work like a donkey or swine for more money and pleasures of senses, but to attain highest perfection towards Self-realization. *Bhagavad Gita* (6.41-43) states that a man who enters upon the path of Self-realization but does not complete the process, despite having sincerely tried for it, is given a chance to appear in the family of *suchi* or *srimat*. *Suchi* means a spiritually advanced *brahmana,* and *srimat* means a *vaisya*, a member of the mercantile community. Such a person who fails to achieve Self-realization is given a better chance in his next life, due to his sincere efforts in this life. With this one can imagine the fates of those who have achieved success. Even attempting to realize God, one is guaranteed birth in a wealthy or aristocratic family. Others who never even attempt and are towards material enjoyments alone are called *asuras* or *atma-sambhavita* in *Bhagavad Gita* (16.17-18), and are certain to enter the darkest regions. One should not only try to solve economic problems on a tottering platform but also try to solve all the problems of material life.

Mantra 4

Although fixed in His abode in one place, the Personality of Godhead is swifter than the mind, can overcome all others running and controls those who supply wind and rain. The powerful demigods like Indra cannot approach Him. He surpasses all in excellence.

Even the greatest philosophers cannot know Supreme Lord through mental speculations, nor the demigods can approach Him. A non-devotee philosopher may travel with the speed of wind or the mind for hundreds of millions of years, yet the Absolute Truth will appear far away. Only a devotee can know Him through His own mercy (*Brahma Samhita* 5.34). Just as a fire situated at one place can spread its heat and light around to some distance, even so by the inconceivable potencies of Lord Supreme, although being in His transcendental abode called Goloka and engaged in His pastimes, He can simultaneously reach every part of His creation and/or diffuse His energies everywhere (*Brahma Samhita*, 5.37).

His innumerable energies can be broadly divided into three principal categories: internal potency, marginal potency and external potency, each category having innumerable divisions again. The material world is a projection of His external potency. Powerful demigods controlling phenomena like air, light and rain; and lesser living beings such as humans correspond to the marginal potency of the Lord. Whereas the spiritual sky, where the kingdom of God is situated, is due to the internal potency of the Supreme Being. Since the personal features of the Lord have been mentioned in so much detail, it suggests that the Absolute Truth is in the form of an Absolute Person.

Since the parts and parcels can never equal its whole, the Lord cannot be fully appreciated through His various potencies. No one can establish the identity of the Lord through mental speculations. One should try to learn the transcendental form of the Lord, who is the source of the *Vedas*, since the Lord alone has the knowledge of His transcendence.

Every part and parcel of the Complete whole has been endowed with a particular energy. One may forget one's designated role under the influence of *maya* or illusion, which can be revived through one's initiative properly utilized, and then one may arrive at the original consciousness lost in association with *maya* or the external energy. Every particular power should be utilized to execute the will of the Lord, who is the source of all powers. Such a submissive service attitude can lead one to know God. Chit or knowledge consists in knowing the Lord in all His features, knowing all His potencies and their working through His will. *Bhagavad Gita*, which is the essence of all the *Upanishads*, has the details of these matters described by the Lord.

Mantra 5

The Supreme Lord walks and does not walk. He is far away, and He is very near as well. He is within everything and yet He is outside of everything.

Contradictions prove the inconceivable energies of the Lord such as walking and not walking at the same time. It means that He has both the features—personal and impersonal. The impersonalist philosophers of Mayavada accept only impersonal activities of the Lord and not the personal ones. Followers of Bhagavata School, who adopt perfect conception of the Lord, accept His inconceivable potencies and understand both features. Since the Lord cannot be seen through the eyes it should not be concluded that He has no personal existence. The material sky itself is not measurable, so what can one say of the spiritual sky that lies further beyond (*Bhagavad Gita*, 15.6). Although the abode of the Lord is so far away, He can descend before us at once, in less than a second. Foolish people consider Him a mortal being, but His body is not of the material nature like an ordinary person, as erroneously understood by the so-called scholars (*Bhagavad Gita*, 9.11). Non-believers in His inconceivable energies say that either He cannot incarnate, or if He does He descends in a material form. Even if He descends in material form, it can be converted into spiritual form through His inconceivable potencies. Since He is the source of all energies, He can accept our service through any sort of medium.

Because of our imperfect material existence including our vision, we cannot see the Lord. Yet for the favor of devotees, He appears in material form to accept their services and is seen. Worship through the idol goes to the Lord and He appears before them in an approachable way. I can vouch for this by my own experiences that are described in the first chapter on autobiography. Lord treats a devotee according to his degree of surrender (*Bhagavad Gita*, 4.11). For a surrendered soul He is always within reach, whereas for unsurrendered soul He is far, far away and is unapproachable.

There are two aspects of the Lord—*saguna* (with qualities) and *nirguna* (without qualities). However, His material form with perceivable qualities is not subject to laws of material nature. He can never be under the influence of material energies even though He uses them at His will. He has an eternal form and is never formless. His impersonal aspect as Brahman is a glow of His personal rays, like the sunrays being the glow of sun-god. He is everywhere and can appear anytime, as in the case of Narsimha—the half-man, half-lion incarnation appearing from the pillar for His devotee Prahlad, and killing his atheist father who was a king. He appears in order to vanquish non-believers and protect believers (*Bhagavad Gita*, 4.8).

According to *Brahma Samhita* (5.35) He remains outside in His *virat* form, and enters and lives within everything as *antaryami*. He witnesses everything that is going on and all actions are awarded with results according to *karma phal* or fruit of karma. We might forget our acts of previous life, but He has in record everything and results are awarded accordingly. When a pitcher is dipped in a pond of water, there is water inside and water outside; even so there is God inside and God outside. Everything is a manifestation of His different energies. The Lord in His personal form through them ultimately enjoys all the pleasures enjoyed minutely by the tiny part-and-parcel living beings.

Mantra 6

He who sees everything in relation to the Supreme Lord, who sees all living entities as His parts and parcels, and who sees the Supreme Lord within everything never hates anything or any being.

Lord's presence is realized in three stages. Lowest stage of realization comes to a *kanistha adhikari* who goes to a place of worship—temple, church or mosque, and worships according to one's faith following scriptural injunctions. He believes the Lord to be present only at the place of worship and nowhere else. They have no judgement of the position of a devotee in respect of realization; they follow routine formulas and even fight among themselves considering one type of devotion better than the other. These are materialistic devotees trying to transcend material boundary and reach the spiritual plane.

Persons with realization of the second stage are called *madhyama adhikaris*, having distinctions between four categories of people: (i) the Supreme Lord; (ii) people devoted to the Lord; (iii) the innocent ones, having no knowledge of the Lord; and (iv) the atheists, having no faith in the Lord and hating the devotees of the Lord. Behavior of *madhyama adhikaris* is different towards the people of these four

The Liberation of Man

divisions: adoring the Lord as object of love; making friends with the devotees of the Lord; trying to awaken the love of God in the simple-minded people and avoiding to meet the atheists.

People of highest realization are called *uttama adhikari*, seeing everything in relation to the Lord, treating everyone as part and parcel of God. He finds no essential difference between a *brahmana* and a dog, believing that the *brahmana* particle of the Lord has not misused his little independence given by the Lord, while the dog particle has misused his independence and is being punished as encasement in the body of dog. Disregarding the respective actions of the two he remains good to both. Being a learned devotee he is not mislead by material bodies and is equally attracted by the two because of having the same spiritual spark in them. False philanthropists who try to imitate an *uttama adhikari* behave only on the bodily platform, without knowing that the individual soul is an expansion of Lord's Supersoul dwelling everywhere. The word *anupasyati* in the *mantra* means that one should not see things as observed by the physical eye but should follow the previous *acharya* or source of knowledge, of which highest is Vedic wisdom coming in discipalic succession from the Lord Himself.

The two most important revealed scriptures are *Bhagavad Gita*, spoken by the Lord Himself and recorded by Vyasadeva and *Srimad Bhagavatam*, which is the natural commentary on *Vedanta sutra* by Vyasadeva. Commentaries by others not belonging to the disciplic succession of Vyasadeva should not be taken as authentic. Only the one who is liberated (*brahma-bhuta*) can become an *uttama adhikari*, looking at everyone as his brother, a vision that cannot belong to a politician seeking only material gains. Imitators of *uttama adhikari* cannot serve the spirit soul but the body for fame and material rewards. *Uttama adhikari* sees the spirit soul inside the physical body and serves him as soul; the material aspect is taken care of automatically.

Mantra 7

One who always sees all living entities as spiritual sparks, one with the Lord in quality, becomes a true knower of things. What, then, can be illusion or anxiety for him?

The sparks of fire have the same qualities of heat and light as the fire itself, but the quantities of heat and light present in the sparks are not equal to those in the fire. As another example, the qualities of salt with regard to chemical composition are the same in a drop of water and the whole ocean, but the quantity of salt in a drop is not the same as that in the ocean. Since there is no difference between the energy and the energetic, there is the sense of oneness. Although heat and light are different from fire analytically, the word fire has no meaning without heat and light. Therefore heat, light and fire are the same synthetically. Even so *jivas* or individual souls that are sparks of Supersoul, the Supreme Lord, are synthetically "one" with the Lord in quality, but not the same in quantity. Not even the powerful demigods can equal the Lord in any respect. Such an "oneness" of the *jiva* and the Lord is rightly understood by the *madhyama adhikari* and *uttam adhikari* only.

According to *Vedanta sutra* (1.1.12) the Supreme Lord and all His parts and parcels are *ananda-mayo-bhyasat* or meant for eternal enjoyment. However, the *jivas* encaged in physical bodies are seeking enjoyment in material pleasures, which is the wrong platform while the Supreme Lord enjoys Himself with all His associates on the spiritual platform. There is always a clash between individuals on material platform because the enjoyment is sought from the wrong centre. There is no clash on spiritual platform because it has no material objects there. As soon as one gets connected to the right centre of spiritual *rasa* dance, that is Supreme Lord, one becomes transcendental and without any clash, and then there is no *moha* (illusion) or *soka* (lamentation). According to *Bhagavad Gita* (7.14) only those who surrender to the lotus feet of the Supreme Lord can get across the stringent laws of nature. Because of its impermanence and vulnerability all the time, the world of politicians is always full of anxiety.

Atma bhuta interest in this *mantra*, which is the same as *brahma bhuta* interest in *Bhagavad Gita* (18.54), is obtained through serving the Lord's interest in everything we do. Supreme *atma* is the Lord and minute *atma* is the *jiva*. Just as the father extends himself through children and maintains them as family to derive pleasure through them, even so Paramatma maintains the *jivas* as a transcendentally arranged family. Neither the *jiva* nor the Lord is impersonal; both are transcendental personalities with eternal life and full of transcendental knowledge and bliss—existence, knowledge and bliss or *sat-chit-ananda*. Transcendental realization is achieved after many life times. Such a *mahatma* or great soul who knows his transcendental position and surrenders unto the lotus feet of the Supreme Lord, Sri Krishna is rarely seen. He breaks the chain of repeated births and transcends to his spiritual home.

Mantra 8

Such a person must know in fact the Personality of Godhead, who is greatest of all, unembodied, omniscient, beyond reproach, without veins, pure and uncontaminated, self-established and self-sufficient philosopher who has been fulfilling everyone's desire since time immemorial.

Personality of Supreme Lord has a form but it is entirely different from the one possessed by us in the material world. Our body, mind and soul are different entities and we have veins. Lord's body, mind and soul are all one and the same and he has nothing like veins. He is not forced to accept a body according to the laws of nature as we are. Even *Brahma Samhita* (5.1) describes Lord's personality as *sat-chit-ananda-vigraha* meaning that He has the eternal form possessing transcendental existence, knowledge and bliss. He does not require a separate body and mind like us and as such his form is entirely different and inconceivable, and because of this difference He is sometimes called formless. *Brahma Samhita* (5.32) also states that through each part of His body He can do the work of other senses. He has different of types hands, legs or eyes and each one of His parts can function like any other part. This property can be summarized as "omnipotence." Lord's worshipable form (*arca-vigraha*) was established in the temples by authorized teachers (*acaryas*) who have realized the Lord as described herein; the original form of Lord is that of Sri Krishna who expands Himself in innumerable forms such as, Varaha, Narsimha and Rama. All these forms and the one worshipped in temples are one and the same Personality of the Lord as His expansions. Worship offered to *arca-vigraha* in the temple goes directly to the Lord. This form may be considered as made of material things as seen by ignorant people or *kanistha adhikaris*, but all such people should remember that the Lord is omnipotent and omniscient, and He can convert matter into spirit and vice-versa, if and when He likes.

Because of forgetfulness of their relations with God the ignorant people may deride Him because He descends in this world as a man. The Lord does not manifest in full to the mental speculators. People come to know Him in proportion to their surrender and devotion to Him. Lord has been supplying things to living entities from time immemorial. However, on demand from people Lord supplies the object of desire in proportion to his qualifications. Wanting to be a high court judge one should be qualified and have consent of the awarding authorities. People are awarded enjoyments by the Lord in proportion to their qualifications and of course, mercy of the Lord. Most people do not know what to ask for. They are attracted by the temporary beauties of the external energy and forget the real aim of life, which is to go back to Godhead. One who wants to go to hell, Lord helps him, and one who wants to go back to Godhead, the Lord helps him too.

The Lord is *paribhuh* (greatest of all) and all others are in fact beggars. However, the right thing to beg is liberation, which in reality means going back to Godhead. Liberation as conceived by an impersonalist is a myth, and begging for sense gratification continues till one realizes one's spiritual position.

Lord Krishna appeared on earth five thousand years ago and He displayed His full manifestation as the personality of Godhead through His various activities. He killed many powerful demons in childhood, lifted Govardhan hill, and danced with *gopis* or milkmaids without social restrictions and without reproach. Although the gopies approached Him with a paramour's feeling of love, but He remained pure, *suddham* (antiseptic) and *apapa-vidham* (prophylactic—the sin cannot touch Him). Antiseptic means that an impure thing becomes pure by His touch, and prophylactic means the power of His association, because of which even an ill-behaved person becomes acceptable as he is on the right path. He may appear to be acting sinfully, but all His actions are good, unaffected by sin. Obnoxious things are purified by virtue of his sterilizing powers.

Mantra 9

Those who engage in the culture of nescience shall enter into the darkest region of ignorance. Those engaging in the culture of so-called knowledge are still worse.

Avidya (ignorance) is certainly dangerous. But the present day knowledge that lays stress on material advancement in the modern civilization is even more dangerous because it is mistaken and misguiding. Since this education excludes the spiritual aspect of life people are unhappier. Forgetfulness of the fact that the Supreme Lord is the proprietor of everything is ignorance. Civilization with such a basis of godlessness becomes more dangerous than a less educated civilization. Among the three classes of men—*karmis, jnanis* and *yogis*—the karmis are the ones engaged in activities of sense gratification under the banners of industrialism, economic development, altruism and politics, since it excludes God consciousness stated in the first *mantra*. *Bhagavad Gita* (7.15) calls such people as *mudhas* or donkeys who are the symbol of stupidity. In *Hari-bhakti-suddhodaya* (3.11-12) advancement of education without God consciousness is like a procession with decorations on a dead body for the pleasure of the lamenting relatives. In rising values we have senses, mind, intelligence and soul; the education therefore should be aimed at Self-realization for knowing the spiritual values of the soul. Education without such realization is *avidya* or nescience, which can lead only to the darkest regions of ignorance.

Bhagavad Gita (2.42, 7.15) states that mundane educators (*veda-vada-rata* and *mayayapahrata jnana*) pose themselves as learned in the Vedas and highlight the fruitive results as attainment of heaven rather than knowing the Personality of Godhead, which is the real purpose of Vedas. The ultimate purpose of all religions is to bring one back to Godhead. The *veda-vada-rata* people should aim at reviving the forgetful soul's relationship with Supreme Lord and not for attainment of heavenly pleasure for sense gratification, which is lust causing material bondage. Such *vidyayam ratah* or "those engaged in study of the *Vedas*" are condemned because of being ignorant of the actual purpose of the *Vedas* and for disobeying the *acharyas* or real teachers. Such people have their own teachers who are not in the chain of transcendental succession. *Mundaka Upanishad* (1.2.12) states that one must approach a bona fide spiritual master.

The *mayayapahrata jnana* class of people are self proclaimed Gods. They think that they are God themselves and there is no need to worship any other God. They are ready to worship a rich man and cannot explain how God can be entrapped by *maya*.

Mantra 10

According to the wise, certainly different result is derived from the culture of knowledge as compared to the result obtained from the culture of nescience.

According to *Bhagavad Gita* (13.8-12) knowledge can be cultured through the following steps:

(1) Becoming a perfect gentleman and giving respect to others.
(2) Not posing as a religionist simply for name and fame.
(3) Not becoming a source of anxiety to others through one's actions of body, thoughts of mind, and by one's words.
(4) Learning forbearance even when provoked by others.
(5) Avoiding duplicity in one's dealings with others.
(6) Searching a bona fide spiritual master who can guide him towards spiritual realization, submitting oneself to such a spiritual master, rendering service to him and asking relevant questions.
(7) Following regulative principles through revealed scriptures to achieve Self-realization.
(8) Fixing one to the tenets of the revealed scriptures.
(9) Refraining from the practices that are detrimental to the interest of Self-realization.
(10) Not accepting more than what is required for the maintenance of one's body.
(11) Not identifying oneself falsely with the gross material body, and not considering those related to one's body as their own.
(12) Remembering that miseries of repeated birth, old age, disease and death are to be faced as long as one has a material body.
(13) Not attaching to more than the necessities of life required for spiritual development.

(14) Not attaching to wife, children and home more than the revealed scriptures ordain.

(15) Not being happy or distressed over desirables and undesirables, knowing that such feelings are only creation of mind.

(16) Becoming an unalloyed devotee of the Personality of Godhead, Sri Krishna, and serving Him with rapt attention.

(17) Liking a residence in a secluded place with a calm and quiet atmosphere favorable for spiritual culture, and avoiding congested places where non-devotees congregate.

(18) Becoming a scientist or philosopher and conducting research into spiritual knowledge, recognizing that spiritual knowledge is permanent whereas material knowledge ends with the death of the body.

No other method except the combination of these eighteen items can lead to real knowledge. Advancement of material knowledge is converting the modern man into a donkey. Some people decry the present system of civilization as satanic, but they do not culture real knowledge as advocated by *Bhagavad Gita*. Thus they cannot change the satanic situation.

The boys and girls in colleges and universities do not respect their teachers and elders, which is causing concern to them. Regulative principles could have led them to *brahmcharya* or celibate life while students, but it is not so. Education and research is developing lethal weapons that might end the world itself one day. Religious principles are taught for name sake only, and animosity is increasing in social and political fields. All these things are happening because education is devoid of spiritual injunctions.

People do not remember that this earth is a tiny particle in the whole universe that has millions of planets like ours. We are proud of our airplane drivers but do not think about the supreme driver of these greater, more gigantic spaceships called planets. We are frustrated by repeated birth and death, old age and disease. The span of human life is decreasing constantly. More than fifty percent of nation's resources are spent on defense against each other, rather than the cultivation of real knowledge. According to *Bhagavad Gita*, knowledge should be acquired from a *dhira*, who is not disturbed by material illusion, is perfectly spiritualized and does not hanker nor laments for anything. He knows that body and mind are acquired through material association and are foreign elements, but he makes the best use of the bad bargain. *Dhira* knows that the living entity or *jiva* or soul has actual functions in the living, spiritual world and not in this dead material world. Politicians pose as *dhiras*, which they are not, since they are after money, power and material gains. One can become a *dhira* (the undisturbed) by submitting to a bona fide spiritual master, like Arjuna who became *dhira* by listening and submitting to Lord Krishna.

Mantra 11

By learning simultaneously the process of nescience and transcendental knowledge one can transcend the influence of repeated birth and death and enjoy the full blessings of immortality.

Laws of nature cannot provide immunity from old age, disease and death and material knowledge cannot provide a solution to it, though it can create a bomb to accelerate the process of death. Notorious king Hiranyakashyap through heavy meditation pleased demigod Brahma, creator and ruler of the planets, and asked him the boon of becoming immortal. Brahma said that he himself is not immortal though having a long life, so the king may ask conditions that may secure immortality. The king asked that any man, animal, god or any other living being within the 8,400,000 species should not kill him. Further he asked that he should not die on land, air or water, or by any weapon; also that he should not die either in the day or night, and neither inside the house nor outside it. Brahma gave him this boon and the king thought that he cannot be killed and has become immortal. But at the right time the Lord incarnated as Narsimha—half man, half lion—and killed the king satisfying all conditions he had received in the boon. Even such a powerful king could not achieve immortality, how can a common man talk about it. The only way to have permanent life is to go back to the spiritual home or Godhead. This transcendental knowledge can be acquired through the study of Vedic scriptures such as the *Upanishads, Vedanta Sutra, Bhagavad Gita and Srimad Bhagavatam*. The Lord has kindly delivered these scriptures in India and other scriptures in other countries to remind the forgetful humans that this material world is not their home. Humans as *jivas* are spiritual entities and they should endeavour to return to their true home that lies in the spiritual sky, for unending happiness.

Lord keeps on sending his bona fide servants and sometimes incarnates Himself to propagate this message. Miseries of the material world indirectly remind us of our incompatibility with dead matter. Intelligent people take the hint and engage themselves with *vidya* or transcendental knowledge. Facilities are available only in human incarnation, for which even the gods keep trying. Unrestricted sense enjoyment through body and material things is the path of ignorance and death. Spiritual senses possessed by the *jiva* are now materially manifested, being covered by the material body and mind. Material activities are perverted reflections of the activities of the original, spiritual senses. Thus removal of material contamination can provide real enjoyment. Since the culture of spiritual knowledge necessitates the help of body and mind, the body and mind should also be maintained as a balanced program. One should lead a healthy life with a sound mind just to realize *vidya* or true knowledge, which is most perfectly presented in *Srimad Bhagavatam*. The Absolute Truth is realized step by step as Brahman, Paramatma and finally

The Liberation of Man

Bhagvan, the Personality of Godhead. The broadminded man who has followed the eighteen principles and attained knowledge and detachment realizes the Truth. Finally, attainment of transcendental devotional service to the Personality of Godhead leads to the goal. Srila Rupa Goswami has presented the path in *The Nectar of Devotion*. *Srimad Bhagavatam* (1.2.14) states:

"Therefore, with one-pointed attention one should constantly hear about, glorify, remember and worship the Personality of Godhead, who is the protector of the devotees."

Unless religion, economic development and sense gratification aim towards the attainment of devotional service to the Lord, they are only different forms of nescience as shown by Sri Ishopanishad in the following *mantras*.

Mantra 12

Those who worship demigods enter into the darkness of ignorance, and still more so do the worshippers of the impersonal Absolute.

Sambhuti in Sanskrit means "having independent existence," referring to Absolute Personality of Godhead. *Asambhuti* therefore means "not independent," referring to demigods, great sages and mystics, whose source is the Lord appearing as Krishna—a man, through His own internal potency (*Bhagavad Gita*, 10.2). Distinguishing the Absolute from relatives, *rishis* and mystics may imagine that the Absolute must be formless and without qualities. However, the definition of Absolute by negation is not complete. Speculating in this way one may utmost reach the impersonal effulgence of God, known as Brahman, and not beyond. Brahman is the glaring effulgence of His transcendental body, and Paramatma—the Supersoul, is His all-pervading plenary representation. Speculators cannot believe the appearance of the Lord as Krishna, having His eternal form with the transcendental qualities of eternal bliss and knowledge.

According to *Bhagavad Gita* (7.20, 23) only the people having a strong desire for sense gratification worship the demigods for relief from problems and/or for getting certain material advantages. It is useless to ask for temporary relief from the dependent demigods; one should aim at spiritual plane where eternal life, knowledge and bliss exist. Worship of all-attractive Krishna can lead us to complete freedom from material bondage by taking us back home, back to Godhead. *Bhagavad Gita* (7.23) states that the spaceship, mystic powers or worship of demigods can lead one to the planets of demigods' up to Brahmaloka, which is the topmost planet in the universe. However, all planets in the material universe are temporary residences; the only permanent planets are the Vaikunthalokas in the spiritual sky, where the Personality of Godhead Himself predominates. According to Lord Krishna in *Bhagavad Gita* (8.16):

"From the highest planet in the material world down to the lowest, all are places of misery wherein repeated birth and death take place. But one who attains My abode, O son of Kunti, never takes birth again."

The whole universe is dark and covered as coconut is covered with a shell and half-filled with water. Sun and moon are therefore needed for illumination. Outside the universe is the vast and unlimited *brahmajyoti* expansion, which is filled with Vaikunthalokas. The biggest and highest planet in the *brahmajyoti* is Krishnaloka, also known as Goloka Vrindavana, where the Supreme Personality of Godhead, Sri Krishna Himself, resides. Although always situated in his abode with His eternal associates, Lord Krishna is present everywhere in the material as well as spiritual cosmic manifestations.

Athiests deny the existence of the Supreme Personality of Godhead, and the impersonalists support them by stressing the impersonal aspects of the Supreme Lord. Since the Lord can run faster than any person, how can He be impersonal? The ignorant pseudo religionists and the manufacturers of the so-called incarnations who violate the Vedic injunctions are liable to enter the dark regions of the universe because of misleading their followers. Such misleading guides call themselves *acharyas* or bona fide teachers, while they do not even follow the principles of *acharyas*. Law because of religious freedom cannot punish them, but the higher court of God is going to throw them in the darkest regions. Lord Krishna states in *Bhagavad Gita* (4.2), "This supreme science of God is received through the disciplic succession." Hence one must follow a teacher of the Vedic discipline. As soon as one reaches the Lord through the only means of devotional service, one attains complete freedom from the bondage of repeated births.

Mantra 13

Different results are obtained by worshipping the Supreme Lord, the cause of all causes and by worshipping what is not supreme. All this is heard from the undisturbed authorities, who explained it perfectly.

One who is not disturbed by the changes of the world is a bona fide *acharya* or teacher. Such a teacher who has himself heard the *sruti-mantras* or Vedic knowledge from his undisturbed teacher, would never present anything that is from outside Vedic literature. One should learn from the *parampara* of "spiritual teachers," the bona fide system of disciplic succession, who will never say that all paths lead to the same goal. According to *Bhagavad Gita* (9.25) different results are obtained by different modes of worship. Worshippers of *pitris* or forefathers attain the planets of the forefathers, worshippers of demigods attain the planets of demigods, those who want to remain on this wretched planet with planning commissions and stopgap political adjustments will be reborn here, and the worshippers of the Supreme Lord will certainly reach Him in His eternal abode. It is like purchasing a ticket for Calcutta will take you only to Calcutta and not Bombay or Delhi. In *Bhagavad Gita* (4.2) Krishna tells His beloved disciple Arjuna:

"This supreme science was thus received through the chain of disciplic succession, and the saintly kings understood it in this way. However, in the course of time the succession was broken, and therefore the science as it is appears to be lost."

While on earth Lord Krishna had to reestablish the disciplic system beginning with Arjuna and correct the distorted principles of *bhakti yoga* or the path of devotion. Arjuna could understand *Gita* because he was a devotee and friend of the Lord. Those having no faith in Krishna and His abode cannot explain *Bhagavad Gita*. Lord says in *Bhagavad Gita* (10.8):

"I am the source of all spiritual and material words. Everything emanates from Me. The wise who perfectly know this engage in My devotional service and worship Me with all their hearts."

Brahma, Vishnu and Shiva were created by Krishna and He enlightened Brahma. Another name for Krishna is Narayana, who created Prajapatis, Indra, eight Vasus, eleven Rudras and twelve Adityas. Impersonalist Sripada Sankaracharya also accepted the identity of Narayana. All Vedic literatures and even *Brahma Samhita* (5.1) confirm that Narayana, Govinda or Krishna is the cause of all causes. Lord Krishna states in *Bhagavad Gita* (7.26) that He is fully conscious of past, present and future and that no one, including demigods such as Siva and Brahma, knows Him fully. Clearly the half educated spiritual leaders who are disturbed by the tides of material existence cannot know Him fully. They compromise by making mass of humanity the object of worship, which is like pouring water on the leaves of a tree instead of the root, which dries up for want of nourishment. Water should be poured on the root, the soul, which is the source that generates different types of bodies according to the law of *karma*. Serving humans through medical aid, social help and educational facilities while at the same time slaughtering animals is no service to the soul, the living being, which is perpetually suffering from the miseries of birth, old age, disease and death.

Although *Upanishads* indirectly draw our attention to the primeval Lord, Sri Krishna, *Bhagavad Gita*, which is the summary of all *Upanishads*, points to Sri Krishna directly. *Srimad Bhagavatam* (1.2.17) states that, "By hearing of the activities of the Lord, the devotee draws the attention of the Lord. Thus the Lord, being situated in the heart of every living being, helps the devotee by giving him proper directions." This is also confirmed by *Bhagavad Gita* (10.10). Lord's inner direction cleanses the devotee's heart of all contaminations produced by the material modes of passion and ignorance. Passions do not allow detachment from material hankerings, and there is no chance of Self-realization, whatever one may do as a religionist. Anyone as a devotee, even a lowborn, can get situated in the quality of goodness, which is the sign of a *brahmana*. And then the science of God is unveiled before him automatically. One gradually becomes free from material attachments, and one's doubtful mind becomes crystal clear by the grace of the Lord. Anyone attaining this stage is a liberated soul, who can see the Lord in every step of life. This is the perfection of *sambhava* in the present *mantra*.

To be more clear, one who believes in Krishna can understand God—His way of working, the way His energies are acting, the way He is manifesting, what is this material world, what is the spiritual world, what are the living creatures, and what is their relationship with God.

Mantra 14

One should know the eternal Personality of Godhead Sri Krishna along with His transcendental name, form, qualities and pastimes; as well as the temporary material creation with its temporary demigods, men and animals. When both kinds of knowledge is acquired, one surpasses death and the ephemeral cosmic manifestation with it, and one enjoys his eternal life of bliss and knowledge in the eternal Kingdom of God.

Scientists are improving the living conditions of humans in various ways but they cannot change the laws of nature according to which one has to pass through six conditions—birth, growth, maintenance, production of by-products, deterioration and finally death. Accordingly, none of the demigods, man, animal or plant can survive forever in the material world. In other words, beginning with the chief living being of this material universe—Lord Brahma, who lives for millions and millions of years—down to the minute germ who lives for few hours only, no one can survive eternally in the material universe. There are millions of Brahmas in different universes, and they are all liable to death one day. Accordingly, the whole material universe is called Martyaloka or the place of death. Scientists and politicians are trying to make the earth's life deathless since they do not know the "deathless spiritual nature" explained in the Vedas and confirmed by mature transcendental experience.

Vishnu Purana (6.7.61) states that Lord Vishnu, the Personality of Godhead, possesses two different kinds of energies—*para* (superior) and *apara* (inferior). The living entities are created by the superior energy while the material creation is due to inferior energy that covers the living entities with *avidya* or ignorance and induces them to perform fruitive activities. Beyond these two energies there is another part of superior energy that creates deathless, eternal abode of the Lord, as also confirmed by *Bhagavad Gita* (8.20).

Innumerable planets like sun, moon and venus are scattered throughout the space that exist only during the lifetime of Brahma. On upper planets twenty-four hours or one day and night equals to one year of earth. Due to different time scale the four ages of earth—Satya, Treta, Dwapara and Kali—equal only twelve thousand years on higher planets. One thousand rotations of the four ages or such lengths of time constitute a day of Brahma, and a similar duration is there for a night of Brahma. 360 days and 360 nights make one year of Brahma, and a hundred such years is the life span of Brahma. At the end of Brahma's life, the whole creation comes to an end. Beings of higher planets like sun and moon, inhabitants of earth, and those living on lower planets—all are merged into the waters of devastation during the night of Brahma. This is material non-existence of all, although their spiritual existence continues. Thus there are two *avyakta* or unmanifested stages—one during every night of Brahma, the other at the end of Brahma's life. Beyond these two unmanifested states there is another unmanifested state, the spiritual atmosphere or nature, having innumerable spiritual planets therein. Life on these spiritual planets exists eternally, even when all the material planets are vanquished at the end of Brahma's life. Cosmic manifestation of a large number of material universes, each under a specific Brahma, occupies only one-fourth of the space, using only one-fourth of Lord's energy (*ekapad vibhuti*), which is *apara prakriti* or inferior. Three-fourth of the Lord's energy (*tripad vibhuti*), which is *para-prakriti* or superior, induces spiritual atmosphere or nature, which is beyond the jurisdiction of any Brahma.

Lord Sri Krishna, the predominating Supreme Person, residing in the spiritual atmosphere, can be approached only by unalloyed devotional service and not by *jnana* (philosophy), *yoga* (mysticism) or *karma* (fruitive action). The *karmis* or fruitive workers can elevate themselves to Svargaloka planets like sun and moon. *Jnanis* and *yogis* can rise to still higher planets like Maharloka, Tapoloka and Brahmaloka; and by becoming more qualified through devotional service they can enter—either the illuminating spiritual sky (Brahman) or one of the Vaikuntha planets, according to the qualifications they have acquired. The Vaikuntha planets are ruled by various expansions of Lord Krishna, called Narayana forms, as also confirmed by *Gopala-tapani-Upanishad* (1.3.21). On the material planets everyone has to be born as a demigod, man or animal and pass through the process of repeated births and deaths, unless one engages into devotional service and enter spiritual sky or planet. Lord's last instruction is, "Give up all the processes and just surrender unto Me alone (*Bhagavad Gita*, 18.66)." Only awakening of God consciousness can pacify the insurmountable material nature (*Bhagavad-Gita*, 7.14).

The present *mantra* teaches that both *sambhuti* or the Personality of Godhead and *vinasa* or the temporary material manifestation should be known side by side. Elevating human life through hospitals and many other useful scientific discoveries cannot save one from devastation; only the complete knowledge of the eternal life of bliss and awareness can save one. Question of liking or disliking does not arise, as this is the bare truth. Devotional service to the Lord is therefore a matter of necessity.

Mantra 15

O my Lord, sustainer of all that lives, Your real face is covered by Your dazzling effulgence. Kindly remove that covering and exhibit Yourself to Your pure devotee.

Lord explains His personal rays (*brahmajyoti*), the dazzling effulgence of His personal form, as follows (*Bhagavad Gita*, 14.27): "I am the basis of the impersonal Brahman, which is immortal, imperishable and eternal and is the constitutional position of ultimate happiness." Brahman, Paramatma and Bhagvan are the three aspects of Absolute Truth. Brahman is the aspect most easily perceived by the beginner; those who have progressed further realize Paramatma, the Supersoul; and Bhagvan realization is the ultimate realization of the Absolute Truth. *Bhagavad Gita* (7.7) confirms this statement when Lord Krishna says that He is the ultimate concept of Absolute Truth. *Brahmajyoti* and Paramatma are plenary expansions of Lord Krishna, for the maintenance of the entire material creation and all manifestations in the spiritual world. This is confirmed in *Bhagavad Gita* (10.42) when the Lord says, "But what need is there, Arjuna, for all this detailed

The Liberation of Man

knowledge? With a single fragment of Myself I pervade and support this entire universe." Material creation, maintenance and destruction are all done by His expansion as Paramatma or Supersoul, who pervades the entire material creation, while Lord Himself remains situated in His abode. Every living entity is *atma* or soul, and the principal *atma* who controls them all is Paramatma or Supersoul.

Sri Krishna is always filled with transcendental bliss (*ananda-mayo-bhyasat*). During His existence five thousand years ago in India He displayed transcendental bliss right from the beginning of His childhood pastimes. Enjoying with His mother, brother and friends, killing of demons, lifting the Govardhan mountain and playing the role of a naughty butter thief—all His activities gave celestial bliss to His associates. These pastimes were the counter acts to attract the dry speculators and acrobatic *hatha yogis* in search of Absolute Truth. According to Sukadeva Goswami in *Srimad Bhagavatam* (10.12.11): "The Personality of Godhead, who is perceived as the impersonal, blissful Brahman by the *jnanis*, who is worshipped as the Supreme Lord by devotees in the mood of servitorship, and who is considered an ordinary human being by mundane people, played with the cowherd boys, who had attained their position after accumulating many pious activities." Thus the Lord is always engaged in transcendental activities with His spiritual associates in various relationships of *santa* (neutrality), *dasya* (servitorship), *sakhya* (friendship), *vatsalya* (parental affection) and *madhurya* (conjugal love).

This system of God Realization is a great science. Beginning with materialistic *sankhya-yogis*, they can only analyze and meditate on twenty-four factors of the material creation, since their information of the *purusa* or the Lord is poor. Next the impersonal transcendentalists end up with bewildering *brahmajyoti*, the glaring effulgence of the Lord. To see the Absolute Truth in full, one has to go beyond twenty-four material elements and penetrate further through *brahmajyoti*. Only after piercing through the dazzling covering of the Lord one can perceive the real face of the personality of Godhead.

Lord's expansion as Paramatma features *visnu-tattavas* or *purusa-avatars*. First of them is Ksirodakasayi Vishnu, who is the Vishnu in the Trinity—Brahma, Vishnu and Shiva—all-pervading Paramatma in each and every individual living entity. The second is Garbhodakasayi Vishnu, the collective Supersoul within all living entities. Beyond these two is Karanodakasayi Vishnu, lying in the Causal Ocean, and the creator of all universes. Through the *yoga* system the serious aspirant should go beyond the twenty-four material elements of the cosmic creation and meet the *vishnu tattavas*. Philosophy then helps in the realization of the impersonal *brahmajyoti*, the glaring effulgence of Sri Krishna (*Bhagavad Gita* 14.27): "In the millions and millions of universes there are innumerable planets, differing with each other in their cosmic constitution. All these planets are situated in a corner of the *brahmajyoti*, the personal rays of the Lord, Govinda, whom I worship." Prayer is offered for the removal of this *brahmajyoti*, which is necessary for seeing the real face of the Lord. *Mundaka Upanishada* (2.2.10-12) describes this *brahmajyoti* effulgence as follows:

> "In the spiritual realm, beyond the material covering, is the unlimited Brahman effulgence, which is free from material contamination. Transcendentalists understand this effulgent white light to be the light of all lights. No other light from sun, moon, fire or electricity is needed in that realm. Illumination that appears in the material world is only a reflection of that supreme illumination. That Brahman is in front and in back, in the north, south, east and west, and also overhead and below. That Brahman effulgence spreads throughout both the material and spiritual skies."

Lord Sri Krishna is the root of this Brahman effulgence. One describes the Supreme Truth as Brahman, Paramatma

The Liberation of Man

or Bhagavan according to one's realization of Him. The *jiva* or individual soul can never equate with the all-powerful Supreme Truth. One who has no knowledge of the potencies of the Supreme Truth will realize the impersonal Brahman. Similarly, on realization of material potencies and having no information about spiritual potencies, one attains Paramatma realization. These are both partial realizations of the Absolute Truth. One who continues the search and realizes the Supreme Personality of Godhead, Sri Krishna, also known as Vasudeva, in full potency, realizes that He is everything—Brahman, Paramatma and Bhagavan. Beginning with the root Bhagavan, one can understand Brahman and Paramatma to be His branches.

Bhagavad Gita (6.46-47) gives a comparative analysis of the three types of transcendentalists—*jnanis,* the worshippers of impersonal Brahman; *yogis,* the worshipers of the Paramatma feature; and *bhaktas,* the devotees of Lord Sri Krishna. *Jnanis,* having cultivated Vedic knowledge are better than ordinary fruitive workers; *yogis* are still greater than *jnanis*; and among the *yogis,* those who have devoted themselves to and served the Lord with their full potential are on the top. In other words, a philosopher is better than a laboring man, a mystic is superior to a philosopher, and of all the mystic *yogis,* those who have followed *bhakti-yoga,* engaging themselves in the service of the Lord, are the topmost. This is the teaching of Sri Ishopanishad.

Mantra 16

O maintainer of the universe, O primeval philosopher, O regulating principle, destination of real devotees, well-wisher of the progenitors of mankind, please remove the effulgence of your transcendental rays so that I can see your most auspicious and blissful form. You are the eternal Supreme Personality of Godhead, like unto the sun, as I am.

Just as the sun and its rays are one and the same qualitatively, even so the Lord and *jivas* or individual souls are one and the same in quality. Just as the sun is one but its molecules are innumerable, even so the Lord is one but His offshoot *jivas* are innumerable. Just as the sun-god lives in the sun and sunrays emanate from him, even so the Lord lives in His supreme spiritual planet, Goloka Vrindavana, wherefrom *brahmjyoti* effulgence is emanating. According to *Brahma Samhita* (5.29): "I worship Govinda, the primeval Lord, the first progenitor, who is tending the cows fulfilling all desires in abodes filled with spiritual gems and surrounded by millions of wish-fulfilling trees. He is always served with great reverence and affection by hundreds of thousands of Lakshmis, or goddesses of fortune." Since the *brahmajyoti* effulgence is very dazzling and blinding, the prayer is offered to the Lord to remove these effulgent rays so that the pure devotees can see His all-blissful transcendental form.

Auspicious aspect of Lord is experienced on realizing the impersonal *brahmajyoti*, even more auspicious enlightenment is experienced on realizing the Paramatma, and the most auspicious feature of the Supreme is experienced on meeting the Personality of Godhead face to face. Since He is the progenitor, maintainer and well-wisher of the universe He cannot be impersonal. Realizing the impersonal brahmajyoti first, then seeing the personal aspects of the Lord and finally seeing the most auspicious eternal form of Lord the Absolute Truth is realized in full by the devotee.

Bhagavat Sandharbha explains that full potency is not realized in *brahmajyoti* and hence it is only partial realization of Truth. In *bhagavan*, *bha* means "one who fully maintains or guardian", *ga* means "guide, leader or creator", and *van* means that "every being lives in Him and He also lives in every being." Thus the transcendental sound *bhagavan* represents infinite knowledge, potency, energy, opulence, strength and influence, without any material inebriety. The Lord fully maintains His devotees and guides them progressively on the path of devotional perfection.

The Liberation of Man

Ultimately the devotee sees the Lord eye to eye by His causeless mercy; and thus the Lord helps the devotee reach the supermost spiritual planet, Goloka Vrindavan. He provides all necessary qualifications to the devotee so that he can reach Him. By His plenary expansions as *purusas*, He creates, maintains and annihilates the cosmic manifestation.

Since the *jivas* or living entities are also differentiated expansions of the Lord's self, some of them desire to imitate the Lord. For this reason the Lord provides all facilities to living entities over the nature, although the ultimate controller is the Paramatma or Supersoul feature of the Lord, who is one of the *purusas*. The difference between *atma* and Paramatma is obviously that *atma* is controlled and Paramatma is the controller. However, due to His full cooperation, He is the constant companion of the living entity. Brahman is all-pervading feature of the Lord that exists in all three states of waking, sleeping and potential activities; and from whom the *jiva-sakti* or living force is generated as both conditioned and liberated souls.

Whenever the pure devotees assemble they glorify the Lord's transcendental activities. Those devotees who are not pure yet, that is the ones who have realized only Brahman and Paramatma features of the Lord, cannot appreciate the activities of the pure devotees. Lord imparts necessary knowledge into the hearts of pure devotees and dissipates all darkness and ignorance. The speculative philosophers and yogis cannot imagine this since they depend more or less on their own strength. *Katha Upanishad* (1.2.23) states that the Lord bestows special favors upon His pure devotees, who alone can know Him, and not others. This is also the message of *Sri Ishopanishad*.

As it can be seen through my autobiography, I got the experiences more or less in the same order, though in gradual and larger number of steps, which confirms the process of realization. To begin with it was materialization of the *jyoti* or flame from Brahman, called *brahmajyoti*. Then it was the manifestation of Aum or Shabda-Brahman or Cosmic Sound inside me. Next it was the "experience of death" (of ego). Then I saw the manifestation of yogic powers in trance, like uprooting a tree, throwing the big stones and breaking the big logs of wood with the gesture of my fingers; flying up and down the sky at will, breaking open the wall of a hall by the force of my body, and so on. Then the manifestation of Kundalini Sakti in female form as the Mother in red clothes, blessing me with her hand on my head, I being in white dress and bowing down to her. This experience repeated about four times in six months. Then I experienced being in front of the palace of Brahma for a while, the crossing of the cosmic river as if moving on a hair-broad bridge, arriving at a group of mountains—the Kailash, the abode of Lord Siva, then suddenly returning to my physical body. In the next experience I entered *brahmajyoti* over and over again, feeling extremely blissful and homely. I would enter the vast body of light and bliss and come out. This happened to me again and again over the years. And then I saw Lord Krishna in front of me as a beautiful child or boy, smiling and looking at me with His full open big eyes. Another time He appeared at a different angle, still smiling and looking at me with open eyes. Appearance of Lord Krishna has taken place many times when I was least expecting it.

Mantra 17

Let this temporary body be burnt to ashes, and let the air of life be merged into the totality of air. Now, O my Lord, please remember all my sacrifices, and because you are the ultimate beneficiary, please remember all that I have done for you.

Bhagavad Gita (2.20) states that no living entity is originally formless, and the entity exists after the annihilation of the material body. Every living entity takes a body suitable to the satisfaction of its desires. One who likes to eat stool is born as a hog, one who wants to eat flesh and blood is born as a tiger or similar animal with

The Liberation of Man

suitable teeth and claws. However, humans are born with teeth suitable to chew and cut fruits and vegetables, although they have two canine teeth that were used by primitive humans to eat flesh. In the course of evolution the bodies are changed one after another. At one time the world was full of water, and then the living entity was born in aquatic form. Eventually the living entity passed to vegetable life, to worm life, to bird life, to animal life and finally to human form, which is the highest developed form possessing spiritual knowledge. At the time of death the air of life will be merged into the eternal reservoir of air. There are different kinds of *prana-vayu* or life giving air in the body that are controlled by the *yogis*, making them pass from one circle to another until the arrival at *brahma-randhra* or crown-centre. From there the *yogi* can transfer himself to any planet of his choice. The key is to enter into the spiritual atmosphere, where one can develop an entirely different kind of body—a spiritual body that has no change or death.

In the material world, bodies vary from lowest germ to highest Brahma or demigods, but the intelligent man sees oneness through the spiritual spark of the Supreme Lord possessed by each one of them. Only when one comes to a point of knowledge of spiritual identity and surrender to the Lord after many, many life times, one may not fall down again to the material world. Indeed, one has to fall down even after becoming one with the *brahmajyoti*. There are innumerable sparks in *brahmajyoti* that are individual entities with full sense of existence. To enjoy their senses these living entities are placed in the material world to have power and position directed by senses, as false lords. The desire for lordship is a material disease that enforces transmigration into different bodies. Hence becoming one with *brahmajyoti* is not a mature knowledge. One has to develop surrender and spiritual service to the Lord in order to reach the highest perfectional stage.

At the time of relinquishing this material body and air, one prays to the Lord to remember his activities and sacrifices during lifetime, in order to enter the spiritual kingdom of God. Those under material influence remember only heinous acts performed during the life, and consequently they get another body after death. According to *Bhagavad Gita* (8.6): "Whatever state of being one remembers while leaving the body, O son of Kunti, that state he will attain without fail." Propensities of the living entity are thus carried by the mind to the next life. Unlike animals with undeveloped mind, human mind remains charged with material desires at the time of death, which does not allow him to enter the spiritual kingdom. Lifetime's practice is needed in order to remember love and surrender to Lord when dying. However, in case of a pure devotee, even if he forgets devotional service to Lord, the Lord does not forget him. *Bhagavad Gita* (9.30-34) states:

"Even if one commits the most abominable action, if he is engaged in devotional service he is to be considered saintly because he is properly situated in his determination. He quickly becomes righteous and attains lasting peace. O son of Kunti, declare it bodily that My devotee never perishes. O son of Partha, those who take shelter in Me, though these be of lower birth—women, *vaishyas* (merchants) as well as *sudras* (workers)—can attain the supreme destination. How much more this is so of the righteous *brahmanas*, the devotees and the saintly kings. Therefore, having come to this temporary, miserable world, engage in loving service unto Me. Engage your mind always in thinking of Me, become My devotee, offer obeisances to Me and worship Me. Being completely absorbed in Me, surely you will come to Me."

A conditioned soul has to act for double functions—maintenance of the body, and Self-realization. The first part includes social status, mental development, cleanliness, austerity, nourishment and the struggle for existence. The second part requires one to be a devotee of the Lord and perform connected activities. The two functions have to run parallel. Until the proportion of devotional service comes to the right point, there is a chance for occasional exhibition of worldliness. However, such imperfections will soon come to an end by the grace of the Lord. Therefore, if one is on the right path of devotional service to the Lord, this occasional worldliness; even if the devotee appears to be of *sudurachara* or a person of loose character; does not hamper one in the advancement of Self-realization.

The impersonalists are attached to the *brahmajyoti* feature of the Lord, they cannot penetrate the *brahmajyoti* because they do not believe in the personality of Godhead, and hence there is no question of devotional service. They are concerned with impersonal fruitless labour with world jugglery and mental speculation (*Bhagavad Gita*, 12.5).

Constant contact with the personal feature of the Absolute Truth can provide all facilities suggested in this *mantra*. This requires nine transcendental activities: (1) hearing about the Lord, (2) glorifying the Lord, (3) remembering the Lord, (4) serving the lotus feet of the Lord, (5) worshipping the Lord, (6) offering prayers to the Lord, (7) serving the Lord, (8) enjoying friendly association with the Lord, and (9) surrendering everything unto the Lord. All or one of these principles at a time can make one remember Lord at the time of death. For example, the desired result was obtained by (1) Maharaja Parikshit of *Srimad Bhagavatam* by hearing of the Lord, (2) Sukadeva Goswami, speaker of *Srimad Bhagavatam* just by glorifying the Lord, (3) Akrura by praying to the Lord, (4) Prahlada Maharaja by remembering the Lord, (5) Prathu Maharaja by worshipping the Lord, (6) Lakshmi, the goddess of fortune by serving the lotus feet of the Lord, (7) Hanuman by rendering personal service to the Lord, (8) Arjuna through his friendship with the Lord, and (9) Maharaja Bali by surrendering everything he had to the lord. Invariably, a single approach involves other principles also in variation.

Vedantasutra summarizes and *Srimad Bhagavatam*, which is the mature fruit of the Vedic tree of wisdom, explains the present *mantra* in greater details. Maharaja Parikshit asked the great spiritual master Sukadeva Goswami, "What is the duty of every man, specifically at the time of death," to which he answered: "Everyone who desires to be free from all anxieties should always hear about, glorify and remember the Personality of Godhead, who is the supreme director of everything, the extinguisher of all difficulties, and the supersoul of all living entities." (*Bhagavad Gita*, 2.1.5)

People sleeping and having sex in the night, and earning money in the day have dismissed God's existence in so many ways. But all the Vedic scriptures declare that Lord is a sentient being and is supreme over all other living beings. His glorious activities are identical with Himself, and hence, once should engage in godly activities only, without hearing or speaking of rubbish activities and world politics. Only when one is used to devotional service sacrifice during his life he can remember the same at the time of death, not otherwise. The art of sacrifice, which means denial of sensual interests, can be practised during one's life by employing the senses in the service of the Lord. Then alone can the results of such practice be used at the time of death.

Mantra 18

O My Lord, as powerful as fire, O omnipotent one, now I offer You all obeisances, falling on the ground at Your feet. O my Lord, please lead me on the right path to reach You, and since You know all that I have done in the past, please free me from the reactions to my past sins so that there will be no hindrance to my progress.

The Lord is addressed as fire since He can burn the sins of the surrendered soul. A conditioned soul is very often apt to commit mistakes, and the only remedial measure is to surrender to the lotus feet of the Lord in order to receive His guidance to avoid such pitfalls. Born as the son of a *brahmana* is no guarantee that one really becomes a *brahmana* unless he acquires brahamanical culture including truthfulness, sense control, forbearance, simplicity, full knowledge and faith in God. By becoming proud as being born in *brahmana* family and neglecting to acquire *brahmanical* qualifications one can fall from the path of Self-realization. Even a man of low caste can become a real *brahmana* by acquiring requisite qualifications while a son of *brahmana* may fall. However, according to *Bhagavad Gita* (6.41-42) a fallen person, known as *yoga bhrastha* is given a chance to rectify himself by taking next birth either in a family of good *brahmanas* or in the family of rich merchants. Such a birth has higher chances of Self-realization, which if missed, the good opportunity offered by the Lord is lost.

Karmakanda or path of fruitive actions may involve many sinful reactions, while the *jnanakanda* or path of philosophical actions involve lesser sinful reactions. However, *bhaktikanda* or the path of devotion to the Lord has practically no chance of incurring sinful reactions. After cultivating transcendental knowledge for many, many life times one achieves perfection and develops an attitude of surrender to the Lord. If this attitude of surrender is from the beginning, one surpasses all preliminary stages through the devotional attitude. Such a person has very little chances of incurring sinful reactions while going through paths of *karma* and *jnana*, which are necessary in that order for a perfect development into a devotee of the Lord. Lord Krishna has said that He loves *Jnanibhaktas* or devotees with full knowledge more than others. Omnipotent Lord sitting in everybody's heart gives directions to His sincere devotees for adopting the right path, even if he desires something else. For others God gives sanction to the doer only at his own risk. A devotee is directed by the Lord in such a way that he never acts wrongly. *Srimad Bhagavatam* (11.5.42) states:

"The Lord is so kind to the devotee who is fully surrendered to His lotus feet that even though the devotee sometimes falls into the entanglement of *vikarma* (acts against the direction of Vedas), the Lord at once rectifies such mistakes from within his heart. This is because the devotees are very dear to Him."

By surrendering oneself unto the Lord and acting according to His directions, the Lord takes charge of the fully surrendered soul. Directions come to the devotee in two ways: one is by way of the scriptures, saints and spiritual master; the other is by way of the Lord Himself, living in the heart. In this way the devotee, fully enlightened with Vedic knowledge, is protected in all respects. Mundane educational procedures cannot make one understand Vedic knowledge, which is transcendental. One requires the grace of the Lord and the spiritual master. A bona fide spiritual master is found by the grace of the Lord; in fact, the Lord appears as the spiritual master. There is no chance of falling again into the mire of material illusion since the devotee has triple guidance from Vedic injunctions, spiritual master and the Lord Himself from within. With such an all round protection, the devotee is sure to reach perfection. *Srimad Bhagavatam* (1.2.17-20) explains that hearing and chanting the glories of the Lord cleanses the devotee of all undesirable things and the devotion gets fixed upon the Lord. Effects of the lower modes of nature (passion and ignorance) vanish completely, and the devotee acquires brahamanical qualifications. Devotional service enlightens the devotee fully, making him pure and he comes to know the way to attain the Lord.

Swami Prabhupada has written very good commentaries on various scriptures. In his book *The Topmost Yoga System* he has highlighted many other useful points. When Arjuna said that *hatha yoga* system is not possible for him, Krishna told him, "Of all different types of *yogis*—*hathayogis, jnanayogis, dhyana yogis, bhakta yogis, karmayogis*—you are the best yogi. Of all *yogis*, the one who is constantly thinking of Me within himself, meditating upon Me within the heart, is the first-class *yogi*." There were different yoga systems used in different yugas or great divisions of time. In Satya Yuga or golden age the method was to meditate on Vishnu. In Treta Yuga the method was of great sacrifices. In the next Dwapara Yuga it was through temple worship. In the present Kali Yuga, the age of quarrel and disagreement, where no one agrees with anyone else, the only method recommended is chanting the holy name. When you are in love you are always thinking of your lover. This is love consciousness. Similarly when you think of Krishna all the time, it is Krishna consciousness, which is the best method of reaching Him.

There are eight kinds of transcendental ecstasies: (i) Being stopped as though dumb, (ii) perspiration, (iii) standing up of hairs on the body, (iv) dislocation of voice, (v) trembling, (vi) fading of the body, (vii) crying in ecstasy, and (viii) trance. First symptom of touching the spiritual platform after chanting for a while is an urge to dance along with chanting of *mantra*. According to Sri Raman Maharishi *sphurana* (a kind of indescribable but palpable sensation in the centre of the heart) when sensed continuously and automatically it is realization.

The way of the world is that as soon as one becomes a devotee of the Lord he finds so many obstacles. But the obstacles will not hinder one or be impediments on the path. One who engages in full devotional service, unfailing in all circumstances, at once transcends the modes of material nature and thus comes to the level of Brahman (*Bhagavad Gita*). If you put an iron rod within fire, it will become like fire. And when the iron rod is red-hot, you can touch it anywhere, and it will burn. Similarly, if you keep yourself in touch with Krishna consciousness, your body will become spiritualized and act spiritually, although it is material. No more material demands. When you desire to gratify your senses that is material life. And when you desire to serve God, that is spiritual life. That is the difference between material life and spiritual life. A mother is more pleased by feeding her son. She does not eat but seeing her son eating nicely she becomes pleased. Similarly, when you desire to please Krishna, spiritual pleasures come to you. The chanting process is purifying, the more you become purified the more you will feel ecstasy. A disciple is one who has voluntarily agreed to be disciplined by the spiritual master. That is austerity, which should be practised even if you do not want it.

Perfection comes when one realizes that he is not this body; he is spirit, soul or atman. That is *brahmabhuta* stage, called Brahman realization. That is perfection after which one engages in devotional service. If one is already engaged in devotional service it means he has the Brahman realization. It is called *samsiddhi*. No more *karma*, no more karmic reaction.

The best devotee does not preach, because he thinks that everyone is a devotee and there is no need of preaching. He is called an *uttamaadhikari* or the one having highest form of realization. However, when he has to preach, he comes to a second-class platform. When one preaches he has many disciples. And then some diseases attack the spiritual master, which is due to the sinful activities of others. Hence the injunction is, "Don't take many disciples." One has to suffer and yet accept these disciples as being the *guru*. "The spiritual master takes responsibility for all the fallen souls. That idea is also in the *Bible*. Jesus Christ took all the sinful actions of the people and sacrificed his life. Therefore he suffered. That is the responsibility of spiritual master. Krishna is *apapavidha*—He cannot be attacked by sinful reactions. But a living entity is sometimes subjected to their influence because he is so small. Big fire, small fire. If you put some big thing in a small fire, the fire itself may be extinguished. But big fire can consume everything[22]."

The solution to all problems is to get out of the conditioned state of life. That is called *yoga*—to link yourself to the Supreme. He who learns to be disillusioned gets free from all encumbrances. If we want freedom from all bonds, then we have to understand God. Ordinarily nobody

The Liberation of Man

enquires; but if a man does, he can make progress and come to the understanding that Krishna is the cause of all causes. Followers of scriptures and higher authorities inquire about Krishna. Those addicted to sinful activities can't inquire. The righteous, pious man inquires and goes to God. If one associates oneself with Krishna consciousness his dormant relationship with Krishna will be evoked.

If by chance one meets a teacher who is a saintly person and a pure devotee, who has sacrificed everything for the Lord, then by such a contact one becomes pure. Krishna is within you, and as soon as He sees that you are very sincere, that you are seeking, He sends a bona fide spiritual master. Hearing and chanting are the waters to be continuously poured on the plant of Krishna consciousness to grow properly. Such a devotee is not satisfied even if he is offered Siddhaloka, where the inhabitants are so powerful and elevated that they can fly in the sky without airplanes, he endeavors for more. Innumerable universes have innumerable suns and many more planets, the highest being Brahmaloka in the material universe. A Krishna conscious person will reject even that. He also neglects the impersonal *brahmajyoti*. The material atmosphere containing all the universes is situated in a corner of *brahmajyoti*. The covering of this universe is ten times the space within, so one has to penetrate that covering, and then reach Viraja, the Causal Ocean. The Buddhist philosophical perfection is to reach that Viraja[23]. When this material existence is completely finished, it is called Viraja in Vedic terms. Krishna conscious person penetrates even the covering of Causal Ocean, which is the neutral position, and continues. The growth of the plant continues from Brahmaloka to Viraja to the spiritual sky, and yet not satisfied with any planet of the Vaikunthaloka. The highest planet in spiritual sky is Krishnaloka, like a lotus flower, where Krishna is standing. As soon as the devotional plant finds Krishna's lotus feet it exclaims, "Now I have found the end of the journey, let me expand here."

To expand means to enjoy Krishna's association and feel satisfied.

An important point highlighted in the last *mantra* is that a *bhaktayogi* or devotee to Lord from the beginning attracts help for the completion of *karmayoga* and *jnanayoga*, which brings him perfection towards the attainment of the Lord. I can say this from my own experiences. As can be seen from my autobiography, I was in the devotional service right from early childhood. In the course of time I got regular help from nature towards yogic exercises and reading literature connected with realized persons round the world. Luckily as a professor at various universities I had plenty of time to give to these practices, after completing the necessary work in mathematics at the university. Whenever I had a question in mind I would come across a book and/ or a saintly person and I used to get the answer. Many times I would get the answer as the first thought in the morning when I would just wakeup. This should be the answer from the Lord.

The present chapter has given various methods for Self-realization and the reader is free to choose the one he or she likes. However, all these methods are based on self-efforts and each one is called *aanavopaya* or "the method of atom." This is so because in self-efforts one uses one's mind and body, which are made of atoms. Such methods take the whole lifetime and even more than one lifetime to achieve the desired results. The other method is based on Shakti or Cosmic Energy and is called *shaktopaya* or "the method of Shakti." In this method Shakti passes from the Guru to the disciple through *initiation* and the results are achieved in a short time, depending on the preparation of the disciple, and in a single lifetime. Referring to my personal experiences I can say that I have initiated about twenty selected disciples in the last three years and all of them have their Kundalini awakened and are having a satisfactory spiritual progress. My recommendation is that one should begin with *bhaktiyoga* or path of devotion with firm faith in

Almighty the God and then introduce *karmayoga* and *jnanayoga* and activities of selfless action and philosophy or scriptural knowledge. One should keep an eye open for a genuine Shaktipat Guru, and as the destiny favors or the grace of the Lord works, one will find a Guru and take initiation from him. With the awakening of Kundalini or dormant spiritual energy one becomes an *initiate* or *twice-born* and then one understands the scriptures and hidden knowledge since the "ring pass-not" is pierced. This is an ideal combination and nothing can beat it to achieve the highest spiritual goal in a single lifetime and that too in a short period. The next chapter describes all the intricacies of the method of Shaktipat.

CHAPTER 5
QUANTUM JUMP INTO DIVINITY THROUGH SHAKTIPAT

Introduction

Shaktipat is an ancient method of awakening and activating the Kundalini. In many cases it is instant. Awakening by a Guru involves a minimum or no risks or side effects. Knowing there is no death comes through intuition and as a result one begins to live more fully and awakens to reality for the first time. Automatic movements in the body reverse the flow of vital fluids, enriching and preparing the brain to receive enlightenment. Accumulated karma from past lives is released and calm, contentment and synchronicity with life prevail. Living in two worlds becomes a reality.

Why there is anxiety about death?

Anxiety about death arises from the transition we believe happens when we die. A shift from being to non-being, one moment we are living, breathing, interacting and the next we don't exist. Understanding the nature of the conscious energy of Shakti can greatly relieve such anxiety. Conscious Energy or Chit-Shakti forms the visible world. Vibrations in Chaitanya, a state of Chit-Shakti, creates all form in the world, such as rivers, mountains, men, women, animals, the sun and moon. All manifested reality exists, like waves on the ocean, until they merge once more with the ocean. The internal awareness of Shakti enables the objective world to exist and as soon as Shakti withdraws its awareness, the objective world disappears and Shakti only remains. Shakti can be understood by thinking about electricity. The fan, refrigerator and computer serve us as long as electricity powers them; the moment electricity is withdrawn, all stop working and become useless. The same is true of human bodies, which are alive as long as the Shakti powers them. The moment Shakti withdraws life force bodies die and are useless. The Shakti connection is responsible for everyday experience in the material world. However, orthodox science has no explanation for this phenomenon, so without understanding, we grieve when our loved ones die, not understanding that they continue to live on in another form and in another reality. Shakti forms the seen world and also forms the unseen world. And because of the uncertainty of when death will come and the mystery of an uncertain afterlife, we are afraid of dying. Accordingly, "the fear of death" is a menace to humanity because it denies us the full enjoyment and experience of life. So why do we continue to teach it? Fear and pleasure cannot occupy the same space, at the same time.

How Shakti replaces the fear of death with a trust in existence?

When Cosmic Energy or Universal Shakti comes into contact with its latent Shakti, called Kundalini or Serpent Power, hitherto lying dormant, it awakens and activates the sleeping Kundalini. The awakening of Kundalini is a sure sign of active Shakti; although, in its inactive state it still supplies the energy, which keeps us alive. The individual consciously feels the oneness of one's own Shakti Kundalini with the Universal Shakti, just as a drop of water feels the union when it contacts the ocean. With the rising of the serpent power comes the intuitive knowledge that there is no death. When this happens the inner state of the aspirant quickly changes; there is calm, inner contentment and synchronicity with life not present before. Accumulated karma from other lifetimes gradually loses potency until all karmic debt is dissolved. The practitioner then experiences Shakti active within him/her as an all-encompassing and expansive energy. The body of the practitioner becomes the entire cosmos, as the cosmos and the practitioner complement each other. The practitioner experiences a unified, eternal flow of life force or energy circulating between he/she and Universal Consciousness. The physical limits of the practitioner are now extended to the cosmic level and all distances come within his/her reach; the third eye is opened, other dimensions can be seen and travel to higher realms becomes a reality. Not only is the "fear of death" gone forever but also one begins living fully, totally awake for the first time. At this level the Self-realized person can do anything on earth except the Divine processes of creation, preservation and destruction. A kind of "mechanical switch" develops enabling the persons to live either in this world or others, as they wish.

Kundalini energy can be awakened through three main practices: (i) Yogic postures, mudras and breath-control exercises, (ii) Grace of the Guru, and (iii) the accumulated results of spiritual practices through several lifetimes. Awakening Kundalini through the grace of a guru is often seen as the best and most natural way of stirring this energy. For the first method there are several rules that need to be adhered to in order for the energy to rise. One has to learn yogic postures, mudras and breath control practices of Hatha-yoga. These may not be easy for everyone, and having embarked on the path of learning these postures and mudras there is no knowing how long they will have to wait before Kundalini rises and the person "awakes." For this reason it is better to find a Guru and receive his/her grace, then there is no need for rules and regulations.

When Kundalini energy awakens through the grace of the Guru, various yogic postures, mudras and breath control exercises do not need to be performed as it often happens that when Kundalini rises through yoga practice, rather, everything unfolds by itself according to the individuals, karmic history. Awakening through the grace of the Guru is a sure and quick way, although finding a Guru is not so easy. When the consciousness of the internal and external Guru is integrated, the physical Guru is not needed for awakening. Where it is not possible to receive grace from a Guru then the first method can also work but may be slower.

Using examples we can compare the three methods of awakening. The first method is comparable to someone who works very hard, tolerating the sun and heat, working relentlessly to earn his/her living. The second method is similar to an individual who receives great wealth from a rich person through an act of compassion. The third method is comparable to someone who suddenly discovers wealth on the way home or while sitting at home, it is instant and without effort. Whatever the method, those who have successful Kundalini Awakening can be recognized by their: healthy body, happy countenance, appearance of "anahat-shabd" or the "inner sound" known as AUM or WORD, beautiful and peaceful eyes, becoming an "urdhvareta" or the one in whom the reversal of the flow of semen has taken place or the one who has attained the power of retaining the semen, and the purification of body and nerves. In my own experience when the Kundalini awakened I used to have some squeezing sensation in my testicles that seemed to be directing the fluid upward to the brain through unseen capillaries.[1] Swami Muktananda[2] and Pundit Gopi Krishna[3] have described similar experiences in their books. Female practitioners have reported similar experiences, for example, a college professor in the Midwest and Siddha-Yoga practitioner Karen felt energy rocket up from her first chakra (Mooladhar), causing her whole body to vibrate and shake. In the case of Beth of Arkansas, there was often a sucking sensation around her cervix, as if vaginal fluid was needed by the energy (4). Thus, whether the person is male or female, it seems that vital sexual fluids are used to enrich the brain to make it strong enough to receive enlightenment.

Shaktipat or Kundalini Mahayoga

Kundalini Maha Yoga is a self-proven and self-perfecting spiritual practice. The power of Kundalini can cause an initiate to perform kriyas (automatic movements) through the power of Kundalini itself. The force of Kundalini is such that the body performs these asanas unconsciously. Another name is Siddhayoga, or the self-proven path of meditation. In all aspects, body, mind and intellect, Shakti uses Kundalini to perform the meditation. The initiate will be drawn into flowing with the energy and must surrender to the process. When and how Kundalini-Shakti manifests is the work of the divine power (Shakti) itself. To practise Siddhayoga one must allow the divine power the opportunity to perform the meditation and yogic postures without interference.

With initiation it is easier to realize the fruits of knowledge, meditation, yoga, japa (chanting), tapa (austerities), devotion, karma and dharma (spiritual duties). Kundalini Maha-yoga (Shaktipat) as a path of initiation is different from other paths of meditation and/or initiation, because on other paths one has to learn certain tasks or master specific techniques. He/she is responsible for doing meditation or they need to learn about different stages in meditation. Ceremonies may be performed or different yogic postures or asanas, or they will have to struggle to eject undesirable thoughts from their minds. In Shaktipat it is not necessary to do any of these things. All the person needs to do is to sit with a complete sense of surrender to the present moment. To be warm and welcoming to all thoughts, feelings and emotions as they occur, allowing inner life to flow effortlessly through the body without interference or judgement. Then, according to the nature and state of spiritual consciousness of each initiate, different meditative experiences - emotional, intellectual or creative in nature - will occur by themselves.

Guru and the Initiate

A Guru is a person who can awaken Kundalini energy in another. The one who receives the energy from the Guru is the initiate. A person in whose presence or by whose touch inner happiness and bliss is felt, is a Guru. In fact, one's Atman or Soul is the authentic and ultimate Guru, there is no one above Atman, but this concept is too abstract for many on the spiritual path, which is why many people seek a physical Guru. One may adopt such a Guru until the realization of Atman (the inner guru) takes place. When not satisfied with a Guru, there is always the freedom to choose another, but this should only be done when following that Guru doesn't feel right intuitively anymore. A Guru is there to reveal and dissolve the ego, which is never easy. Vigilance as to why there is discomfort working with the Guru is vital, because the ego, when feeling threatened, will find any number of reasons to get rid of the Guru to stop any further spiritual advancement. Just as a bee goes from one flower to another in search of honey, a practitioner can also go from Guru to Guru in search of knowledge, but one needs to be aware that superficial flitting from one Guru to another will not aid spiritual development.

In an initiation if the initiate does not feel inner happiness or bliss, and certainly if one year after initiation and having rigorously followed instructions and been vigilant with the ego one does not receive bliss and intuitive knowledge, then it may be time to look for another Guru. Finding a self-declared Guru who is ready to work for money is easy, but finding somebody authentic is difficult. An authentic Guru has the power to transform suffering and provide bliss and intuitive knowledge.

Just as the Guru must be proper, so the initiate needs to be prepared. For the initiate this means that the mind and body must be made as strong as possible. One can understand this through an example. If cement is put on mud, it also becomes powerless like mud; but if it is put on a brick, it becomes strong like stone. Similarly, if the practitioner has prepared himself/herself through prior Hatha Yoga training and has renounced the world before Shaktipat initiation, he/she should attain a high state of spiritual development soon after initiation. However, Gurus normally do not insist on prior preparation. In cases where the initiate is unprepared, some of the Shakti is used for improving and transforming the neo-initiate, strengthening body, mind, and bringing physical changes. After initiation, one should build better foundations for spiritual advancement by taking on spiritual practices. Yogic postures provide stability to the body, mudras give the body strength, and pranayama or breath-control provides subtlety to the body, cleansing the nerves and prompting withdrawal from the outer world. This aids in turning attention inward; determination and meditation provide single-pointed concentration to the consciousness, and samadhi (inner absorption) provides the final absorption of consciousness. The Vedanta pointed out that simple knowledge without practical application in the form of spiritual practice is insufficient for Self-realization. According to the Vedanta, "One whose consciousness has become quiet and single-pointed through sadhana, who has controlled one's senses, whose karma has been burnt through tapas or austerities, who is ready to act and serve according to one's dharma, who is virtuous and willing to follow the directions given by the Guru, such a practitioner alone deserves the teachings of Brahmajnana or the knowledge of Brahman."

Building strong spiritual foundations results in practitioners acquiring two qualities. One is Non-attachment, a state of controlled Chitta (mind-stuff) containing no movement towards desire or taking away desire. This does not mean there is a physical disassociation with the objects of the world, but a sense of detachment at the mind's level, breaking the cycle of desire and attachment. When this happens the second quality of renunciation follows. Discarding (attachment to) things completely is renunciation. A practitioner develops non-attachment first and renunciation follows naturally. Non-attachment and renunciation are the result of a meditative and contemplative life and are the pillars for the highest good. They are called Parmarth. These two things are very important for the initiate to possess, in order to experience a successful and effective Shaktipat.

To understand the above and the suffering that arises when these qualities are lacking, one has only to look at the average person and how they suffer because of their attachment to the worldly goods. The physical body is everything and "the fear of death" is paramount in that person's consciousness. Little spiritual progress is made when the mind is consumed with a fear of death. By controlling the Chitta (mind) and making it dispassionate in gradual steps, non-attachment can be achieved. Slowly one understands the world is transitory, changing constantly and ultimately decaying. The pursuit and satisfaction of desire cannot lead to inner happiness, since one desire leads to another in an unending chain of dissatisfaction. Combining this understanding with the study of spiritual literature and contemplation and meditation increases detachment from the objective world. This results in corresponding gains in spiritual advancement. An initiation at this stage can produce wonderful direct experiences with Shakti.

Also important is the relationship between the path of knowledge and the path of yoga. Those on the path of knowledge experience Yoga (joining the Soul with Supersoul, or Self-realization) after many lifetimes. A yogi on the other hand acquires knowledge through the practice of Yoga and becomes liberated in a single lifetime. Therefore

Yoga is the only certain method by which results can be achieved in a single lifetime. Just as a monkey jumps from one branch to another to finally reach the desired tree laden with fruits so the yogi moves from one chakra to another. He/she gradually crosses the first six chakras until he/she finally arrives at the seventh-crown center, where consciousness and prana are anchored. At this stage the yogi acquires intuitive knowledge and liberation at the same time. An ideal way for spiritual advancement is to pursue the path of knowledge and the path of yoga simultaneously, so they complement each other. This may also be the fastest.

In some cases a yogi may not achieve liberation because of an inability to control the senses. Also a devoted yogi might leave this world before complete results are achieved and enlightenment attained. Lord Krishna, in the *Bhagavad Gita*, has discussed the plight of such yogis. According to Krishna, a fallen yogi is never destroyed either in this world or in others. One who has worked for the good of all is never abandoned. One who has progressed on the path of yoga but has gone astray before achieving the end result, because of the pull of senses or because the consciousness has turned towards materialism, after death such a person lives in heavenly worlds for a long time, because of the good deeds performed by him/her. Rebirth will be into pure and rich families, where much pleasure will be experienced. It is likely the person will take up yoga in this reincarnation because of the seeds sown in the past life. Where a dedicated practitioner of yoga dies before achieving the end result. He incarnates into a family of yogis. Such a birth is rare. The seeds of yoga sown in a past life are germinated again in this life and the individual is unknowingly forced towards the perfection of yoga. (*Bhagavad Gita*, 6, 40-44)

According to "yogshikhopnishad", if a person dies of bad karma before achieving the final result of yoga, then he has to take a body according to the way that life has been lived. Because of the good karma of yoga he/she cultivates the company of a true Guru and because of his/

her "grace" prana enters the central nerve Sushumna and the individual achieves final success in yoga, that is, liberation. One should remember that such quick success in yoga is only possible because of yoga practices in a previous life. Such a process is called "kakmat": just as a crow (kak) focuses on his target with both eyes concentrated on it (mat) and then gets it, so, a superior practitioner concentrates both jnana (knowledge) and yoga on the single target of "liberation" or "salvation" and achieves it.

It is important to understand that a yoga practitioner never suffers in this life or any other. Therefore everyone is advised to attempt yoga. It opens the gates to the knowledge of everything else. After studying all scriptures and their meanings one becomes convinced that yoga is the superior way of achieving liberation. That is why Lord Krishna said that a yogi is superior to all and advised his dearest disciple and friend Arjun to become a yogi. A Yogi is considered superior to those who observe austerities, those who study scriptures, and those who rigorously follow dharma. A yogi bypasses the dharma prescribed in the Veda. One who is dedicated to yoga is understood to have bypassed all the duties of dharma already.

Shaktipat Initiation

The method of awakening through a Guru is called "Shaktipat". In this method "divine energy" passes directly from the Guru to the initiate. This saves the initiate from lengthy and mechanical yogic practices. Energy is transmitted from the Guru to the initiate immediately when the Guru accepts him/her. The initiation can be performed in four ways: through touch, sight, mental concentration or a mantra. The easiest way of understanding how these four processes work is through an example. A bird affects the growth of the chick inside an egg by sitting on it or touching it with its body, in the same way; the Guru awakens the power of the disciple by his/her touch. As a fish nourishes its children through its sight, so, the Guru passes the energy to the disciple by his/her sight or look. As a tortoise brings out the children from the eggs under the ground by concentration and determination, so, the Guru awakens the energy in the disciple through mental concentration. A Guru can also awaken the energy by speaking and passing on a mantra to the disciple. A mantra contains the subtle seeds of divinity and is not just a combination of words or letters. The divine power of mantra is realized when it passes from the Guru to the initiate.

It is the duty of the Guru to determine the ability of the practitioner, in terms of their prior preparation with Hatha Yoga and the degree of their faith and surrender, before initiation. The desirable effects in the practitioner are brought forth through Shaktipat – the transmission of energy from the Guru. Once activated, the Shakti will first purify and transform the practitioner, and then the automatic movements will come into manifestation. Sometimes Kundalini Shakti is activated but its manifestation takes time. Activation and manifestation are two different things. To make Kundalini manifest either the Guru has to impart additional Shakti or the practitioner has to engage in spiritual discipline. Inactive Shakti can be caused by a number of reasons. (i) Nervous disorders or the continuous loss of seminal fluid can cause inactivation. Energy activates quickly in a sound body. (ii) Since the organs and senses become weak with age, activation is faster among younger practitioners. Because women are more emotional they have a greater chance of activating the energy. (iii) Indifference or annoyance on the part of the Guru towards the disciple can impede the process. (iv) Higher moral values and a pure heart trigger activation. Impurities of any kind will slow the process down. (v) Evil deeds or impure thoughts such as, theft, murder or determination to harm someone in any way will impede the process of activation. However, the practitioner has no reason to worry if he/she has truly surrendered to the Guru, since the Guru's additional supply of energy will guide the practitioner through. But ultimately the practitioner is responsible for his/her own actions and intentions. A Guru can only act as a catalyst for what is ready to be reborn, given the initiate's karmic history. No Guru can short-circuit karma and for this reason each person who is intending to awaken Kundalini either with or without a Guru must take the responsibility and karmic consequences of such actions.

Sometimes Shakti may manifest more intensely, affecting how a person behaves in public. There may be imbalances in walking, trembling and weeping or maybe crying at holy places. Where this happens, body movements should be stopped and the Guru consulted. The Guru has the power to regulate slower as well as faster movement. The practitioner should continue to practise yoga and avoid going to public places since the transmigration of energy into non-initiates can result in automatic movements that may become manifested in others and need hospitalization. In a house where many people are living, the practise of yoga should be carried out in a separate room where non-initiates do not come. However, if the people are living in the house permanently and they are likely to keep intruding, it is better to either initiate them into the process or to explain the situation to them so they will respect the need for privacy.

If the Guru dies there is no need to be afraid that the grace of the Guru will be lost, since the activation of Shakti in the practitioner is permanent and will always be a part of his/her experience. The power comes from God since the Guru; inner Guru, Universal Consciousness and God are one. If the practitioner dies before the achievement of the final result, the activated Kundalini continues in the next incarnation, and the process continues as explained earlier, until the achievement of 'samadhi,' that is, oneness with Ultimate Reality. The spiritual force then merges into the cause, that is, the Soul. In some cases the successor of the Guru, usually appointed by him before his death, continues to help practitioners towards the goal.

Liberation

Shakti Kundalini, when awakened, transforms the seeds of the past actions into automatic movements, which consequently reduces passions. The thought currents of Chitta (mind-stuff) transform themselves from disturbing ones to calm ones and ultimately lose their power. Similarly, the mind is also freed of desires. The vices of lust, anger, passion, attachment, pride and jealousy are transcended. These vices are the veils of ignorance, which delude the mind. The awakened Shakti destroys the veil of Maya (illusion). Shakti, originates in the Soul, by which Chitta appears to be conscious and is responsible for the creation of the veil of Maya, which when shattered returns and reunites with the Soul. Thus, the identification of Chitta with the Soul is broken, and with the destruction of Chitta activity, the state of Self-realization is attained. In this way the individual soul attains the state of superconsciousness.

As the automatic movements become progressively subtler, the aspirant experiences greater joy from these movements, though there are no outward signs of them. For example, one may experience jerking, vibrating, rolling or rigorous yogic postures in the beginning, with little or no peace or bliss. In later stages, vibrations become rhythmic and soft, with experiences of light and sound and entering into trance states. The aspirant is inwardly absorbed in bliss and after the initiate's mind has been purified the movements disappear. The practitioner is now in touch with the beyond and experiences oneness with Ultimate Reality.

Experiences on Awakening

Because Yoga is such a widespread activity and produces results felt by everyone, it is not surprising that the personal experiences of hundreds are being recorded as their

Kundalini Shakti awakens and becomes active. Through "pranayama" (breath control) or meditation or through the Shaktipat of an able Guru the inner power awakens and the following symptoms are observed. However, no two practitioners experience the same symptoms. The symptoms are not permanent; and their intensity is proportional to the karmic debt of the practitioner. They fade away on acquiring maturity. A practitioner who has less karmic debt is likely to have milder symptoms than one who has more karma to work through. But at the end of the process, only the feelings of inner bliss and intuitive knowledge are left, everything else vanishes.

I witnessed the manifestation of "kriyas" or automatic movements at the annual conference of the Kundalini Research Network in Philadelphia in 1995 for the first time. The person was a male practitioner from Rishikesh, India. For almost one minute he called out the name of the holy river Ganges and started movements with his hands, while he was seated on the ground. Immediately his movements appeared to be controlled by an invisible force and he began to perform various yoga postures, one after the other. Many of the postures he performed were not ordinarily possible and he demonstrated pain while performing them. The genuineness of the performance was felt and appreciated by everyone present. Practitioners will automatically go into those movements, which are necessary for his/her development. They have no control or authority over them; they take place automatically. After about half-an-hour the practitioner came back to normal and reported feeling fine. The next demonstration I saw was in India by practitioners in the presence of their Guru.

There are many kinds of movements known to manifest in practitioners when the Kundalini-Shakti is awakened. Below are some examples where the wakening of energy can be identified.

The body of the practitioner begins to vibrate. Because of prana (life energy) establishing in mooladhara (root centre) the practitioner fills with bliss and begins to dance. Since Kundalini Shakti resides in the root centre, the base of creation is also there and one begins to see the whole world there. All gods reside in the base. On the left side of the base are the three nerves – Ida, Pingala and Sushumna, which are united. Concentration at this point opens the mouth of Sushumna and eventually frees the practitioner from bondage to the world.

If the root centre becomes activated the body begins to vibrate. There is a holding in or out of the breath, which becomes automatically strong. Inhalation and exhalation become very forceful, and it may become difficult to hold the body still. This is proof of an awakened Kundalini and one should sit quietly and observe the process.

When one is established firmly on the ground with crossed legs; root, naval and chin locks are applied automatically. The tongue turns backward forcefully, it may become difficult to sit with the rush of energy and hands and legs are pulled forcefully by themselves. One should then understand that Kundalini has been activated.

When the person is seated firmly on the ground and the inner sight is concentrated between the eyebrows and the pupils of eyes begin to rotate, the breath is held spontaneously and one's thinking becomes free from the worldly thoughts. Then one should understand that the Kundalini is activated.

When one feels prana or life-energy moving from the root centre to the crown centre, the chanting of a mantra begins automatically, and one feels bliss in different ways. Then the Kundalini is activated.

When one begins to hear the unstruck sound or word in different forms, the spinal chord appears to vibrate, feelings of numbness or non-existence are experienced with regard to the body, everything appears void, one becomes unable to open one's eyes even with sustained effort or the flow of electric currents may appear to be coming out of the body, then the Kundalini has been activated.

When one feels an upsurge of energy and the feeling that someone enters the body, and performs various yogic postures, without feeling any kind of uneasiness (some practitioners experience pain, if they have not practised Hatha Yoga before), rather one may have a feeling of happiness or bliss (some pranayama may also be accompanied with it) then the Kundalini is activated.

When one continuously feels these activities in the body, wherever one concentrates one's thoughts immediately, that part of the body begins to vibrate or move, even while asleep one may feel the motion of prana in the sahasrara or crown centre, and even if this remains active in dreams, then it indicates the awakening of Kundalini.

When one sits and sees one's subtle body just by sheer will, one may lose the sensation of the physical body, even with open eyes one may feel the void, and the sense of time may be lost, then Kundalini is awakened and active.

The following examples are from people who have experienced an awakened kundalini and show how the symptoms differ.

Nan was a mid-western college student in the 60s. She had been a drug addict but later lived in an ashram in India, where she meditated for up to eight hours a day and ate little. Nan frequently experienced kriyas such as making sounds, humming, jerking her body, rolling around on the floor and falling over. She said, "I experienced twisting-snaking energy that was blissful, moving from my lower back or base of the spine upward, that caused my body to writhe around, moaning and groaning, twisting, swaying, falling forward or backward and then having a sudden backward jerk of the head accompanied by the sound of 'hum'. There was also an arching backward until falling over." Sometimes she fell over and rolled on the ground or moved into asanas or mudras, and once she danced in a trance of ecstasy[5].

Chris was born in California in 1941 and raised Catholic by a devout mother and non-Catholic father. Once while meditating she felt intense awareness of a column of brilliant light running through her. She would go into intense kriyas during the sessions, shaking, jerking, doing asanas (yogic postures), and feeling a loss of conscious awareness.

Karen a college professor, slim and graceful in her 50s studied Self-realization Fellowship courses of Yogananda and practised Kriya Yoga. She began Jungian analysis, and had lucid dreams. One night she began breathing rapidly and felt like jumping into an abyss. She saw an image of a door opening and energy passing through her. Another time, vibrations and tremors passed through her legs, spine and face and she performed yoga asanas (postures) spontaneously for three hours. Energy streamed upwards and vibrations shook her entire body. She felt the energy wanted to do things with her body she was unable to do, and her body felt like clay. She was pulled into extreme postures – underneath, backward and curled forward, and then began rocking. Then she fell entirely backward and upside down, her fingers rigid. Next she performed a headstand against the wall with her head between her knees. Then she stood up with a full body vibration and went forward to the ground. She heard the words "siddha yoga" and her head jerked from side to side. She did not know if she was laughing or crying. She had a sense of a butterfly body living within her as if her body was its cocoon. It seemed to break out as a new body through her back, with still wet wings beginning to unfold. She began laughing and crying at the same time. An unusual breathing pattern took over. Then she had phlegm in her throat and began growling and pawing at the floor. She found herself saying, "I am a leopard; I'm a South-American leopard." She felt completely embodied as this animal, growling and moving to clear her energy. Her body went into postures, some of which choked her, and she felt like vomiting but held it back[6].

These examples demonstrate how Kundalini energy varies according to the individual and their karmic history. There are three categories of practitioners – superior, middle and low. A practitioner of the superior category is someone devoted from the beginning and who is happy to receive initiation. They are overwhelmed with joy after receiving the initiation. These people receive the results of initiation immediately. A practitioner who doesn't know about initiation or yoga, but who becomes devoted after initiation and feels inner peace, belongs to the medium category. This individual will receive results in time. A practitioner of the third category is ignorant of the initiation procedure and yoga, and doesn't experience devotion and inner peace immediately after initiation. Such practitioners are the lowest in the hierarchy, and knowledge and devotion are slow to develop in them. The fruits of initiation grow with different speeds in practitioners according to their category, although Shakti and Guru are the same in each case.

Every experience whether pleasant or unpleasant leaves its impression in the Chitta (mind). Unless the consciousness is cleared of such past impressions and sensual attractions, sadhana (yogic practices or Shaktipat initiation) cannot achieve completion.

Prana is the life energy experienced by practitioners who have cleared their Chitta from the past. Kundalini carries prana, dwelling in the body of the practitioner according to the four elements of earth, water, fire or ether (akash). During daily practices following Shaktipat, prana will work differently in different practitioners. When prana dwells in earth the practitioner sits firmly on the ground with crossed legs, in the state of water one experiences a flow of tears, in the state of fire one experiences surprise, and in the state of ether (akash) one experiences catastrophe, samadhi, senselessness, trance or sleep. By observing these symptoms in daily practice, one can know the degree of prana in the practitioner. By this the Guru will know how committed the initiate is.

Order of Experiences of Realization

When the awakening of Kundalini is first experienced, the practitioner feels that the body, mind and prana have become powerless, since all activities are stilled. Next when Kundalini receives light from Shakti, the practitioner feels the active energy of prana in one's consciousness. Later, one hears an internal sound but cannot find the origin of the sound. When Kundalini assumes the form of nada (unstruck continuous sound) then one begins to hear its form very faintly. Next the practitioner begins to see divine lights that gradually take the form of a fine flame, whereupon the nada takes the clear form of sounds from the violin, flute, humming bees and other similar sounds. Finally nada takes the form of OM or AUM, which is Brahman Itself, and then whatever one determines comes to pass. The subtle form of OM eradicates sin and the deeper form of OM provides liberation. All other forms of automatic movement cease and only the sound of OM remains. One is sightless, only the state of peacefulness and single-pointed concentration remain. On physical death one attains the Brahma-lok or the plane of the residence of Brahman, the final achievement.

Divine Light is seen in various forms and colors, such as the lustre of electricity, lightening, stars, moon, sun, fire and the flame of light. Divine light is also seen in the form of points of light, and diamond-like groups, such as glow-worms. The subtleties of this Light are seen in proportion to the quality of fineness of one's consciousness.

As the consciousness becomes pure one sees the Guru, Brahman and various demi-gods or saints clearly. One may also have visions of the spiritual personalities one is most familiar with, such as Krishna, Buddha, Jesus, Mother Mary, formless Light or any other representation of pure and compassionate energy – they are seen by the practitioner either in dreams, visions or in trance. Their appearance indicates successful spiritual practice. One may witness such things while walking, sitting or in spiritual practice.

Sounds too have various forms, such as the sound of blowing a conch shell, ocean waves, a water fall, a burning fire, a peacock, buzzing bees, a flute, the humming sound of a high tension wire, voices singing and crowd noises. There are ten sound forms of the unmanifested OM – chin sound, chin chin sound, bell, conch, violin, a pair of striking metal pieces, flute, drum, pipe organ and clouds. On the first appearance of the chin sound the body experiences fine vibrations, the second chin chin sound produces feelings of body breaking down, the third bell sound produces feelings of giddiness, the fourth sound, of the blowing conch, produces vibrations in the head, the fifth violin sound produces nectar that trickles down from the palate, the sixth sound, of striking metal pieces, produces the taste of nectar, the seventh sound of the flute, brings intuitive knowledge, the eighth sound of the drum brings the power of speech, the ninth sound, of the pipe organ produces physical beauty, paranormal powers and divine insight and the tenth sound of clouds brings the state of samadhi and oneness with Brahman.

Mahayoga or the great yoga in the theory of Shaktipat, so called because it involves all kinds of yoga in one, has for stages of development that are found in all kinds of yoga.

Stage1 (arambhavastha): The *kriyas* or automatic movements following the awakening of Kundalini are the beginning of real yoga. It induces the form of *Hathayoga* or yogic postures that are necessary for the development of the practitioner. *Asanas* or yogic postures give stability to the body, *bandha* or locks and *mudras* or gestures give strength, *pranayama* or breath-control gives subtlety, and the purification of nerves gives perfection and balance in everything. Thus the first stage brings automatic perfection in *Hathayoga* for the practitioner.

Stage2 (ghatavastha): Body becomes purified and full of *sattvic* (pure and spiritual) qualities; greed and lust are destroyed; remembering God becomes continuous; *Hathayoga* and *Layayoga* (yoga of absorption) become easy and smooth.

One remains zealous and uncomfortable due to separation from God. The first two stages run together as stage one unifies the body while stage two unifies the mind. Both body and mind become purified and strong. *Kundalini* finds its path unobstructed and travels easily and smoothly to the crown centre. *Prana* or life energy becomes static and mind becomes stable at the second stage.

Stage 3 (*parichayavastha*): *Prana* is absorbed in the inner sky or *akasha*. *Kundalini Shakti* on establishing *prana* in heart centre or *anahata-chakra* gets united with Shiva in the crown centre or *sahasrara*. As long as *prana* remains static, the practitioner's body becomes motionless and gives the appearance of being lifeless, although he is fully alive internally. *Atman* is united with *prana* and the practitioner is now called a *siddha* or adept, who attracts power from beyond and acquires unworldly capabilities. *Prana* crosses all the seven chakras and rests in the crown. Semen converts into energy and the practitioner finds intuitive knowledge flowing into him. Practitioner becoming an adept or *siddha* can pass over energy to others and awaken their *kundalini*. Karma is burnt, all doubts are removed and the knot at the level of heart is opened by the grace of God Almighty. He is absolved and has the power of absolving others too. Even if such a person appears without morals outwardly, his knowledge cannot be camouflaged by anything whatsoever. Those who criticize him take these sins with them, and those who praise him take these virtues with them. He has seen the way to the realm of *Brahman* and when he leaves this world he will arrive straight into the realm of *Satya* or Truth. The Lord conveys that such an adept is acquainted with Him and now he can show the way to Him, to anyone he likes.

Stage 4 (*nishpatti-avastha*): The practitioner-turned-adept or *siddha* witnesses himself as the soul or *Atman*. He has reached the level of Shiva-ness, *Kundalini Shakti* is absorbed in Shiva, and he is known as *jivan-mukta* or liberated-while-living. He experiences the universe being absorbed in his own *Atman*.

In the words of Yogendra Vigyani, Shaktipat Guru and author in the Tirth lineage:

"Sound, touch, beauty, taste and smell are the five sense-objects in the world that attract and absorb the mind and heart of a person; and getting involved in these objects the individual ends up with destruction and downfall. All scriptures say the same thing, but the enjoyment of these five objects and getting involved in them after successful completion of yoga and meditation does not lead the individual to downfall, rather one progresses upwards. Therefore, without knowing the knowledge given by Lord Maheshwara (Shiva) the ignorant people end up with destruction through enjoyment of the sense-objects; but enjoyment of these sense-objects by the God-loving and wise people leads to happiness and success under all conditions[7]."

My Own Experiences

I have passed through the experiences described above which were first published in the Academy of Religion and Psychical Research, New York, as a series of research papers. Later they appeared in chronological order in my book *Kundalini for Beginners*[8]. However, they have now been presented in complete details in the first chapter on autobiography. One can be successful in yoga while living a practical conventional life. These two things are inclusive and they do not interfere with each other. On the contrary, yoga practices generate the energy necessary for success in the world while also enjoying life more fully. By enjoying life's experience in full one achieves liberation and breaks the cycle of death and rebirth, once and for all.

I have seen the manifestation of kriyas or automatic movements in practitioners in the presence of their Guru. This same Guru initiated me, although I had my Kundalini awakened many years ago. The Guru told me, when I asked for the reason this initiation should be taken even though I had an awakened Kundalini, that continuous activation of Kundalini is required after its awakening. It is like a person awakened from sleep in the morning but sitting quietly in bed. It is important to recognize the difference between an awakened and active Kundalini. It is only after activation that full results manifest. The Guru passed his power into me by his touch. For the next three days I also underwent automatic movements of my body, although the movements were gentle and rhythmic, and not as violent and varied as in the case of some beginners. I also experienced fast and deep inhalations and exhalations accompanying the movements. After 30 to 45 minutes of movement I went into a trance, witnessing inner bliss and oneness with the Reality. For the rest of the day I was filled with an inner happiness and was indifferent to the outer world. Afterward and for the next two weeks I had an itchy back and burning in my spine. Gradually these symptoms subsided.

When Kundalini is both awake and active for sometime, Shaktipat becomes stabilized in the practitioner; he/she is now a Guru him/herself, and begins to help others to raise their Kundalini. I saw some practitioners, who had spent time preparing themselves, would go into samadhi when I touched their third eye. An Australian couple came to see me after reading the book *Kundalini for Beginners*. The man had been practising Hatha Yoga and Pranayama (breath-control) for several years. In the morning he came for a lesson. I gave him instruction in performing asanas (yogic postures) and touched him. He began to perform several yogic postures perfectly and effortlessly, which he could not do earlier. His eyes were closed all the time, and he did not see what he was doing. After half-an-hour of this performance he became still and normal, and looked peaceful and happy. He told me he had some kriyas in the past but not as intensely as that day. Later I initiated about twenty selected people in about three years' time, and almost all of them have their Kundalini awakened and activated. They are now living an entirely different life since then.

Although the art of Shaktipat is the easiest and most direct method of awakening Kundalini, its use is uncommon and rare in the present age. The reasons are two-fold: the practitioners do not prepare themselves through detachment, renunciation and Hatha Yoga practices; and, because of a lack of faith and surrender in Guru and God, the Guru chooses only a few practitioners as his/her disciples. Also, the teachings of Shaktipat had been from mouth to ear and hence, they were lost in antiquity. To find a Master, practitioners have been searching Himalayan caves, with little success. Nevertheless, for some, there has always been and will continue to be the Guru-initiate Shaktipat.

What help is offered?

The theory of Kundalini and the Integral Path of yoga has been described in detail, and a practical formula, called Integral Path has been presented in the book, *Kundalini for Beginners*[9]. Greater discussion has been given in my next book, *Secrets of Kundalini Awakening*[10], in which the process is described through pictures. Yet more complete details have appeared in the next book, *The Kundalini Book of Living and Dying*[11]. In the three books mentioned above I have given details of other worlds, I have discussed the power of Soul and have elaborated on various possible ways of achieving higher consciousness. Finally, *Secrets of Shaktipat*[12] presents all intricacies related to this hidden art of Shaktipat. Thus, these books have self-help programs, which practitioners can follow to prepare themselves for initiation. We have established centres in New Delhi, Copenhagen, London and Bradenton (Florida) for practical spiritual growth. It is advisable for practitioners to practise the integral path of yoga for a period of six months to one year. Depending on the personal progress and wishes of the individual during this period, practitioners are accepted as disciples for Shaktipat initiation.

AFTERWORD

If this book was helpful to you, we recommend that you visit the Academy sometime and take the membership. Academy of Kundalini Yoga is a non-profit organization that provides services in two directions: numerology and self-realization. When I was in Greece some 2600 years ago Master Pythagoras was my Guru. I learnt from him in all the three directions of his specialization – mathematics, numerology and spiritual practices to achieve oneness with the Lord. He has been helping me in other incarnations as well since then.

Through numerology you can know your past, present and future; and get remedy for your problems. In spirituality, a disciple is trained through yoga, pranayama and meditations so as to receive Shaktipat initiation for quick awakening of Kundalini Shakti. I work with a very small group of disciplines at a time, till his or her Kundalini is awakened, which normally takes a few months time. About a hundred people have received Initiation successfully in the past three years from different parts of the world. We have rooms to stay and all other facilities. You may contact as follows for appointment.

Ravindra Kumar
(Now Swami Ravindranand)
Academy of Kundalini Yoga and Quantum Soul
Tel: 9891467723, Email: kumarravi@mail.com
Website: www.quantumsoulaware.com
Europe: Email: jytteravi.kumar@mail.tele.dk

Glossary

Aarti	–	a ceremony for greeting the Lord with chanting and offerings of food lamps, fans, flowers and incense.
Abhinivesha	–	blind tenacity in believing the validity of material creation
Adhivahikas	–	bearers in transit
Aditi	–	primordial light
Ahan	–	day
Ahamkara	–	ego
Akash	–	sky
Alaya	–	soul of the world
Ananda-maya-loka	–	realm of bliss
Ananta	–	timeless
Ananta-shesha	–	great serpent of eternity
Aniyamsam	–	smallest of small
Ankh	–	life
Ant mati so gati	–	placement of a person after death according to one's last thoughts
Aparokshjnana	–	real comprehension through direct experience
Ardhanari	–	hermaphrodite goddess
Artha	–	cessation of all sufferings
Arupa	–	formless

Glossary

Asana	–	steady and pleasant physical posture
Achyuta	–	unfallen
Asita	–	dark
Asu	–	breath
Asuras	–	demons/spiritual divine beings
Atma/Atman	–	Soul
Avastha	–	state
Avatar	–	a descent, or incarnation of the Supreme Lord
Avikara	–	undifferentiated
Avyakta	–	unrepresented
Bhakta	–	one who is given to the yoga of love and devotion, in which intense love for a Divine incarnation or some other embodiment of God leads to merging with the chosen ideal.
Bhastrika Pranayama	–	control of prana with rapid movements of breaths
Brahma	–	neuter, unmanifested first cause
Brahmaa	–	manifested first cause
Brahman	–	the eternal, imperishable Absolute; the supreme non-dual Reality
Brahmajyoti	–	effulgence from the Lord that lights all the material and spiritual worlds
Brahmanidhan	–	baptism or absorption/merging of Self in the Holy Sound
Brihaspati	–	Jupiter
Budha	–	Mercury
Buddhi	–	spiritualized mind or intelligence
Chit	–	universal knowledge

Chitta	–	Mind-stuff, calm state of mind
Chit-Shakti	–	Conscious Energy
Chaitanya	–	A state of Chit-Shakti
Chohans	–	gods, angels or devas
Chyuta	–	fallen
Daitya-guru	–	guru of primeval giants
Devas	–	Angels
Dhyani-Chohans	–	creators, angels, devas
Dvija	–	twice-born
Dwesha	–	aversion from objects of repulsion that give hatred or pain
Ekanekarupa	–	many
Grahastyashrama	–	domestic life
Gunas	–	modes of nature—Sattva, Rajas and Tamas
Hamsa-vaahana	–	one who uses swan as vehicle
Jiva	–	the embodied Self that exists in the realm of duality
Jivanmukta	–	liberated while living
Jnani	–	one having the *jnana* or knowledge that leads to God through intellectual discrimination between the false and transitory and what is true and has lasting value
Jyotsna	–	dawn
Kalahansa	–	eternal swan
Karana	–	cause
Karma	–	action, which leads to the chain of cause and effect operating in human relationships and individual moral evolution
Kirtana	–	the devotional process of chanting

Glossary

		the names and glories of the Supreme Lord
Kriya Shakti	–	yoga power
Kriyas	–	Automatic movements of different parts of the body after the awakening of Kundalini
Kruralochana	–	evil-eyed
Kumbhak	–	retention of breath
Kundalini	–	Dormant Serpent Power or Sleeping Spiritual Energy, lying coiled like a snake at the base of spine, metaphorically. When awakened, it rises through and vitalizes the chakras, bringing spiritual knowledge, mystical vision, psychic powers, and ultimately enlightenment, if one has achieved the condition of an *urdhvareta* or the one in whom the flow of semen is reversed towards the brain. The process can lead to insanity if it goes awry. The goddess who personifies this energy is also called Kundalini
Kurta Pyjama	–	dress for the night
Kutastha Chaitanya	–	Omniscient Holy Spirit
Lila	–	amusement
Linga	–	phallus
Lohitanga	–	fiery bodied
Mahamantra	–	the great chant for deliverance: Hare Krishna, Hare Krishna, Krishna Krishna, Hare Hare; Hare Rama, Hare Rama, Rama Rama, Hare Hare
Mahatma	–	the highest adept

Mala	–	set of beads woven around a thread for chanting of a mantra.
Manas	–	mind, intellect
Mantra	–	a transcendental sound or Vedic hymn, which can deliver the mind from illusion
Manus	–	the thinkers, mental beings in terrestrial body
Manushyas	–	humans
Manvantara	–	duration of the universe from the beginning to the end
Martanda	–	Sun
Maya	–	cosmic illusion or ignorance, based on misinterpretation of a partial aspect of Reality
Mooladhara Chakra	–	the first chakra or the root centre, located at the lowest part of the central nerve *sushumna* between the genitals and the anus. Kundalini in unawakened state is supposed to be lying coiled in *mooladhara*
Mulaprakriti	–	Root-Nature
Nathas	–	Lords
Nirmankayas	–	body makers
Nitya	–	eternal
Niyama	–	religious rules
Ojas	–	spiritual energetic conversion of the seminal fluid, preparing the brain to receive enlightenment
Padma	–	lotus
Parmarth	–	the highest good

Parabrahman	– Lord Absolute above his expansion as Brahman.
Paramatma	– Supersoul or Oversoul, taking care of all the souls in existence
Paramartha	– complete cessation of sufferings with no chance of recurring
Parokshajnana	– matter of inference, true comprehension of nothingness of the world
Pitris	– ancestors, progenitors
Pradhan	– soul of the world/primordial matter
Pralaya	– dissolution (of universe)
Prana	– life energy from cosmos penetrating and maintaining the body and that is most overtly manifest in the breath. In Hinduism there are five different pranas: *prana* itself, the pure life force; *vyana*, guiding the circulation; *samana*, controlling the intake and metabolism of nutrients; *apana*, governing elimination and active in the lower part of the body; and *udana*, working in the upper body and creating a bridge between the physical and the spiritual. It is the combusting agent that converts physical energy into radiation, as mental activity and sexual energy.
Pranayama	– control over prana or life energy, fourth stage of the eight-fold yoga system.
Pranidhan	– persevering ceaseless devotion

Pratyahara	–	withdrawal of the senses from the external world
Prembijam chit	–	Omniscient love
Puranas	–	eighteen of the kind, written parallel to the Vedas about spiritual truth
Purusha	–	the son of God, the spiritualized atom, jiva or individual soul
Purvaja	–	pregenetic
Radha	–	divine spark, luminous body sent by God
Raga	–	attraction or attachment for things of pleasure
Rajas	–	action, worldly activities, goal orientation
Ratri	–	night
Rupa	–	with form
Sach Khand	–	the highest division of spiritual realms
Sadaikrupa	–	changeless
Sadhu	–	one who has renounced the world for God's Realization, holy person or monk.
Sahasrara	–	the seventh chakra located at the crown of the head, above the upper end of *sushumna*. Physically the brain corresponds it
Samadhi	–	inner absorption, true concentration
Samyama	–	restraint
Sadhana	–	Yogic practices
Sandhya	–	evening twilight
Shani	–	Saturn

Sat	–	reality
Satsang	–	a religious gathering for talking and singing about God.
Sattva	–	pure knowledge, goodness, religious activities, spirituality
Shaktipat	–	transmission of Cosmic Energy from Guru to Initiate, resulting in instant awakening of Kundalini
Shiva	–	belongs to the Hindu trinity of gods: Brahma (creator), Vishnu (preserver), and Shiva (destroyer of illusion or ignorance). He is the symbol of higher consciousness. Kundalini rises and travels to sahasrara, which is the union of Shiva and his consort Shakti
Shoonyata	–	voidness, which is everything in reality
Shraddha	–	heart's natural love
Soma	–	moon
Smriti	–	memory of one's divinity
Sthula Sarira	–	physical body, outer covering
Shukra	–	Venus
Sukshma Sarira	–	subtle body
Sushumnadwara	–	door of the inner worlds where cosmic sound is heard
Sutraman	–	thread doctrine
Svabhavat	–	plastic material filling the universe
Swadhyaya	–	study with deep attention
Tamas	–	ignorance, inertia, unproductive
Tapa or tapas	–	austerities, patience or equanimity under both favorable and adverse circumstances

Trikuti	–	centre between the eyebrows
Uddiyan Bandha	–	naval lock
Urdhava retas	–	reversal of the seed—the reproductive system and the flowing of the seminal essence or nerve energy is reversed, travelling upward to the brain through the spinal chord. It is the basis of Kundalini yoga and ultimate aim of every kind of yoga for the attainment of the transcendental state of consciousness.
Vach	–	voice
Vaikunthalokas	–	the spiritual planets beyond material universe, free of anxiety
Varaha	–	boar
Vedas	–	the books of the knowledge, the earliest Indian scriptures. Though originally one Veda, it was divided into four parts: Rig Veda, Yajur Veda, Atharva Veda and Sam Veda
Vedanta	–	culmination of the Vedas and Upanishads, a summary of philosophy and spiritual discipline especially for intellectuals and philosophers.
Viratvam	–	magnanimity of the heart
Virya	–	moral courage, semen
Vishnu	–	Logos incarnate
Vyakta	–	manifested, represented
Yama	–	morality or self-control
Yoga	–	meaning yoke, a way to achieve "union" with Cosmic Consciousness. It implies union of soul with Oversoul and the method of doing

	it. Yoga accelerates the natural process of evolution, which is already at work to open the supersensory perception in the brain that can manifest a transhuman state of consciousness capable of receiving revelation. Main kinds of yoga are bhakti, karma, jnana, raja, kriya and kundalini yoga.
Yogi	– one who practices yoga
Yoni	– vulva, the female generative organ

REFERENCES

Chapter 1

1. Kumar, Ravindra, 2001. *All You Wanted to Know about Dreams.* Sterling Publishers, New Delhi.
2. ———————1992. *Secrets of Numerology—A Complete Guide to the Layman.* Sterling Publishers, New Delhi.
3. Saraswati, Swami Satyananda. 1984. *Kundalini Tantra.* Bihar School of Yoga, Munger, India.
4. Kumar, Ravindra, 2000. *Kundalini for Beginners.* Llewellyn Worldwide Ltd., MN, USA.
5. Saraswati, Swami Satyananda. 1984. *Kundalini Tantra.* Bihar School of Yoga, Munger, India, p.152.
6. Twitchell, Paul. 1971. *The Far Country.* IWP Publishing, Menlo Park, CA, USA.
7. Newton, Michael 1994. *Journey of Souls.* Llewellyn Publications, St. Paul, MN, USA.
8. ——————— 2000. *Destiny of Souls.* Llewellyn Publications, St. Paul, MN, USA.
9. Muktananda, Swami. 1972. *Chitshakti Vilas.* (*The Play of Consciousness*) Gurudev Siddhapeeth, Maharashtra, India.
10. Radha, Swami. 1993. *Mantras.* Motilal Banarsidass Publishers Ltd., Delhi, India.
11. Svoboda, E. Robert 1986. *Aghora.* Brotherhood of Life, Inc., USA. & Rupa & CO., New Delhi, India.

12. Guiley, Rosemary E. 1998. *Dreamwork for the Soul*. Berkley Books, New York.
13. Kumar, Ravindra 2000. *All You Wanted to Know About Hatha Yoga*. Sterling Publishers, Delhi.
14. —————————2000. *All You Wanted to Know About Kundalini Yoga*. Sterling Publishers, Delhi.
15. ————————— 2000. *All You Wanted to Know About Kriya Yoga*. Sterling Publishers, Delhi.
16. ————————— 2000. *All You Wanted to Know About Chakras and Nadis*. Sterling Publishers, Delhi.
17. ————————— 2001. *All You Wanted to Know About Dreams*. Sterling Publishers, Delhi.
18. ————————— 2001. *All You Wanted to Know About Aura*. Sterling Publishers, Delhi.
19. —————————2001. *All You Wanted to Know About Mantras*. Sterling Publishers, Delhi.
20. ————————— 2001. *All You Wanted to Know About Psychic Development*. Sterling Publishers, Delhi.
21. ————————— 2002. *All You Wanted to Know About Karma Yoga*. Sterling Publishers, Delhi.
22. ————————— 2002. *All You Wanted to Know About Jnana Yoga*. Sterling Publishers, Delhi.
23. ————————— 2002. *All You Wanted to Know About Bhakti Yoga*. Sterling Publishers, Delhi.
24. ————————— 2002. *All You Wanted to Know About Tantra Yoga*. Sterling Publishers, Delhi.
25. Tanner, Wilda B. 1988. *The Mystical Magical Marvellous World of Dreams*. Sparrow Hawk Press, Oklahoma, p 157.
26. Kumar, Ravindra 2002. "How Shakti-Kundalini Conquers Death-Anxiety and Achieves Liberation." JRPR, April 2002.
27. Greenwell, Bonnie. 1990. *Energies of Transformation*. Shakti River Press, Cupertino, CA.

Chapter 2

1. Blavatsky, H.P.B. 1979. *The Secret Doctrine—Vol. I*, The Theosophical Publishing House, Adyar, India, 1888, Preface, p. viii.
2. ———p. 13
3. ———p. 63
4. ———p. 50.
5. ———p. 285
6. ———p. 342
7. ———p. 349
8. Movers. 1841. *Die Phonizier.* Vol. I, p. 268.
9. Blavatsky, H.P.B. 1979. *The Secret Doctrine—Vol. I*, The Theosophical Publishing House, Adyar, India, 1888, p.350
10. Blavatsky, H.P.B. 1979. *The Secret Doctrine—Vol. II*, The Theosophical Publishing House, Adyar, India, 1888, p.77
11. Franck, A. 1843. *La Kabbale.* P. 173.
12. Blavatsky, H.P.B. 1979. *The Secret Doctrine—Vol. I*, The Theosophical Publishing House, Adyar, India, 1888, p.347
13. Blavatsky, H.P.B. *Isis Unveiled.* Vol. 1, p. 341.
14. Hippolytus. (ed. P. Cruice, 1860). *Philosophumena.* Book VI, ch. 43.
15. Blavatsky, H.P.B. 1979. *The Secret Doctrine—Vol. I*, The Theosophical Publishing House, Adyar, India, 1888, p. 352.

16. Hippolytus. (ed. P. Cruice, 1860). *Philosophumena.* Book VI, ch. 43.
17. Blavatsky, H.P.B. 1979. *The Secret Doctrine—Vol. I*, The Theosophical Publishing House, Adyar, India, 1888, p. 351, footnote.
18. *Ibid* p. 89.
19. *Ibid* p. 90
20. *Ibid* p. 90
21. *Ibid* p. 90
22. Blavatsky, H.P.B. 1979. *The Secret Doctrine—Vol. II*, The Theosophical Publishing House, Adyar, India, 1888, p. 70.
23. Blavatsky, H.P.B. 1979. *The Secret Doctrine—Vol. I*, The Theosophical Publishing House, Adyar, India, 1888, p. 170.
24. *Ibid* p. 311
25. *Ibid* p. 285
26. Blavatsky, H.P.B. 1979. *The Secret Doctrine—Vol. II*, The Theosophical Publishing House, Adyar, India, 1888, p. 70
27. *Ibid* p. 43
28. Blavatsky, H.P.B. 1979. *The Secret Doctrine—Vol. I*, The Theosophical Publishing House, Adyar, India, 1888, p. 245.
29. *Ibid* p. 653.
30. *Ibid* p. 655
31. Mackey, S.A. 1822-23, *The Mythological Astronomy of the Ancients Demonstrated,* Part-II—*The Key of Urania*, pp. 23-24.

Chapter 3

1. Blavatsky, H.P.B. 1979. *The Secret Doctrine—Vol. II*, The Theosophical Publishing House, Adyar, India, 1888, p. 1.
2. *Ibid* p. 3
3. *Ibid* pp. 6-12.
4. *Ibid* p. 11
5. *Ibid* p. 25
6. *Ibid* p. 25
7. *Ibid* p. 29
8. Blavatsky, H.P.B. 1979. *The Secret Doctrine—Vol. I*, The Theosophical Publishing House, Adyar, India, 1888, p. 684
9. Blavatsky, H.P.B. 1979. *The Secret Doctrine—Vol. II*, The Theosophical Publishing House, Adyar, India, 1888, p. 68.
10. Blavatsky, H.P.B. 1979. *The Secret Doctrine—Vol. I*, The Theosophical Publishing House, Adyar, India, 1888, pp.611-612.
11. *Ibid* p. 610.
12. *Ibid* p. 612.
13. *Ibid* p. 620.
14. *Ibid* p. 622.
15. *Ibid* p. 63.
16. *Ibid* p. 625.
17. *Ibid* p. 632-633.

18. Bjerregaard, C.H.A. 1887. *The Path.* January 1887, pp. 321-322.
19. Blavatsky, H.P.B. 1979. *The Secret Doctrine—Vol. II,* The Theosophical Publishing House, Adyar, India, 1888, p. 31.
20. *Ibid* p. 34.
21. *Ibid* p. 70.
22. Chatterji, Mohini.M. 1932. *Vivek-Chudamani.* The Theosophical Publishing House, Adyar, India.
23. Blavatsky, H.P.B. 1979. *The Secret Doctrine—Vol. I,* The Theosophical Publishing House, Adyar, India, 1888, p. 245.
24. Blavatsky, H.P.B. 1979. *The Secret Doctrine—Vol. II,* The Theosophical Publishing House, Adyar, India, 1888, pp. 78-79.
25. *Ibid* p. 41
26. *Ibid* p. 42
27. Blavatsky, H.P.B. 1979. *The Secret Doctrine—Vol. I,* The Theosophical Publishing House, Adyar, India, 1888, p. 245.
28. Blavatsky, H.P.B. 1979. *The Secret Doctrine—Vol. II,* The Theosophical Publishing House, Adyar, India, 1888, pp. 50-51.
29. *Zohar,* III, fol. 292 a & b, Brody ed.; Cremona ed. III. Fol 142 a & b, col. 566-67.
30. *Bereshith Rabbah,* Parsha p. ix.
31. Cory. 1832. *Ancient Fragments.* p. 25.
32. Blavatsky, H.P.B. 1979. *The Secret Doctrine—Vol. II,* The Theosophical Publishing House, Adyar, India, 1888, p. 58.
33. *Ibid* p 59.
34. Kumar, R. 2000. *Kundalini for Beginners.* Llewellyn Publications, St. Paul, Minnesota.

35. Kumar, R. and Larsen, J.K. 2004. *The Kundalini Book of Living and Dying*. Weiser Books, Boston.MA/York Beach.
36. Kumar, R. and Larsen, J.K. 2005. *Secrets of Shaktipat*. New Dawn Press, Inc. India.
37. Blavatsky, H.P.B. 1979. *The Secret Doctrine—Vol. II*, The Theosophical Publishing House, Adyar, India, 1888, p. 60.
38. *Ibid* p. 61
39. *Ibid* p. 63
40. *Zohar: Idra Zuta Qaddisha* (Lesser Holy Assembly). Cf. Macgregor Mathers, *Kabbalah Unveiled*, p 302.
41. *Zohar*, Brody ed., III, 135a; Cremona ed., iii, fol. 64b, col. 255, and fel. 142a, col 566. Cf. I. Myer, *Qabbalah*, pp. 386-87.
42. *Zohar*, III, 290a, Brody ed.; Cremona ed., III, fol. 141a, col. 562. Cf. I. Myer, *Qabbalah*, pp. 387-88.
43. Blavatsky, H.P.B. 1979. *The Secret Doctrine—Vol. II*, The Theosophical Publishing House, Adyar, India, 1888, p. 85.
44. *Ibid* p. 88
45. Benfey. *Sacred Books of the East, Vol. IV*. The Zend-Avesta tr. by J. Darmesteter), *Introduction* IV, p. viii.
46. Aurobindo, Sri and Mother. 1989. *The Psychic Being*. Sri Aurobindo Ashram, Pondicherry, India.
47. Blavatsky, H.P.B. 1979. *The Secret Doctrine—Vol. II*, The Theosophical Publishing House, Adyar, India, 1888, p. 95.
48. Francois de Foix. 1579. *Le Pimandre de Mercure Trismegiste de la Philosophie Chretienne*. Bishop of Ayre, Bordeaux.
49. Bourbourg, Brasseur de. *Popul-Vuh*, Part III, ch. I; pp. 199.

50. Max Muller. 1881. *Review of the Popul-Vuh.* Chips, etc., Vol. I, p. 331.
51. Darmester, James. *Sacred Books of the East.* Vol. IV, p. 209, footnote.
52. Woodroffe, Sir John. 1981. *The Serpent Power.* Ganesh & Co., Madras, India.
53. Krishna, Gopi. 1971. *Kuindalini—The Evolutionary Energy in Man.* Shambhala, Boston & London.
54. Saraswati, Swami Satyananda. 1984. *Kundalini Tantra.* Bihar School of Yoga, Munger, India.
55. Radha, Swami Sivananda. 1992. *Kundalini Yoga.* Motilal Banarsidass Publishers, Delhi.
56. Goel, B.S. 1985. *Third Eye and Kundalini.* Third Eye Foundation of India, Haryana, India.
57. Kumar, Ravindra. 2000. *Kundalini for Beginners.* Llewellyn Publications, Minnesota, USA.
58. ————————— 2003. *Secrets of Kundalini Awakening.* Sterling Publishers Pvt. Ltd., Delhi.
59. ————————— 2004. *The Kundalini Book of Living and Dying.* Weiser Books, Boston, USA.
60. ————————— 2005. *Secrets of Shaktipat—Awakening of Kundalini by the Guru.* New Dawn Press, Inc. UK, USA, India.
61. Wagner, W. *Asgard and the Gods.* p. 305.
62. Blavatsky, H.P.B. 1979. *The Secret Doctrine—Vol. II,* The Theosophical Publishing House, Adyar, India, 1888, p. 100.
63. Everard, Dr. John. 1650. *The Divine Pymander.* Bk. II, verse 22, pp. 10-11.
64. *Chaldean Account of Genesis,* p 92.
65. *Ibid,* p 91.
66. *Poimandres,* I, 6 (Chambers, pp. 2-3); or II, 8 (Everard, p. 8).

67. Blavatsky, H.P.B. 1979. *The Secret Doctrine—Vol. II*, The Theosophical Publishing House, Adyar, India, 1888, p. 107, footnote.
68. *Ibid* p 107.
69. *Ibid* p 108.

Chapter 4

1. Josephus *History of the Jewish war*, Book. II, chap viii, p. 11.
2. Judaeus, Philo. *De Gigantibus*, article 2; *De Somniis*, I, article 22.
3. Paul, St. *1 Corithians vi*, 3.
4. Luria, R. Isaac. *Sephr M'vo Shearim*, translated by Isaac Myer, *Qabbalah*, p 110.
5. Blavatsky, H.P.B. 1979. *The Secret Doctrine—Vol. II*, The Theosophical Publishing House, Adyar, India, 1888, p. 124.
6. Kumar, Ravindra. 2000. *Kundalini for Beginners*. Llewellyn Publications, St. Paul, Minnesota, pp. 26-27.
7. Blavatsky, H.P.B. 1979. *The Secret Doctrine—Vol. II*, The Theosophical Publishing House, Adyar, India, 1888, p. 81.
8. Paul. *I Corinthians*, xv, 47.
9. Blavatsky, H.P.B. 1979. *The Secret Doctrine—Vol. I*, The Theosophical Publishing House, Adyar, India, 1888, p 245.
10. ——— p 135.
11. Yukteswar, Swami Sri 1984. *The Holy Science*. Self-realization Fellowship, Los Angeles, California.
12. ——— pp. 64-67.
13. Kumar, Ravindra 1999. *The Journey Back to our True Home through Spiritual Energy-KUNDALINI*. Sterling Publishers Pvt. Ltd., New Delhi.

14. ———2005. *Secrets of Shaktipat*. New Dawn Press, UK.
15. Geeta Press, Gorakhpur. *Srimad Bhagavata Mahapurana*. Geeta Press, Gorakhpur, India.
16. Acharya, Pandit R. V. and Acharya, R. Venkataraman. 1990. *A Synopsis of Srimath Bhagavatam."* Tirumala Tirupati Devasthanams, Tirupati, India.
17. Venkataramiah, M. 2000. *Talks with Sri Ramana Maharishi.* Sri Ramanasramam, Tiruvannamalai, India.
18. Chatterji, Mohini M. 1932. *Vivek-Chudamani (The Crest Jewel of Wisdom)*. The Theosophical Publishing House, Adyar, India.
19. Krishna, Gopi. 1993. *Living with Kundalini*. Shambhala Publications, Boston, p. 378.
20. Prabhupada, A.C.Bhaktivedanta Swami. *Sri Ishopanishad*. The Bhaktivedanta Book Trust, Mumbai, India.
21. Venkataramiah, Munangala. 2000. *TALKS with Sri Ramana Maharishi.* Sri Ramanasramam, Tiruvannamalai, India, p. 70.
22. Prabhupada, A.C.Bhaktivedanta Swami. 1972. *The Topmost Yoga System.* The Bhaktivedanta Book Trust, Mumbai, India.
23. *Ibid* p 107.

Chapter 5

1. Kumar, Ravindra, 2000. *Kundalini for Beginners*. Llewellyn Worldwide Ltd., MN, U.S.A.
2. Muktananda, Swami 1972. *Chitshakti Vilas (The Play of Consciousness)*. Gurudev Siddhapeeth, Maharashtra, India.
3. Krishna, Gopi 1975. *The Awakening of Kundalini*. New York, NY: Kundalini Research Foundation, U.S.A.
4. Greenwell, Bonnie 1990. *Energies of Transformation-A Guide to the Kundalini Process*. Shakti River Press, Cupertino, CA, p 203.
5. *Ibid.* pp 189-190.
6. *Ibid.* pp 208-209.
7. Vigyani, Yogendra 1938, 1997. *Mahayoga Vigyan*. Vigyan Bhawan, Rishikesh, India, p 152.
8. Kumar, Ravindra, 2000. *Kundalini for Beginners*. Llewellyn Worldwide Ltd., MN, U.S.A.
9. *Ibid.* p 256.
10. Kumar, Ravindra. 2003. *Secrets of Kundalini Awakening*. Sterling Publishers Pvt. Ltd., Delhi.
11. ——————— 2004. *The Kundalini Book of Living and Dying*. Weiser Books, Boston, USA.
12. ——————— 2005. *Secrets of Shaktipat*. New Dawn Press, Inc., UK, USA, India.

BIBLIOGRAPHY

Acharya, Pandit R. V. and Acharya, R. Venkataraman. 1990. *A Synopsis of Srimath Bhagavatam.* Tirumala Tirupati Devasthanams, Tirupati, India.
Aurobindo, Sri and Mother. 1989. *The Psychic Being.* Sri Aurobindo Ashram, Pondicherry, India.
Benfey. *Sacred Books of the East, Vol. IV.* The Zend-Avesta (tr. By J. Darmesteter), Introduction IV, p. viii.
Bereshith Rabbah, Parsha ix.
Bjerregaard, C.H.A. 1887. *The Path.* January 1887, pp. 321-322.
Blavatsky, H.P.B. 1979. *The Secret Doctrine—Vol. I,* The Theosophical Publishing House, Adyar, India, 1888.
———————1979. *The Secret Doctrine—Vol. II,* The Theosophical Publishing House, Adyar, India, 1888.
Bourbourg, Brasseur de. *Popul-Vuh,* Part III, ch. I; pp. 199.
Chaldean Account of Genesis, p. 92.
Chatterji, Mohini M. 1932. *Vivek-Chudamani (The Crest Jewel of Wisdom).* The Theosophical Publishing House, Adyar, India.
Cory. 1832. *Ancient Fragments.* p. 25
Darmester, James. *Sacred Books of the East.* Vol. IV, p. 209, footnote.
Everard, Dr. John. 1650. *The Divine Pymander.* Bk. II, verse 22, pp. 10-11.
Franck, A. 1843. *La Kabbale.* p. 173.
Francois de Foix. 1579. *Le Pimandre de Mercure Trismegiste de la Philosophie Chretienne.* Bishop of Ayre, Bordeaux.
Geeta Press, Gorakhpur. *Srimad Bhagavata Mahapurana.* Geeta Press, Gorakhpur, India.
Goel, B.S. 1985. *Third Eye and Kundalini.* Third Eye Foundation of India, Haryana, India.
Greenwell, Bonnie 1990. *Energies of Transformation-A Guide to the Kundalini Process.* Shakti River Press, Cupertino, CA.
Guiley, Rosemary E. 1998. *Dreamwork for the Soul.* Berkley Books, New York.
Hippolytus. (ed. P. Cruice, 1860). *Philosophumena.* Book VI, ch. 43.
Josephus. *History of the Jewish war,* Bk. II, viii, p. 11.
Judaeus, Philo. *De Gigantibus,* article 2; *De Somniis,* I, article 22.

Bibliography

Krishna, Gopi. 1971. *Kundalini—The Evolutionary Energy in Man*. Shambhala, Boston & London.
——————1975. *The Awakening of Kundalini*. New York, NY: Kundalini Research Foundation, U.S.A.
——————1993. *Living with Kundalini*. Shambhala Publications, Boston, p. 378.
Kumar, Ravindra. 1992. *Secrets of Numerology—A Complete Guide to the Layman*. Sterling Publishers, New Delhi.
——————1996. *Destiny, Science and Spiritual Awakening*. Sterling Publishers, Delhi.
——————1999. *Kundalini-Journey Back to our True Home*. Sterling Publishers, Delhi.
——————2000. *Kundalini for Beginners*. Llewellyn Worldwide Ltd., MN, U.S.A.
—————— 2000. *All You Wanted to Know About Hatha Yoga*. Sterling Publishers, Delhi.
——————2000. *All You Wanted to Know About Kundalini Yoga*. Sterling Publishers, Delhi.
—————— 2000. *All You Wanted to Know About Kriya Yoga*. Sterling Publishers, Delhi.
—————— 2000. *All You Wanted to Know About Chakras and Nadis*. Sterling Publishers, Delhi.
—————— 2001. *All You Wanted to Know About Dreams*. Sterling Publishers, Delhi.
—————— 2001. *All You Wanted to Know About Aura*. Sterling Publishers, Delhi.
——————2001. *All You Wanted to Know About Mantras*. Sterling Publishers, Delhi.
——————2001. *All You Wanted to Know About Psychic Development*. Sterling, Delhi.
—————— 2002. *All You Wanted to Know About Karma Yoga*. Sterling Publishers, Delhi.
—————— 2002. *All You Wanted to Know About Jnana Yoga*. Sterling Publishers, Delhi.
—————— 2002. *All You Wanted to Know About Bhakti Yoga*. Sterling Publishers, Delhi.
—————— 2002. *All You Wanted to Know About Tantra Yoga*. Sterling Publishers, Delhi.
—————— 2003. *Secrets of Kundalini Awakening*. Sterling Publishers Pvt. Ltd., Delhi.
—————— 2004. *The Kundalini Book of Living and Dying*. Weiser Books, Boston, USA.
——————. 2005. *Secrets of Shaktipat*. New Dawn Press, Inc., UK, USA, India.

Luria, R. Isaac. *Sephr M'vo Shearim*, translated by Isaac Myer, *Qabbalah*, p. 110.
Mackey, S.A. 1822-23, *The Mythological Astronomy of the Ancients Demonstrated*, Part-II—*The Key of Urania*, pp. 23-24.
Max Muller. 1881. *Review of the Popul-Vuh*. p. 331.
Movers. 1841. *Die Phonizier*. Vol. I, p. 268.
Muktananda, Swami 1972. *Chitshakti Vilas (The Play of Consciousness)*. Gurudev Siddhapeeth, Maharashtra, India.
Newton, Michael 1994. *Journey of Souls*. Llewellyn Publications, St. Paul, MN, USA.
Paul. I Corinthians xv, 47.
Poimandres, I, 6 (Chambers, pp. 2-3); or II, 8 (Everard, p. 8).
Prabhupada, A.C.Bhaktivedanta Swami. 1972. *The Topmost Yoga System*. The Bhaktivedanta Book Trust, Mumbai, India.
Prabhupada, A.C.Bhaktivedanta Swami. n.d. *Sri Ishopanishad*. The Bhaktivedanta Book Trust, Mumbai, India.
Radha, Swami Sivananda. 1992. *Kundalini Yoga*. Motilal Banarsidass Publishers, Delhi.
——————————— 1993. *Mantras*. Motilal Banarsidass Publishers Ltd., Delhi, India.
Saraswati, Swami Satyananda. 1984. *Kundalini Tantra*. Bihar School of Yoga, Munger, India.
Skinner, J. Raltson 1885. *Masonic Review*. Vol. 63, July 1885. See "Hebrew Mythology."
Svoboda, E. Robert 1986. *Aghora*. Brotherhood of Life, Inc., USA. & Rupa & CO., New Delhi, India.
Tanner, Wilda B. 1988. *The Mystical Magical Marvelous World of Dreams*. Sparrow Hawk Press, Oklahoma, p 157.
Twitchell, Paul. 1971. *The Far Country*. IWP Publishing, Menlo Park, CA, USA.
Venkataramiah, Munangala. 2000. *TALKS with Sri Ramana Maharishi*. Sri Ramanasramam, Tiruvannamalai, India, p. 70.
Vigyani, Yogendra 1938, 1997. *Mahayoga Vigyan*. Vigyan Bhawan, Rishikesh, India.
Wagner, W. *Asgard and the Gods*. P. 305.
Woodroffe, Sir John. 1981. *The Serpent power*. Ganesh & Co., Madras, India.
Yukteswar, Swami Sri 1984. *The Holy Science*. Self-realization Fellowship, Los Angeles, California.
Zohar: *Idra Zuta Qaddisha* (Lesser Holy Assembly). Cf. Macgregor Mathers, *Kabbalah Unveiled*, p. 302.
Zohar, Brody ed., III, 135a; Cremona ed., iii, fol. 64b, col. 255, and fel. 142a, col 566. Cf. I. Myer, *Qabbalah*, pp. 386-87.
Zohar, III, 290a, Brody ed.; Cremona ed., III, fol. 141a, col. 562. Cf. I. Myer, *Qabbalah*, pp. 387-88.

INDEX

Acadmey of Kundalini Yoga and Quantum Soul (AKYQS), 77
Academy of Religion and Psychical Research (ARPR), 3, 70, 82, 297
Acharya Rajneesh, 26
Adi-Shakti, 103
Adi Guru Shankaracharya, 101, 145, 230
Africa, 125
Ananda, 8
A. R Wallace, 125
Arjuna, 46, 231, 249, 253, 254, 258
Asia, 126, 179
Atharva Veda, 100, 231
Atlantic Ocean, 126
Atul, 42
AUM, 39, 64, 99, 183, 190, 191, 192, 195, 210, 264, 279, 294
Australia, 125

Baghdad, 117
BAPU, 10, 70
Bhakti Yoga, 91, 94
Bhagalpur, 158
Bhrigu Rishi, 63, 74, 131
Bible, 106, 109, 117, 123, 142, 165, 180, 181, 182, 188, 272

Bombay, 253
Brahman, 4, 29, 95, 108, 118
'brahmajyoti', 29, 66, 89, 252, 258, 260, 262, 265, 267, 273
Brahmalokas, 95, 190
Buddhism, 102, 114, 169

Calcutta, 253
California, 26, 291
  Mt. Madonna Yoga Centre, 63
Chaldean, 102
Chandigarh, 16
China, 179
Chit, 8, 43, 182, 184, 185, 189, 195, 196, 209, 210, 288
Chitshaktivilas, 29
Christianity, 102, 110, 143
Cleopatra, 98
Creation of Universe and Man:
  Cosmic Evolution, 123-174
  God, monad and atom, 135-142
  nature of Gods and seven rounds, 128-134
  seven races, 123-127
  variety of, process of creation of man, 158-174
  Venus, 143-158

Daksha, 147, 155
Death (of ego), 2, 3, 4, 10, 11, 33, 35, 264
Delhi, 9, 15, 17, 41, 49, 50, 60, 61, 62, 63, 67, 73, 74, 76, 77, 78, 83, 90, 117, 253, 299
   University of Delhi, 17
Denmark, 23, 24, 73, 74, 90
Destiny, Science and Spiritual Awakening, 48
Devaki, 148, 230
Doug Scot, 34
Dr. B. Bhattacharya, 63
Dr. B. S. Goel, 9, 26, 41, 42, 44, 50, 167
Dr. Carl Jung, 29, 44, 95
Dr. Elizabeth Kubler Ross, 33, 96
Dr. Juno Jordan, 26
Dr. Khandelwal, 73
Dr. Michael Newton, 56
Dr Narayan Datt Srimali, 27
Dr. W. Wagner, 169

Eckankar, 25, 40, 46, 55, 59, 68, 210
Egyptian, 102, 114
Elizabeth, 27, 29, 30
England, 13, 14
Ethiopia, 24, 51, 60
   University of Addis Ababa, 51, 60
Europe, 126, 179

Fiji, 24, 61, 125
Florida 73, 76, 299

Ganga Singh, 71
Gautam Buddha, 13
George Smith, 170, 171
Goddess Durga, 62, 98, 116

Goddess Kali, 62
Goddess Lakshmi, 132
Goloka Vrindavana, 252, 262, 263
Greenland, 117, 127
Guru Deepak Yogi, 9, 83, 85
Guru Kirpal, 72, 73

Harare, 48, 50, 55
"Hare Krishna, Hare Krishna, Krishna Krishna Hare Hare, Hare Ram Hare Ram Ram Ram Hare Hare", 63
Hatha Yoga, 91, 94, 278, 286, 299
Hinduism, 108, 110, 111, 112, 118, 120, 173
Hindus, 43, 52, 102, 104, 105, 108
Holi, 13
How I Learned Soul Travel, 59
H. P. B. Blavatsky, 102, 118, 123, 192

India, 9, 12, 13, 15, 16, 19, 24, 26, 27, 41, 62, 70, 73, 74, 76, 90, 92, 107, 108, 111, 113, 118, 125, 159, 160, 168, 178, 179, 180, 259, 289, 291
Indian Ocean, 125
Inner turmoil, 2
Iraq, 24
ISKCON (International Society for Krishna Consciousness), 27, 79, 175, 229
Islam, 39, 102, 158
Italy, 79

Jiva (Monad), 9, 40, 45, 46, 52, 53, 74, 95, 106, 135, 136, 140, 141, 146, 156, 159, 176, 224, 225, 242, 243, 250, 251, 263

Jnana Yoga, 91, 94
John F. Kennedy, 229
Judaism, 102, 111
Jytte Larson, 73, 75, 76, 83, 88, 89

Kailash Mountain, 11, 264
Karma Yoga, 91
Karna, 116
Kashmir, 79
King Parikshit, 220, 267, 268
Kundalini (Mother Kundalini), 2, 3, 5, 6, 9, 10, 11, 14, 18, 20, 22, 27, 30, 41, 44, 46, 53, 55, 57, 60, 62, 64, 67, 68, 69, 73, 76, 80, 82, 84, 86, 87, 89, 94, 98, 116, 153, 167, 168, 264, 274, 276, 277, 278, 279, 280, 286, 287, 288, 289, 290, 291, 293, 294, 297, 298, 299
Kundalini for Beginners, 5, 71, 81, 297, 298, 299
Kundalini Research Network (KRN), 67, 70, 73, 289
 conference of, 67
Kundalini Tantra, 58
Kunti, 116, 252, 266
Kuran, 117

Liberation of Man, 175-275
 Blavatsky, 175-181
 goal, 193-197
 desire for emancipation, 193
 invocation, 232
 mantras, 233-275
 patanjali's yoga sutras, 215-216
 procedure, 197-209
 process of meditation, 227-229
 revelation, 209-215
 Sri Ishopanishad and Swami Prabhupada of ISKON, 229-232
 Srimad Bhagavata Mahapurana, 216-227
 Swami Sri Yukteswar, 181-192
Living with Kundalini, 66
Llewellyn Worldwide Ltd, 18, 71
London, 6, 25, 43, 52, 57, 61, 77, 299
Lord Buddha, 92, 99, 117, 121, 179, 294
Lord Ganesh, 28, 89
Lord Jesus Christ, 7, 8, 10, 33, 34, 92, 97, 98, 99, 116, 117, 136, 178, 192, 198, 209, 210, 272, 294
Lord Krishna, 4, 6, 28, 33, 35, 44, 53, 69, 95, 99, 117, 147, 148, 192, 210, 230, 231, 232, 235, 244, 245, 248, 251, 252, 253, 254, 255, 258, 259, 260, 264, 269, 271, 272, 273, 274, 284, 285, 294
Lord Shiva, 11, 12, 23, 28, 30, 33, 42, 44, 62, 92, 110, 116, 120, 226, 254, 260, 262, 264, 297
Lord Vishnu, 105, 110, 112, 121, 123, 132, 135, 147, 160, 168, 173, 223, 226, 236, 254, 256, 260
Lu Kuan, 57

Man and His Symbols, 44
Mahabharata, 114, 116, 117, 231
Mahatma Gandhi, 98, 229
Mahanta Sri Harold Klemp, 63
Magnolia, 126

Margaret Dempsey, 81
Maya, 94, 103, 185, 187, 193, 194, 195, 205, 209, 229, 238, 288
Meerut, 43
Mexico, 126
Minnesota, 25
Mohammad, 92, 97
Mona Lisa, 98
Mother Goddess, 5, 38, 42, 69, 99
Mother Mary, 92, 98, 294
My Journey to Godhood, 1-99
   life in Africa, 26-56
   observation, 56-99
      list of dreams, 56
   introduction, 1-12
   historical background, 12-26

Narada, 147, 148, 155, 178, 230, 232
New Jersey, 22
New York, 3, 297
Nigeria, 3, 24, 26, 27, 31, 75

"Om Hrim Shrim Govindaya Namah", 63, 88
"Om Namoh Bhagavate Vasudevaya", 63

Pacific Ocean, 125
Pandit Gopi Krishna, 26, 66, 167, 179, 221, 279
Patanjali Yoga, 2
   asana, 2, 159
   dharna, 2, 159
   dhyana, 2, 159
   niyama, 2, 159
   pranayama, 2, 159
   pratyahara, 2, 159
   samadhi, 2, 159
   yama, 2, 159
Paul Twitchell, 47, 60
Philadelphia, 70, 76, 289
P. L. Sclater, 125
Port Harcourt, 27, 29
   University of Port Harcourt, 27
Priyavarta, 221
Professor Max Muller, 146
Professor S. D. Bajpai, 29, 75
Puranas, 106, 117, 124, 126, 131, 138, 139, 145, 148, 149, 160, 161, 167, 180, 231

Quantum Jump into Divinity through Shaktipat, 276-300
   experiences on awakening, 288-293
   guru and initiate, 281-285
   how shakti replaces fear of death with trust in existence, 277-280
   introduction, 276
   liberation, 288
   my own experiences, 297-299
   order of experiences of realization, 294-297
   shaktipat initiation, 285-288
   shaktipat or kundalini mahayoga, 280-281
   what help is offered?, 299-300
   why there is anxiety about death?, 276-277

Index

Ravindra Kumar, 4, 33, 41, 68, 89
Ray Olsen, 68
Resurrection, 2
Richard Alpert, 26
Richard Maurice Buck, 27, 179
Richard Wilhelm, 44
Rig Veda, 100, 110, 114, 149, 152, 162, 170, 231, 236
Rishikesh, 9, 289
Roman Catholic Church, 116
Romance in Your Name, 25
Rome, 79

S. A. Mackey, 122
Sadhana, 65
Sahaj Yoga, 91
Saint Guruma, 83
Saint Kabir, 40, 53
Saint Mansoor, 100
Sama Veda, 100, 231
San Francisco, 3, 10, 67, 71
Sarah Miles, 34
Sat, 8
Scotland, 117
Secrets of Kundalini Awakening, 73, 78, 299
Secrets of Numerology, 26, 60
Secrets of Shaktipat, 9, 210, 299
Shaktipat, 9, 18, 83, 90, 99, 153, 275, 280, 282, 283, 285, 286, 289, 295, 297, 299, 300
Shwetketu, 101, 276
Sir Fred Hoyle, 34
Sir John Woodroffe, 26, 44
Sir Walter Scott, 215
Sir William Jones, 138
Sonepat, 83
Southern Africa, 54
    University of Malawi, 54
Sri Aurobindo, 76, 164, 203
Sri Herald Klemp, 25, 65, 210
Sri Ramana Maharishi, 86, 221
Sri Sathya Sai Baba, 8
Sri Suka, 221
Srimad Bhagavad Gita, 7, 35, 46, 53, 114, 117, 231, 232, 233, 234, 235, 236, 237, 238, 239, 241, 242, 243, 246, 247, 248, 249, 250, 252, 253, 254, 255, 256, 258, 260, 261, 264, 266, 267, 268, 271, 284
Srimad Bhagavat Mahapurana, 175, 216, 218, 223, 232
Srimad Bhagavatam, 7, 232, 241, 250, 251, 255, 259, 267, 268, 269, 270
Srila Rupa Gosawmi, 236
Sterling Publishers, 71, 78
Suva, 61, 62
Svastika, 132, 168, 169, 170
Swami Dayananda Saraswati, 118, 134
Swami Devendra Vigyani, 9
Swami Dr. Krishnananda Saraswati, 9
Swami Muktananda, 26, 29, 57, 279
Swami Narayan Tirth, 9
Swami Prabhupad, 79, 175, 229, 270
Swami Satyananda Saraswati, 26, 39, 46, 54, 58, 167
Swami Shivananda Radha, 65, 167
Swami Shivom Tirth, 9, 40
Swami Sri Yukteswar, 7, 175, 201, 215
Swami Vishnu Tirth (Saint Sheel Nath), 40, 83

Swami Yogananda Paramahansa, 175
Swami Yogendra, 26

TantraYoga, 91, 218
Tanzania, 23, 24, 38, 62, 67
　University of Dar-Es-Salaam, 23, 62
Taoist Yoga, 57, 559
Terrill Wilson, 59, 60
The Far Country, 55, 60
The Journey Back to Our True Home through Spiritual Energy, 210
The Kundalini Book of Living and Dying, 34, 299
The Nectar of Devotion, 236
The Secret Doctrine, 102
The Secrets of Golden Flower, 44
The Serpent Power, 44
The Spiritual Notebook, 47
The Topmost Yoga System, 270
Third Eye and Kundalini, 9, 41

U K (United Kingdom), 13, 24, 25, 77, 81
Upanishad, 7, 231, 238, 246, 250
　Chhandogya, 100
　Katha, 263
　Mandukya, 103, 260
　Shri, 252, 256, 263

USA (United States of America), 18, 20, 22, 24, 41, 67, 82, 90
Uttarkashi, 9

Vaikuntha Lokas, 7, 95, 252
Varanasi, 9
Vasudeva, 178, 218, 230, 261
Vedas, 7, 139, 152, 218, 246
Vivekchudamani, 101
Vyvasvatha, 221

We are all Gods in making, 100-122
　initiation and natures of Gods, 116-122
　introduction, 100-103
　spiritual hierarchy, 103-116
Wilda B. Tanner, 50, 84, 85, 88, 90
William Henry Belk, 22, 70, 71

Yajur Veda, 100, 231, 233

Zambia, 126
Zimbabwe, 24, 31, 42, 47, 48, 55, 60, 68
　University of Zimbabwe, 31, 32
Zoroastrian, 102